Bioethics and Women

Bioethics and Women

Across the Life Span

MARY BRIODY MAHOWALD

OXFORD
UNIVERSITY PRESS
2006

OXFORD
UNIVERSITY PRESS

Oxford University Press, Inc., publishes works that further
Oxford University's objective of excellence
in research, scholarship, and education.

Oxford New York
Auckland Cape Town Dar es Salaam Hong Kong Karachi
Kuala Lumpur Madrid Melbourne Mexico City Nairobi
New Delhi Shanghai Taipei Toronto

With offices in
Argentina Austria Brazil Chile Czech Republic France Greece
Guatemala Hungary Italy Japan Poland Portugal Singapore
South Korea Switzerland Thailand Turkey Ukraine Vietnam

Published by Oxford University Press, Inc.
198 Madison Avenue, New York, New York 10016

www.oup.com

Oxford is a registered trademark of Oxford University Press

Library of Congress Cataloging-in-Publication Data
Mahowald, Mary Briody.
Bioethics and women : Across the Life Span / Mary Briody Mahowald.
p. cm.
Includes bibliographical references and index.
ISBN-13 978-0-19-517617-9
ISBN 0-19-517617-0
1. Medical ethics. 2. Bioethics. 3. Feminism—Moral
and ethical aspects. 4. Women—Health and hygiene. I. Title.
R725.5.M34 2006
176—dc22 2006040004

2 4 6 8 9 7 5 3 1
Printed in the United States of America
on acid-free paper

In loving memory of my mother and my sister

and for all of our daughters

ACKNOWLEDGMENTS

My thanks are due first to Anne Drapkin Lyerly, who might have been my coauthor if other obligations hadn't intervened in the task. Annie was, in a sense, my inspiration for writing the book. Later on, Lisa Harris, another obstetrician-gynecologist, reviewed a great deal of the manuscript, and provided me with extremely helpful suggestions.

Thanks too to various members of the faculty in the Department of Obstetrics and Gynecology and the MacLean Center for Clinical Medical Ethics at the University of Chicago, which has been my academic home since 1990. These include but are not limited to Sarah Adams, Daniel Brauner, David Cohen, Ismail Mahmoud, Ernst Lengyel, William Meadow, Maura Quinlan, Jaideep Singh, and Diane Yamada. The willingness of these clinicians to review material, discuss cases, and answer my questions has surely made the book more clinically credible than it would otherwise be. Kenneth Iserson, from the University of Arizona College of Medicine, has also been helpful in this regard. Other members of my department who performed tasks for which they had better expertise than I include Steve Gadzinski, Gail Isenberg, and Beatrice Merigold.

I am grateful to members of the Center for Biomedical Ethics at Stanford University, with whom I spent most of the academic year 2001–2002 working on the book and enjoying my interactions with them. During this time, I also benefited by detailed and thoughtful suggestions from anonymous reviewers at Oxford University Press.

Because I spent the first part of my academic career in a philosophy department, the content of *Bioethics and Women* has undoubtedly been influenced by philosophers whose work I read, especially those who have dared to focus on issues of particular relevance to women. I have long counted Alison Jaggar, Rosemarie Tong, Joan Callahan, and Laura Purdy in this group. In addition to Laura, Jennifer Parks, Nancy Snow, and Sara Goehring have been generous enough to review parts of the manuscript and give me helpful feedback.

Jeffrey House was my first contact at Oxford, and as with previous books, he handled the project wisely and efficiently, particularly when I worried about losing a coauthor and being unable to meet Oxford's deadline. Peter Ohlin, who picked up the baton from Jeff, has proved a worthy successor, ably assisted by Lara Zoble. Cynthia Garver did an excellent job of copyediting, and Linda Donnelly, the production editor, facilitated the project not only through her helpful suggestions but also through ease of contact. Two people offered relevant photos or sketches for the book's jacket: Annette Mendola, whom I hope someday to thank in person, and Germaine Wieman, a longtime friend, whom I will thank in person sometime soon.

Last but definitely not least, I want to thank Tony, my life partner and best friend, who has not only contributed to the book through his loving support of me, our children, and my work, but also by helping me to avoid mistakes in his area of expertise, developmental biology and genetics.

PREFACE

At its conception, this book was intended for practitioners who provide health care for women. The goal was to offer a helpful guide to them on the numerous ethical issues that arise in treatment of women across the life span. Issues relevant to this goal include many that are unrelated to reproduction. With regard to those that are related, however, my aim was to write the book in a way that showed respect for the different convictions of those involved, whether women or men, practitioners or patients, about the moral status of the human embryo or fetus. I wanted to track how these convictions may also have implications for nonreproductive decisions, particularly those made at the end of life. And because the book would be devoted to women's health care, I hoped to facilitate recognition of women's own standpoints as central to ethical decisions by and about us.

Since the book was intended for clinicians, I invited a young obstetrician/gynecologist to join me in the project. Her expertise, experience, and youth were complementary to the input I could provide. Together we felt able to write a book on bioethical issues that had not yet been available to clinicians who care for women: one authored by women themselves at different ends of their own life spans. To be useful to practitioners, we wanted the book to accentuate the clinical as well as ethical complexity of cases rather than the theoretical arguments and analyses that academic bioethicists bring to their work.

Fortunately or unfortunately, as often happens in the lives of those who nurture others' lives, family-building events prevented my intended coauthor from finishing the project. At that point, my editor and publisher advised me to go ahead on my own, which I have done.

Going ahead on my own meant broadening the targeted audience to include students and teachers of bioethics. To be useful to this wider readership, I have expanded the theoretical chapters (part I) and reduced the amount of clinical complexity or specialized language in the chapters devoted to practical topics (part II). I have also added a chapter addressing the plausibility and desirability of an ideal of justice in health care and gender justice in women's health care.

While reorienting the book to a broader range of readers, I did not attempt either of two tasks that could be well accomplished by others, or perhaps addressed in my next book: examination of each topic, issue, and case with as full academic rigor as it deserves, and development of a well-reasoned argument from well-supported premises to a definitive conclusion or position on each of the ethical questions raised. Doing this adequately would require an entire book or at least a full article for every topic and issue identified. Because the book offers rich fodder for these analyses, I look forward to reading and learning from others who provide them. In the meantime, the material presented here can be fruitfully used to provoke ongoing, thoughtful discussion not only by students and scholars of bioethics but also by practitioners and the public at large. Fueling and focusing such discussions on women's health care is long overdue.

CONTENTS

Introduction 3

PART I: A BIOETHICS FOR WOMEN

1. An Egalitarian Overview 9
    Diverse approaches to bioethics 10
    Verities, variables, and maxims 15
    Conceptions of justice 18
    Standpoint theory and its implications for just caring 24
    Privileging women's standpoint in our health care 26
2. Distinguishing Features of Women's Health Care 30
    Some sex and gender differences 31
    Models of the practitioner-patient relationship 35
    Possible modifications of principlist and casuistic methods 37
    Who is the patient? 40
    Patients and "dependent moral status" 44
    Guidelines and regulations 47

3. Different Starting Points, Standpoints, End Points 50

Key terms 51

Meaning and significance of moral status 54

Moral relevance of the gestational tie and other relationships 56

Personhood and potential for personhood 58

Thresholds of development and moral status 62

Intermediate positions about moral status 66

PART II: TOPICS, ISSUES, AND CASES

4. Preconception and Prenatal Decisions 73

Preconception counseling 74

Preimplantation genetic diagnosis 78

Prenatal testing 81

Misattributed paternity and carrier testing 85

Sex selection 88

5. Medically Assisted Reproduction 92

Criteria for patient selection 93

Gamete "donation" and "surrogacy" 97

Disposition of in vitro embryos 101

Multiple gestations 104

6. Noncompliance during Pregnancy 109

Refusal of hospitalization 110

Dietary noncompliance 114

Refusal of cesarean section 117

7. Decisions at Parturition and Birth 123

Mode of delivery 124

Cesarean sections for nonmedical reasons 126

Decisions for impaired or very premature newborns 130

Sex assignment at birth 134

8. Treatment of Minors 140

Teenage pregnancy and motherhood 141

Confidentiality issues 145

Ritual female genital surgery 149

Eating disorders 153

9. Preventing Pregnancy and Birth 158

Contraception and sterilization 159

Abortion 163

10. Violence and Discrimination toward Women and Children 172

Child abuse and neglect 173

Elderly abuse and neglect 176

Violence against women 179

Gender discrimination and sexual harassment 182

11. Nonreproductive Health Issues 186

HIV testing and AIDS 187

Breast and gynecological cancers 190

Menopause and hormone replacement therapy 194

12. Care of the Elderly and End-of-Life Care 198

Health-related issues 199

Caregiver issues 203

End-of-life decisions 207

13. Research Issues 214

Women as research subjects 215

Maternal-fetal surgery 220

Cloning and stem cell research 223

PART III: AN EGALITARIAN IDEAL

14. Virtue and Gender Justice in Health Care 233

Recapping the perspective 233

Obligations, virtues, and ideals 235

Individual decision-making and an egalitarian ideal 237

Virtue in women's health care 238

Notes 241

Index 267

Bioethics and Women

Introduction

Work in bioethics requires both theoretical and empirical considerations relevant to each topic, issue, and case examined. This is true regardless of whether the work is done in classrooms or in clinical encounters. The format of this book, therefore, joins both types of considerations. Part I (chapters 1–3) provides an overview of theoretical considerations relevant to women's health care and Part II (chapters 4–13) adds empirical considerations to these while addressing bioethical questions that arise throughout the life span. Part III (chapter 14) offers theoretical considerations that complement those covered in the body of the book.

Chapter 1 sketches the egalitarian perspective I have brought to my work in bioethics for many years and explains how this is different from, as well as similar to, alternative approaches. After introducing the relevant ethical principles, I argue that justice is the central principle from which questions involving disparate impact on people must be addressed, with gender justice as the necessary subset of justice from which issues in women's health care should be scrutinized. Drawing on classical pragmatism and feminist standpoint theory, I explain how the input of minorities and women is crucial to overcoming the fallibility of decisions and policies formulated by those who hold positions of dominance or power over those who are less dominant or less powerful.

Chapter 2 identifies unique features of women's health care, examines various models of the practitioner-patient relationship, and critiques mainstream approaches to bioethics for their overall inattentiveness to relevant differences between men and women. Where there is such attentiveness, I suggest that it is sometimes misguided, as in the tendency to view each pregnant woman as two separate patients. In a society in which there is widespread disagreement on various moral questions, individuals must make their own moral decisions without having adequate guidance from laws or policies that are applicable to everyone. Foremost among areas of disagreement is the question of requirements for moral status or personhood. Many people have developed cogent arguments for different answers to this question; I do not regard any of these as definitively proved or refuted. When some ethical quandaries involving women are addressed, however, an answer to the question of moral status is unavoidable, at least implicitly, and different answers have different ethical implications for the decisions of individuals. In chapter 3, therefore, I consider a range of positions about moral status, from the minimal criterion of genetic humanness that occurs in the zygote to the maximal criterion of moral agency that occurs years after birth. Through this discussion, I hope to facilitate examination of topics covered in Part II in a manner that respects the moral integrity of individuals who disagree about this pivotal issue.

Chapters 4–13 cover a wide range of topics involving women's health care across the life span. Obviously, not all of these relate to reproduction, and some topics involve health risks raised by social circumstances such as caregiving responsibilities and domestic violence. Each chapter is subdivided into issues encompassed by the topic addressed, and each of these is introduced by cases that illustrate ethically relevant variables. Empirical and theoretical considerations about the issues and cases are then discussed. The theoretical considerations include conceptual clarifications and discussion of the principles and perspective delineated in Part I. The empirical considerations include clinical variables such as diagnoses, prognoses, and treatment alternatives as well as psychosocial variables such as the patient's age and competence, costs of treatment, societal or cultural influences, and relationships with others. All of the cases are based on the experiences of women and clinicians who care for them. A few have been reported in the media. Where the cases have not been reported elsewhere, particulars have been altered to protect the confidentiality of the individuals and institutions involved.

No matter how thoroughly and carefully one examines, elaborates, and analyzes conceptual and ethical questions raised by specific cases, the nuances of actual, ongoing cases cannot be wholly captured through narration or discussion of them by those who are not directly involved. The actual cases in which patients, family members, and practitioners are required to make ethical decisions always entail more variables than descriptions of them can identify and analyses can address. Moreover, the ethical questions raised and the variables associated with them often change as a case progresses. Those who personally or professionally participate in a case have different standpoints as well as rights and responsibilities regarding the questions raised.

Because it is impossible to identify and examine all of the potentially relevant variables, or consider all of the standpoints relevant to each case or issue, I do not attempt to delineate all of the questions raised or provide definitive answers to all of those addressed. My goal is simply to facilitate ethical decision-making on issues in women's health care through fuller and more critical consideration of the ethical complexity that arises in particular cases. Policies and legislation about specific issues are only adequate or justifiable to the extent that they take account of this complexity.

Part III returns us to the more theoretical concerns of Part I, but with a focus on virtue or supererogation instead of obligation. I was motivated to write this concluding chapter by the belief that most of the moral quandaries that people face in health care, as in other areas of life, are questions about what is the morally better or best thing to do rather than what is morally or legally obligatory. Women and practitioners alike, I believe, want to do more than simply meet a minimal standard of morality or legality. In this final chapter, therefore, I examine how the egalitarian perspective developed in Part I supports an ideal conception of virtue that is applicable to the issues addressed in Part II.

Although the perspective I bring to the pages that follow is consistent with the standpoint I have brought to my other work in bioethics, I believe it is also consistent with the standpoint of those who agree with its starting point and end point, as discussed in chapters 1 and 14. The starting point is the belief that every person has the same value, and the end point is the ideal of justice as human flourishing for each person, based on her or his unique capabilities. Admittedly, this approach is not free of flaws or inadequacies, both theoretical and empirical. Other variables and other standpoints could lead to different conclusions. However, I attempt to reduce the fallibility of my standpoint by attributing central importance to the standpoints of those whose views tend to be ignored, who nonetheless experience the consequences of decisions and policies fashioned by others. In women's health care, those most affected are obviously the women themselves. Throughout the book, therefore, I try to impute privileged status to women as patients. I do not expect my effort to be sufficiently egalitarian and inclusive to yield certainly true or totally persuasive conclusions; I do, however, think it is moving in that direction, and thus is more ethically and epistemologically desirable, than other attempts to settle ethical questions about women's health.

PART I

A Bioethics for Women

1

An Egalitarian Overview

The majority of people involved in health care are women. Not only do women outnumber men as patients; they also outnumber men as caregivers of the young, the aged, the ill, and the impaired. Often, women enter the health care system not because they themselves are ill or impaired but because of a capacity that men lack—namely, the capacity to bear children. Were it not for this capacity, many women might not seek health care in their own behalf. Another reason women outnumber men as patients is that they tend to live longer than men. Although this suggests that women in general are healthier than men, some studies indicate that the reduced quality of women's extended life span mitigates this advantage considerably.[1] Many of women's contacts with the health care system are initiated and sustained on behalf of others, especially children and ill or impaired relatives who depend on them for care. In professional caregiving roles, women are likely to occupy less prestigious and less remunerative positions than their male counterparts.

In light of these and other gender differences, this book considers ethical issues that arise in the health care of women across the life span from an egalitarian perspective. Preliminarily, I sketch the background against which other well-known approaches to ethical issues in health care have developed, and explore how these may or may not be helpfully incorporated into an egalitarian approach to ethical issues involving women's health. The approach I recommend starts with recognition that gender justice is a necessary subset of justice, requiring explicit and deliberate attention to the impact of health care decisions on women. Because gender justice is central to consideration of issues in women's health care from an egalitarian perspective, this approach is also a feminist perspective. However, different meanings of "justice" and "equality" may lead to different positions on what constitutes gender justice in specific circumstances. This leads me to elaborate and defend specific meanings of both terms. I also describe a strategy by which injustice related to gender differences in health care may be reduced.

Diverse approaches to bioethics

Van Rensselaer Potter coined the term "bioethics" in 1971 to refer to the study of ethical questions raised by the impact of advances in biology on the world's environment.[2] Gradually, the term acquired a narrower and different meaning, that is, the study of ethical issues raised by human biology, involving medical research and practice.[3] Within this still-burgeoning, interdisciplinary field, some bioethicists devote most of their time to writing, teaching, and lecturing about specific issues; others work primarily with patients and clinicians who are facing the issues. The first group, sometimes called medical ethicists, typically deals with policies that might influence future decisions; cases are examined in retrospect to provide guidance in the development of recommendations. The latter group, sometimes called clinical ethicists, deal with ongoing cases, where decisions with immediate impact are unavoidable.[4] Some individuals belong to both groups, and their dual involvement tends to enrich their contribution in both arenas. However, the majority of medical ethicists, even those trained as clinicians, devote the bulk of their time to what may be called academic bioethics: research, teaching, and writing that, if successful, facilitates ethical decisions by those who are actually facing bioethical dilemmas.[5]

Theoretical and practical approaches to issues in bioethics are distinguishable through their association with traditional philosophical theories and critiques of these theories. In some quarters, the former set of approaches has been dubbed "principlism," that is, a methodology by which general rules are applied to particular cases or issues. The latter set of approaches has been called "casuistry," that is, a mode of reasoning that examines the particularities of cases without appeal to principles. Casuistry has been more explicitly described by Albert Jonsen and Stephen Toulmin as a method recovered from ancient and medieval practice, but consistent with their experience as members of the President's Commission for the Study of Ethical Problems in Medicine and Biomedical and Behavioral Research.[6] When they met as members of the commission in the 1980s, Jonsen had been a Jesuit priest, trained in religious ethics; Toulmin was an analytically trained philosopher of science. Despite their different academic backgrounds, they found that they agreed on specific positions while disagreeing about theoretical approaches to the issues. Their effort to reinstate casuistry as a preferred method of ethical or moral reasoning is intended to facilitate resolution of complex ethical questions that arise for individuals as well as policy makers.[7]

Similarly, Tom Beauchamp and James Childress, the best-known elaborators of principles in medical ethics, initially approached their subject from different backgrounds. Beauchamp, trained in philosophy, championed a rule-utilitarian approach—one in which the applicable rules are derived through consideration of which would produce the best consequences for most people. Childress, trained in religious ethics, was a rule-deontologist—one for whom the applicable rules are construed as laws of nature, God, or reason, without the need to appeal to consequences. When they joined forces to write the first edition of *Principles of Biomedical Ethics* in 1978, Beauchamp and Childress found they agreed on the relevant applicable principles despite their different theoretical backgrounds.

Principle-based approaches to bioethics may appeal to consequences, as in utilitarian theory, or to a priori principles and rights, as in Kantian theory; in addition, they may draw on natural law, virtue theory, or communitarian accounts of ethics.[8] Case-based approaches are exemplified not only by the casuistry of Jonsen and Toulmin but also by various versions of care-based ethics and narrative theory, both of which enrich a case-based approach. The contribution of care-based ethics is its emphasis on relationships, the examination of which is indispensable to ethical decision-making and analysis of cases.[9] The contribution of narrative theory is mainly epistemological because it stresses the need for attention to different "stories" told by different authors from different standpoints about specific cases.[10] Attention to these stories is crucial to the knowledge base required for ethical decision-making.

Principle-based methods have been stereotypically interpreted as relying solely on "top-down" or deductive reasoning, and case-based methods have been stereotyped as relying on "bottom-up" or inductive reasoning. In fact, however, particularities mix with generalities in both contexts. Some approaches, such as pragmatism and Marxism, explicitly mix the two, insisting that theory and practice are inseparable.[11] Various versions of feminism also stress the necessity of attention to context as well as principles.[12] More recent criticisms of principle-based methods of moral reasoning come from moral particularists such as Margaret Olivia Little, who, while insisting that "no one (sensibly) rejects principles that tell us to 'respect autonomy' or to 'be kind,'" also insists that no one "can unpack those very abstract principles into generalizations that are both accurate and contentful enough to be action-guiding."[13]

The concept of autonomy is particularly difficult, if not impossible, to unpack. Some bioethicists simply equate the term with "self-determination," without further specification of its meaning. In clinical practice, autonomy is often equated with the ability to provide "informed consent" to treatment. The prerequisites for informed consent include competence, voluntariness, and adequate understanding of the information relevant to the contemplated decision. Circumstances abound, however, in which one or more of these elements may be lacking or only questionably present in an individual. Clinicians are most likely to question whether a patient is autonomous when she refuses to follow medical recommendations, and they are least likely to question this when the recommendation is accepted. But nonmedical factors sometimes figure more heavily in patient's decisions than medical factors; clinicians are often unaware of these, or they weigh them less heavily than patients weigh them. Relationships to others are as important here as they are in other contexts. Recent work on "relational autonomy" has challenged views of the self as an isolated agent, arguing that women in particular do not make their choices in a contextual vacuum, as if relationships with other people are not integral to the choices they make.[14] Not only are these relationships, including the physician-patient relationship, relevant to autonomy; they may promote or limit its exercise.

In light of a tendency to exclude other morally relevant considerations, and difficulties encountered in determining whether or to what extent a patient is autonomous, bioethicists and clinicians alike have argued against uncritical affirmations of the primacy of patient autonomy in clinical decision-making. In some cases, morally relevant considerations or principles are so intertwined that it may be impossible to assign priority to any of them. Carl Schneider seems to recognize this when he proposes an "optional" model of patient autonomy, by which patients are entitled but not obliged to direct their physicians to make medical decisions in their behalf. Unlike the mandatory model, this model allows the physician to make decisions based on the physician's own understanding of what is best for the patient.[15] Schneider's proposal thus supports a practice described as voluntary paternalism. As discussed in chapter 8, this construal is at odds with the usual understanding of paternalism—as impeding autonomy for the sake of some other good.

Because cases are the mainstay of their daily practice, clinicians find casuistry and other case-based methods particularly appealing. Nonetheless, the principle-based approach of Beauchamp and Childress has dominated the field of bioethics, perhaps because it suggests a systematic approach comparable to a thoroughgoing patient work-up. Just as various bodily systems (e.g., neurological, respiratory, digestive) need to be checked out to determine the treatment plan for a particular patient, the four principles proposed by Beauchamp and Childress need to be considered when a particular ethical question is raised. Accordingly, the principles they introduced in the first edition of *Principles of Biomedical Ethics*—autonomy, beneficence, nonmaleficence, and justice—are routinely cited in defense or refutation of ethical positions on various issues. Subsequent editions have expanded on the first and include interesting modifications. For example, the principle of "autonomy" is called "respect for autonomy" in subsequent editions, and the four principles are referred to as "clusters" of principles in the fifth edition.

As already mentioned, the meaning of autonomy is subject to different interpretations. This makes it difficult at times to determine whether or to what extent an individual is autonomous in her decision-making. The concept of "respect" also means different things to different people. To some, for example, respect for autonomy implies compliance with the autonomous decision of another; to others, it simply means that someone's autonomous decision should be given at least as much weight, and sometimes more weight, than is given to other moral considerations. Beauchamp and Childress support the latter view. Respect for autonomy, they claim, "involves acknowledging decision-making rights and enabling persons to act autonomously," and "disrespect for autonomy involves attitudes and actions that ignore, insult, or demean others' rights of autonomy."[16] On that account, autonomy can always be respected, even when overridden by other morally relevant considerations.

"Rights" are often asserted in the context of claims about autonomy, but this is another term for which different meanings have different ethical implications. The general definition of "right" as a justifiable entitlement or claim on another doesn't address questions regarding who has rights, the extent to which rights are associated with responsibilities, or whose rights should prevail in situations of conflict. Neither does it identify that to which individuals are alleged to have rights—for example, a right to life, a right to choose, a right to health care. A crucial clarification relevant to health care involves the distinction between positive and negative rights. A positive right implies another's responsibility to support or facilitate its expression, whereas a negative right implies another's responsibility not to interfere with the expression of that right. Negative rights are generally more binding on others than positive rights, but either type of right may assert an obligation on the part of others to act in accordance with the principles of beneficence and nonmaleficence toward other individuals.

Although literal meanings of beneficence and nonmaleficence are clear and distinctive, the relationship between the two is subject to different interpretations. Most people are familiar with "Do no harm" as the primary ethical imperative of medical practice, more compelling than the imperative "Do good." In some cases, however, whether a particular act (e.g., removing a respirator) involves "doing" or "not doing" may be questioned, and some scholars view nonmaleficence as a subset of beneficence. If avoiding harm and doing good occur along a single spectrum of moral obligation, the two principles may be collapsed into one. However, Beauchamp and Childress argue that the distinction between nonmaleficence and beneficence should be maintained. While doing so, they distinguish three forms of beneficence: preventing harm, removing harm, and promoting good.[17] By this account, removal from a respirator may be viewed as a form of beneficence in some circumstances (e.g., when it is the only means through which continuing, intractable pain can be ended). Whether one form of beneficence outweighs other forms or nonmaleficence in a particular case depends on how other goods or harms are weighed.

Many scholars have questioned the grounding and meaning of the principles; others seem to take them and the meanings attributed to them by their authors as canonical. Consistent with this regard, the principles have been called the "Georgetown mantra." (Georgetown is the home institution of Beauchamp and of the Kennedy Institute of Ethics, an influential and well-respected center for research and teaching in bioethics.)

While the "mantra" is prevalently invoked by clinical ethicists, some are more enamored of an approach developed by Jonsen, Mark Siegler, and William Winslade. (Jonsen and Siegler refer to their approach as casuistry; Winslade refers to it as contextual or pragmatic ethics.) This method identifies four "topics" to be considered in resolving ethical issues in the clinical setting: medical indications, patient preferences, quality of life, and contextual features.[18]

Quality of life is construed as applicable to the patient alone, and contextual features are delineated as "the social, legal, economic, and institutional circumstances in which a particular case of patient care occurs."[19] Siegler defines the goal of clinical ethics as optimal care of the patient and believes that the great majority of issues in clinical ethics are resolved without having to consider quality of life or contextual factors. Consideration of medical indications (i.e., health burden vs.

health benefit) often suffices to settle questions, but patient preferences (i.e., the voluntary decision of an adequately informed, competent adult) sometimes override medical indications.

The topics proposed by Jonsen, Siegler, and Winslade are relatable to the principles proposed by Beauchamp and Childress. Consideration of medical indications, for example, combines the meanings of beneficence and nonmaleficence because it requires clinicians to weigh the burdens and benefits of alternative treatments or nontreatment for particular patients. Quality of life factors also involve concerns about beneficence and nonmaleficence, but the benefits and harms considered within this topic are nonmedical as well as medical.[20] The patient herself may indicate what quality of life factors are important to her, or clinicians may make that determination paternalistically. Although consideration of patient preferences suggests respect for patient autonomy, "preferences" may refer to unexamined or inadvertent desires rather than autonomous choices. The topic of contextual factors necessarily includes (but is not limited to) issues of justice or responsibilities to others besides the patient.

The casuistic topics of medical indications, patient preferences, and quality of life refer only to patients, whereas the principles of respect for autonomy, beneficence, and nonmaleficence may apply to others as well, including family members and clinicians. In most cases, the principles apply to patients, but occasionally—for example, when a patient is permanently comatose—they may apply to others such as family members, who are included in the contextual category of Jonsen, Siegler, and Winslade. Because the principles are applicable beyond the clinical setting, they provide a more adequate framework than the topics for dealing with ethical issues whose ramifications extend beyond clinical encounters. Accordingly, Beauchamp and Childress claim that their principles are based on a "single, universal, common morality"—that is, norms that all rational persons can and should support in all circumstances toward one another.[21]

Consideration of generalities (principles) and particularities (cases) inexorably mix in practice. If Aristotle was correct that knowledge occurs through abstraction of universals from particular experiences,[22] the principles of Beauchamp and Childress are only understood by individuals through the experiences from which they derive their meanings. Each person's conception of beneficence, for example, is based on her specific observations of people who "do good" to her or others; each one's understanding of justice is based on particular experiences of fair or unfair treatment.[23] Because each one's experiences are unique, conceptions of justice or beneficence or other moral principles may differ even when the same terms are used.

As in other areas of life, communication in the health care setting involves an inadequate but indispensable exchange of concepts or generalizations, often conducted more meaningfully nonverbally than verbally. When a patient moans or grimaces during a procedure, for example, this is typically interpreted as a sign of pain. For each of us, the meaning of pain is inevitably derived from her own experience of pain, and an obligation to relieve pain is a prima facie duty of clinicians. Occasionally, however, some patients prefer a lesser level of pain relief than is available so that they can remain as alert as possible through the course of their treatment or recovery. From their different standpoints, patients inevitably differ about what constitutes harms or benefits to themselves.

Unfortunately, busy practitioners are prone to interpret mere verbal or signed consent to treatment as adequate expression of a patient's autonomy. In fact, though, a patient may sign a form or give oral consent without adequately understanding the consequences of treatment, without time to think about it, without being told of alternatives, or while experiencing fear or pain or the effects of medication or pressure from others to agree to the recommended treatment. In such circumstances, whether the patient's consent is truly or adequately autonomous is highly questionable. In light of these unavoidable limitations, none of the (clusters of) principles of the Georgetown mantra has adequate meaning independently of particular cases or experiences from which those who use or hear or read the terms have developed the conceptions they attach to them.

Verities, variables, and maxims

If thinking is in fact inseparable from experience, stereotypic interpretations of principle-based or case-based approaches to bioethics are not just mischaracterizations of these approaches but inadequate guides to resolution of the questions they address. To the extent that principlism and casuistry are adequate approaches, they combine consideration of particulars and generals, cases and principles.[24] This is as true of clinical decisions as it is of ethical decisions. Case-based reasoning emphasizes consideration of the variables or circumstances of specific cases, while principle-based reasoning stresses consideration of generalities or principles that might also be referred to as "verities" because they are held to be true (from the Latin *veritas* = truth), although not necessarily applicable, in all cases.

The term "verities" suggests a more basic meaning than the term "principles." Consistent with its etymology, it is used for moral values that remain true and are recognized as such by most if not all moral agents. When the term "principles" is used for lesser levels of generality, such as guidelines or specific interpretations of abstract principles, they are challengeable on grounds that they do not conform to the more basic principles. "Beneficence," for example, is an abstract term, whose meaning (to do good) is universally supported as a basic moral value. But less general "principles" (e.g., privacy and confidentiality) are encompassed by the more general ones, and guidelines that specify how good should be done in specific circumstances may well be controversial.[25]

Explicit, careful consideration of both the verities and the variables of cases obviously constitutes a more adequate approach to clinical and policy dilemmas than either approach pursued separately (if that were possible). But even when both variables and verities are considered, they seldom lead to resolution of a dilemma unless a third set of considerations is employed. Recent editions of *Principles of Biomedical Ethics* attempt to provide this by proposing "specification" as a means by which to reduce the vagueness or abstractness of the principles, and "balancing" as a means by which to address the incompatibility of the principles in some situations.[26] However, the verity of justice can also be enlisted to serve these functions. Justice fulfills the balancing function desired by Beauchamp and Childress by mediating among conflicting principles or interests, and justice facilitates the specifying function by providing grounds by which to develop guidelines applicable to similar cases.[27]

In casuistry, paradigmatic cases or issues that have already been resolved satisfactorily provide "maxims" applicable to new cases or issues with which they may be compared. Identifying the applicable paradigm may generate controversy in its own right (e.g., whether an innovative procedure should be considered research or therapy for a particular patient). The definitiveness of conclusions reached through this method depends on how closely the new case resembles the paradigmatic case. The maxims of casuistry offer the specification that Beauchamp and Childress propose, without acknowledgment of the basic principles that underlie them.[28] Consider, for example, the following statement as both a casuistic maxim and a specification of the principle of respect for autonomy: "Surgeons should not operate on competent patients without their free and informed consent." Just as wise sayings or proverbs are intended to facilitate moral reasoning and behavior in specific situations, maxims are also intended to do this. Philosophers from Aristotle through Kant and onward have invoked moral maxims based on principles assumed to hold for everyone.[29]

The early years of medical training involve a greater emphasis on the principles of good medical practice than on cases involving actual patients.[30] In contrast, clinical practice typically employs a casuistic mode of reasoning, taking as "maxims" the protocols that have generated successful outcomes in previous paradigmatic cases, applying these to the case at hand. Whether advertently or not, however, the principles learned earlier generally underlie the maxims followed. In other words, greater generality gives way to lesser generality by including more particulars in its scope, and the process by which more and more particulars are embraced eventually leads to the specific set of variables that identify each case as a unique occurrence. Because no two cases are exactly alike, there are always variables that may augment or thwart the effectiveness of the maxims learned from the paradigmatic case.

Paradigmatic thinking is not only the province of clinicians. Patients often have paradigmatic cases from which they have learned how they want to act in future circumstances. And people in general have a store of paradigmatic cases gleaned from their own experience or through stories told by others. The paradigms that are meaningful to patients often epitomize values drawn from religious or cultural or family traditions. At times, these are at odds with the paradigms inculcated in practitioners from the tradition of medicine. Unless patients and practitioners appeal to a common paradigm for ethical guidance, the casuistic method cannot provide an adequate means by which to reach agreement about a treatment decision.

The term "maxim" may be used in a more limited sense than that of casuistry—to refer to prioritizing guidelines or rules for resolution of problematic ethical cases. Although the maxims generated by paradigmatic cases are often more specific than these, in neither case do they provide definitive solutions to ethical questions addressed by individuals. As Jonsen and Toulmin observe, maxims are analogous to "clues" a detective follows in solving a case.[31] *All* of the relevant variables applicable to specific cases can rarely if ever be identified and addressed, but this flaw does not negate the usefulness of maxims in ethical decision-making any more than it negates the usefulness of those generated by paradigmatic cases in health care decisions. Moreover, recognition of the relevant variables can be maximized through a strategy I shall subsequently explain: standpoint theory.

In the principlist model of bioethics, the term "guidelines" conveys more flexibility than "principles" and is often used to specify their meanings.[32] In other words, the guidelines of principlist approaches are comparable to the maxims of casuistry. The term "maxims" may therefore used for a third set of considerations by which principlist and case-based approaches are both used to determine which verity has precedence and toward whom it should be upheld, in light of the relevant variables. More specific guidelines such as those formulated by professional health care organizations are generally consistent with these maxims.

The egalitarian approach of this book involves both the principles elaborated by Beauchamp and Childress as verities applicable to specific questions and the particularities that casuists emphasize as variables to be examined in light of the verities. The meanings of the verities are also subject to clarification and modification through consideration of the variables. Maxims or guidelines for determining how to prioritize the principles in particular cases illustrate the specification and balancing advocated by Beauchamp and Childress. These are consistent not only with the common-morality theory of Beauchamp and Childress but also with the common sense of the general public. The following maxims are broadly recognized as central to the prioritizing of the principles of respect for autonomy, beneficence, nonmaleficence, and justice in health care:

Maxims

1. The interests of the patient count most (interests = autonomy + beneficence + nonmaleficence).
2. Respect for the patient's autonomy outweighs beneficence and nonmaleficence toward the patient.
3. The interests of others may outweigh respect for the patient's autonomy.
4. If harms and benefits are proportionate, duties of nonmaleficence outweigh those of beneficence.

With regard to maxim 1, the interests of the patient ordinarily count more than those of surrogate decision makers (e.g., family members) or practitioners because she is the one most affected by health care decisions, and social utility is best served by maximizing respect for individual choices. Equality is usually promoted by giving priority to the patient's interests because this will reduce the disadvantage that attaches to her need for health care. Equality may not be promoted if the interest served is likely to advantage the patient rather than restore her health—for example, some cases of cosmetic surgery.

Although maxim 2 does not imply that respect for a patient's autonomy demands implementation of her choices, there is an important epistemological rationale in support of this priority in many cases—namely, that competent, informed patients are in a better position than others to identify their own interests.[33] Further support for this maxim comes from a generally accepted construal of the clinician's primary responsibility: to optimize care for the patient. Optimization of care can only be accomplished by those who attend to nonmedical as well as medical concerns of the patient. Even with optimal care, however, the autonomy of competent, informed patients is occasionally at odds with their health interests. As in other areas of health care, most ethical conflicts for practitioners who care for women arise from the contrast between respect for the patient's autonomy and beneficence or nonmaleficence toward the patient.

Maxim 3 addresses situations in which the welfare of others may be jeopardized by giving priority to the autonomy of a single individual. In the health care setting, such situations arise when patients themselves have competing interests or preferences that cannot be met simultaneously. Moreover, the interests of nonpatients, including family members and clinicians, are occasionally more compelling. If a patient requests treatment that is not medically indicated, for example, a physician is not obligated to provide it, and in some cases it may be wrong to do so.

In general, duties of nonmaleficence outweigh those of beneficence. Maxim 4 takes this into account while indicating that exceptions should be based on calculation of the benefits lost through the avoidance of harm.[34] For example, it would be wrong for a surgeon to perform elective surgery on a patient for whom the risk of the required anesthesia is life-threatening, whereas performing it on a patient whose risk is minimal would be morally acceptable. Similarly, whether a physician may justifiably perform a cesarean section on behalf of a potential child depends not only on its expected benefit to the newborn but also on the degree of risk that the surgery involves for the pregnant woman.

The principal criterion by which the above maxims may be justified coincides with the fourth principle of the Georgetown mantra—justice—which serves a mediating function in an egalitarian approach to health care. Justice also figures among the features that Jonsen, Siegler, and Winslade accommodate within their fourth topic (contextual factors), which calls for examination of the impact on others of decisions for patients.[35] In the next section I examine the meaning of justice in more detail because this principle is indispensable to resolution of ethical conflicts in health care, as it is in other areas of life and public policy. Ethical conflicts would not arise, after all, unless there were competing interests. When the interests of individuals must be prioritized because all of them cannot be satisfied, justice is the overarching principle to be followed. In the language of Beauchamp and Childress, it serves a balancing function by which to address the incompatibility, at times, of the other principles.[36]

Conceptions of justice

Although justice is broadly recognized as a cardinal principle of ethics, its meaning has long been debated by philosophers. In common parlance, "justice" is often used interchangeably with "fairness," "equity," and "equality," but these terms have sometimes been assigned different meanings by classical and contemporary thinkers. For Plato, as articulated through Socrates, justice is the fundamental virtue of society, crucial to the proper ordering of our lives through reason.[37] To Aristotle, justice is a virtue that requires equals to be treated equally and unequals unequally; philosophers refer to this as the formal principle of justice.[38] For Aristotle, people are not all equal to one another; they do not have the same value. However, he does not view equality as implying that people who are equal are the same; in other words, equality does not mean "sameness." Opponents of an egalitarian perspective sometimes conflate these terms—for example, by assuming that gender equality means that differences between men and women are to be disregarded. Those who champion an egalitarian ethic without acknowledging at least some unchangeable differences between men and women are as wrong, I believe, as their opponents.

The contrast between *sameness* and *same value* is clear in mathematical use of the sign for equality. The arithmetical equation $2+3=4+1$, for example, does not mean that $2+3$ is the same as $4+1$, but only that $2+3$ has the same value as $4+1$. Or in algebraic terms, $x=y$ does not mean that x *is* y but only that x and y have the same value. The algebraic formulation lends itself nicely to an expression of gender equality through the different chromosomal arrangements typically found in males and females—that is, XY and XX. To say that XX = XY does not mean that females are the same as males but only that males and females have the same value, despite their differences. This formulation also lends itself to a conception of genetic equality that applies to nontypical chromosomal arrangements such as XO and XXY. A woman with Turner syndrome (XO) is different from one who does not have this condition (XX), but the two surely have the same value, even as they have the same value as males who may or may not have Klinefelter syndrome (XXY). The extended equation XX = XY = XO = XXY shows that anyone who has any of these chromosomal arrangements has the same value as anyone with a different chromosomal arrangement.

Attributing the same value to different people doesn't mean that they should all be treated in the same way. Given the inevitable limitation of resources, however, justice in health care requires prioritization in distribution of health care goods when all needs or desires of patients who are equal to one another cannot be met.[39] Different theorists of justice suggest different approaches to this problem. John Rawls, for example, proposes a theory consistent with liberalism, in which inequality refers to the disparities that exist in people's opportunities to fulfill their own interests. Although inequality is to be curbed, equality is nonetheless subordinated to individual liberty.[40] In other words, Rawls is talking about social inequality, which doesn't necessarily imply that individuals themselves are equal to one another. Amartya Sen and Ronald Dworkin defend a more robust notion of social equality, as do Michael Walzer, Michael Sandel, and Alasdair MacIntyre, whose theories have been called communitarian.[41] In contrast to all of these, Robert Nozick gives priority to individual liberty even if this leads to more disparate distribution of opportunities or capabilities; his theory illustrates libertarianism.[42]

Both liberalism and libertarianism are individualistic in their emphasis on the rights of individuals. For the libertarian, however, the focus is on the right to choose;

liberals support this as well as other basic rights, with different views on how and to what extent the liberty of individuals may sometimes be abridged to accommodate other rights or others' rights. With regard to distribution of health care goods, some liberals support a minimal standard of government funding, whereas others argue for a single-payer system. The greater the opposition to government involvement in health care, the closer the liberal moves to a libertarian framework.

The egalitarian perspective of this book is at odds with Nozick's but consistent with the construal of, and emphasis on, social equality in the other theories. Rawls's liberalism, while more egalitarian than Nozick's, doesn't adequately address the injustice of social inequality. As already suggested, the crucial premise of an egalitarian ethic is that all persons, while different from each other, have the same value. Like Aristotle's basic premises, this is neither proved nor provable but is widely if not universally held to be true.[43] Schemes of distribution that follow from this premise may or may not take account of variables that impede the ability of some people to pursue their goals in life.

According to Nobel laureate Sen, justice requires not only equal distribution of goods (with respect to different needs) but also promotion of equal capability for those whose use of goods is thwarted for irrelevant or inadequate reasons.[44] Impediments to justice as equal capability include those based on characteristics such as gender, class, ethnicity, ability, race, culture, religion, and sexual orientation. Obviously, these characteristics often overlap in the same individual. Sexism, classism, and racism, for example, all impede the capability of poor, African-American women to enjoy the goods that their white, affluent, male counterparts prevalently enjoy because of their dominance. As these examples also illustrate, dominant characteristics are associated with power over others, while nondominant characteristics are associated with disempowerment.

Implementation of justice according to Sen's model of equal capability requires identification of differences associated with social inequality so that the inequality can be eliminated or at least reduced. Being "associated" with social inequality does not necessarily mean that inequality is unjust or that injustice occurs whenever one group is regarded or treated differently than another. It is not unjust, for example, that older people typically have a wider range of experiences and a more extended life span than younger people. Nor is it unjust that some people are more talented, more intelligent, more attractive, or more athletically gifted than others. But disregard of differences, which many advocates of political correctness recommend, runs the risk of exacerbating or masking unjust inequality. Injustice occurs when the differences of one group are interpreted as implying their inferiority, or lesser value, in comparison with the other group, and they are treated accordingly. Using the chromosomal designations mentioned above, for example, gender injustice may be formulated as a situation in which XY>XX or XY<XX: that is, as one in which either men or women are regarded or treated as having lesser value than the other.

Unfortunately, the reference point to which women are often compared is men, rather than the common humanness in which men and women participate equally. In *The Second Sex*, Simone de Beauvoir described this phenomenon as one in which "man defines woman not in herself but as relative to him"—that is, as "the

Other" who is "the incidental, the inessential as opposed to the essential."[45] In contrast, gender justice occurs when men and women are judged according to the standard of their common humanness, respecting the differences that they embody as gendered individuals without imputing inferiority to one or the other on that basis.

While considering unequal distributions of natural abilities or assets among individuals, H. Tristram Engelhardt suggests that such differences are due to failures of fortune rather than fairness.[46] It is unfortunate, he says, that some people are disabled while others are fully able, but it is not unfair that this is so. From an egalitarian perspective, a major flaw in Engelhardt's account is that it says nothing about what should be done or not done about naturally occurring social inequality. It is true that good health is often a matter of luck or good fortune, but changeable circumstances such as economic and social disparities often exacerbate the risks of becoming sick or disabled, or more sick or more disabled, and these inequalities are neither fortunate, nor fair, nor unchangeable.

Engelhardt would probably not claim that it is unfortunate for women that they are not born male, but such a statement is empirically supportable by his libertarian account because women are more likely than men to be poor and dependent on the health care system for themselves and others, and women are less likely than men to be well-educated or to enjoy positions of power and prestige. The fact that women rather than men tend to be the principal caregivers of children and others who need care obviously contributes not only to this discrepancy but also to the health risks associated with it.[47]

In general, a libertarian theory of justice gives priority to the liberty or autonomy of individuals in choosing procedural mechanisms for the distribution of health care and other resources. The economic system thus supported is capitalistic and individualistic. As Nozick paraphrased Marx, the libertarian criterion for distributive decisions is "From each as they choose, to each as they are chosen."[48] On this account, the material gaps of opportunity and capability between some people and others are inevitably widened through maximization of individual liberty in an environment that ignores differences that reduce or enhance autonomy. Affluent patients, for example, can purchase optimal or elective health care, while poor patients cannot. Admittedly, a libertarian perspective endorses choices that are morally praiseworthy, but it also seems to support choices that are morally reprehensible, such as those based on racism, sexism, and classism.

The liberal theory of justice elaborated by Rawls involves two basic principles. First, individual liberty should be limited only to the extent that it is necessary to ensure the same liberty for others; second, social and economic inequalities should be arranged so that they benefit the least advantaged in a situation of equality of opportunity for all. Susan Okin endorsed these principles of justice but criticized Rawls for ignoring injustices that occur in domestic relationships.[49] She refuted Rawls's assumption that families are just by using data illustrating the inherently patriarchal structure of the family and the economic disparities triggered by family-related practices and attitudes.

Norman Daniels has applied Rawls's notion of "equality of opportunity" to bioethics by arguing that health care benefits should be arranged to ensure for everyone, to the extent possible, the "normal opportunity range" of "species-typical function"—that is, the range of function that reasonable persons in a given society are likely to construct for themselves.[50] Key but problematic terms in this account are "normal" and "species-typical." To some scholars, use of these terms undervalues those who cannot or choose not to meet the "normal" or "species-typical" standard, however this is defined. They argue, for example, that this approach has "the coercive potential of medicalizing people's departures from typical or customary functioning."[51] Respect for differences, which is central to the egalitarian framework of this book, is obviously incompatible with that interpretation.

Equality of opportunity is also problematic because of ambiguity and controversiality regarding its meaning in particular cases. In general, this Rawlsian principle supports a right to basic health care and to an environment free of contaminants that might damage one's health; but what constitutes *basic* health care and what type or degree of damage to health is at stake are neither clear nor uncontested. Whether equality of opportunity requires universal access to elective procedures such as cosmetic surgery and infertility treatment is also unclear. The tie between these procedures and basic health care is widely disputed, and some circumstances seem to call for their provision more than others.[52] Moreover, the extent to which society is obliged to pay for the health care of those who cannot pay for it themselves is a matter on which liberals disagree. Some support a minimal level of government subsidies, leaning closer to a libertarian approach; others support a maximal level, with more egalitarian implications.

Communitarian and egalitarian thinkers are the principal critics of both liberal and libertarian accounts of the relationship between autonomy and equality. Communitarians tend to emphasize familial or affective relationships and the cultural or religious contexts in which people live their lives, while egalitarians are more likely to focus on political relationships and the importance of equality as a social goal. Both critiques start with a concept of human beings not as isolated agents but as individuals whose meaning and reality are definable and sustainable only in the context of their interactions with others. As Michael Sandel puts it, human beings are not independently autonomous selves, as Kantians and Rawlsians assume, but "subjects constituted in part by our central aspirations and attachments, always open, indeed vulnerable, to growth and transformation in the light of revised self-understandings."[53] Admittedly, the ethical relevance of relationships has been incorporated into most accounts of special duties to others, including those that arise from a Kantian perspective. But other philosophical traditions make relationships more central to their analyses. To existentialists such as Martin Buber and Gabriel Marcel, for example, relationships are integral to our humanity as such; to classical pragmatists such as William James and Charles Sanders Peirce, relationships are not mere abstractions but practical realities.[54] More recently, feminist scholars have provided diverse and extensive accounts of relationships as indispensable to moral decision-making.[55]

Sandel's emphasis on attachments or particular, duty-related ties to others is consistent with the ethics of care or caring that Carol Gilligan and Nel Noddings developed. Noddings claimed the relationship between mother and child as ethically paradigmatic and argued for a broader application of the care embodied in that relationship.[56] She considered "care" antithetical to "equality" or a justice ethic, as she construed them. Gilligan based her model of moral reasoning on studies of girls and women confronting ethical dilemmas in their own lives.[57] Women, she found, typically reached their decisions through consideration of responsibilities derived from relationships to others rather than consideration of their own or others' rights as individuals. They were more likely than men to be influenced by concerns of caring for those with whom they had established ties than by concerns of justice toward those they did not know.

Just as men and women are not necessarily incompatible or unequal because they are different, a care-based ethic and a justice ethic are not necessarily incompatible, and one of them is not necessarily invalid because they are different. Unlike Noddings, Gilligan acknowledges liabilities in both approaches. The potential error of a justice focus, she says, is "its latent egocentrism, the tendency to confuse one's perspective with an objective standpoint or truth, the temptation to define others in one's own terms by putting oneself in their place." The liability of a focus on care is that it tends "to forget that one has terms, creating a tendency to enter into another's perspective and to see oneself as 'selfless' by defining oneself in others' terms."[58] Historically, these liabilities have given rise to two common distortions of justice and care. In an ethic of justice the distortion is that human is equated with male; in an ethic of care the distortion is the equation of care with self-sacrifice. The liabilities are avoided and the distortions are corrected in an ethic that incorporates both justice and care.

While questioning whether either orientation is adequate from a moral point of view, feminist philosophers have argued persuasively for the compatibility of care and justice.[59] If justice means giving people their due, it demands determination of what constitutes due care for each. The application of this concept to health care professionals is obvious: the practitioner must recognize and respond to different needs or interests on the part of each patient. At times the needs of different parties are at odds with each other. An ethic of care in clinical practice is thus different from an ethic that focuses solely on the individual patient because it involves care for all of those affected by the caregiver's decisions. A *just* caring ethic requires efforts to distribute burdens and benefits fairly. On the account of equality developed here, this means treating every individual as having the same value.

As we have seen, the verity of justice is open to different interpretations, but the maxims mentioned earlier provide clues or guidance regarding its application to the variables that occur in health care. They also offer justifiable guides to resolution of conflicts that arise in applying the other verities or principles to specific cases or issues. However, decision makers are often unable to accurately identify or weigh burdens and benefits to others (cf. beneficence and nonmaleficence), or determine whether others are fully informed, competent, and autonomous (cf. respect for autonomy). Unfortunately, they occasionally make decisions affecting others without recognizing this inability. An obvious, ethically necessary strategy by which to improve the knowledge base of such decisions is to seek and listen to the input of those most affected by them. From an egalitarian perspective, a related and just as necessary strategy is to elicit input from people who stand in positions other than those of the usual policy makers.

Standpoint theory and its implications for just caring

Justice is often portrayed as blind, but blindness to differences brings risk of injustice by ignoring factors associated with inequality.[60] All of us are probably blind, or at least nearsighted, with regard to some of those factors. To overcome this limitation or reduce our nearsightedness, we need to listen to those who see the world differently precisely because they see it from a different place. John Stuart Mill recognized this need when he objected to paternalistic interferences with freedom on grounds that individuals have a better understanding of what promotes their own interests than others have in making decisions for them.[61] Nonetheless, many ethicists seem to believe they are capable of determining the interests of others without their input. The history of ethics is replete with thinkers who claim that impartiality is indispensable to ethical judgments and consider their own ethical positions as exemplars of such impartiality. Thomas Nagel, for example, maintains that ethics begins with the ability "to think about the world in abstraction from our particular position in it."[62] Like others, he apparently purports to prescind from his own standpoint in developing positions on moral matters.

In contrast to Nagel and his ilk, classical pragmatists have lent support to a perspectival view of knowledge that feminist scholars have recently dubbed "standpoint theory." Peirce, for example, recognized the inevitable limitations of individual standpoints and argued for collaborative inquiry as a means by which to overcome them. Because collaboration reduces the nearsightedness of separate perspectives, Peirce considered it illogical and unscientific to be antisocial in the quest for knowledge. "Logic," he wrote, "is rooted in the social principle," requiring that the interests of investigators not be limited to their interests as individuals or even to their own area of research.[63]

More recent critics of demands for impartiality in ethics include John Ladd, who distinguishes between objective and subjective standpoints. Ladd equates the "God's eye point of view" of "social engineers" who see themselves, and whose supporters describe them, as "sincere and dedicated public servants selected on the basis of their professional expertise."[64] Although their approach is inevitably speculative, these social engineers regard their perspectives as overwhelmingly superior to those of ordinary individuals whose lives are affected by their decisions. As "objectivists," they think that their own "formal organizations of expert administrators" are indispensable to achievement of their goal, a true and adequate account of "the way things are."[65] Participation by those who see the world subjectively—from their own different but nondominant perspectives—can only impede that achievement. For paternalistic practitioners, this rationale is not only appealing but justifiable.

From Ladd's perspective, which is essentially egalitarian, the preceding rationale ignores the fact that the individuals who formulate decisions and policies are fallible human beings who, as such, recurrently lack knowledge relevant to the issues they address. Another crucial flaw is that dominant individuals often "lack the kind of involvement in the outcome that is forced on the recipients of the decision," who are nondominant. While the latter are fallible, too, they have a personal moral stake in what is decided, which in itself constitutes a moral argument for their participation. On democratic as well as utilitarian grounds, the input of those who are nondominant should be weighed more heavily than that of those who are less affected precisely because of that differential impact.[66]

For Ladd the critical question that so-called objectivists fail to identify, let alone address, is "Who is to decide?" This question, he says, is even more important today than in the past because those who make decisions are further removed than ever from those to whom their decisions apply. As proof of a longstanding tendency to ignore the question, Ladd offers examples of old men who decide that young people should kill innocent people in war, rich men who decide what kind of welfare the poor should receive, and white men who decide who should police the streets in a black neighborhood.[67] All of his examples are pertinent to standpoint theory, as are two not mentioned: men in general decide what women in general may do, and physicians in general decide what treatments to offer to which patients.

Aware that the "objective approach" threatens the autonomy of less powerful or nondominant groups, Ladd maintains that participation in decision-making is a means of reducing the alienation they often experience. He credits minorities, students, and workers for contributing to "disalienation" through their demands for participation in the communities to which they belong, at home, school, or their places of employment,[68] imputing to them a position of ethical as well as epistemological privilege.

On the issue of privilege, Nancy Hartsock has developed an interpretation of standpoint theory that focuses on the disparities that often arise between those who occupy different positions vis-à-vis one another.[69] Members of the nondominant groups, she maintains, are capable of seeing beneath the surface of the social relations they experience, and the standpoint thus achieved allows them to see beyond present structures to possibilities that the members of the dominant group, which designed the structures according to their lights, are unable to envision. Like Ladd, Hartsock would reverse the status of the parties involved by privileging the standpoint of those who are nondominant as a means of overcoming the inevitable limitations of the dominant view. Both groups are advantaged through the reversal of privilege: members of the dominant group are empowered to correct and expand their vision; members of the nondominant group are empowered to liberate themselves.

The epistemological rationale for standpoint theory is thus based on two factors: recognition that the experiences on which knowledge depends are incomplete and partial, and desire to reduce this limitation through collaborative inquiry. Implementation of the theory cannot totally overcome epistemological limitations or liabilities because nondominant individuals are not only subject to nearsightedness themselves but also subject to distortive influences on their perspectives, for example, through socialization and cultural pressures. Imputing privileged status to them does not imply that their views are immune to critique by the dominant groups or by others who are nondominant. The input of nondominant others as well as the dominant group remains necessary to minimize epistemological limitations. Moreover, the perspective of those who are not personally subject to experiences that nondominant individuals have often facilitates knowledge that might not otherwise be available, especially when it is based on long-term observations and interactions with them.

The ethical warrant for standpoint theory derives from prima facie obligations to respect the autonomy of, and practice beneficence toward, those who are nondominant as well as those who are dominant. It thus facilitates the ethics of authenticity that Charles Taylor proposed as crucial to the moral integrity of diverse individuals.[70] If democracy is understood as requiring participation, or at least representation, of nondominant individuals in the development of policies affecting them, this provides an additional warrant for standpoint theory. While its liberating potential is morally desirable, its potential for reducing inequality is just as desirable and crucial to actualization of the potential for liberation of all members of society. Accordingly, the arguments of Peirce, Ladd, and Hartsock are most persuasive to those for whom justice has priority in political as well as ethical decision-making.

As Albert Camus observed, both oppressors and oppressed are diminished through oppression. "I rebel," he wrote, "therefore we exist."[71] Applying that remark to the practice of health care, clinicians and patients alike may be liberated by imputing privileged status to the standpoint of those who are nondominant. Patients in general are nondominant vis-à-vis clinicians, but many clinicians (e.g., medical technicians and nurses) are nondominant vis-à-vis other clinicians. Standpoint theory is thus applicable to different groups within the health care setting. For all of those involved, it offers a means by which to promote justice while reducing moral, epistemological, and political limitations.

Privileging women's standpoint in our health care

Many men are patients, many women are doctors, and socioeconomic inequality based on differences in race, education, and class abounds at least as much in clinical encounters as in other areas of life. Empirical signs of inequality also abound in these encounters—for example, the doctor standing before the prone or sitting patient, the undressed patient being examined by the fully clothed doctor, the waiting time of patients versus the time spent with them by their doctors, the tendency in some quarters to refer to doctors by title and last name while referring to (adult) patients and nurses by their first names. To the extent that either sex occupies a less privileged or nondominant position in comparison with the other, standpoint theory argues for reversing their privileged status. In comparison with men, however, women tend in much greater numbers to occupy less privileged positions as patients and caregivers. Granting them privileged status in decisions regarding their health serves to reduce the inevitable limitations of practitioners' standpoints in their regard.

Most patients depend on their doctors for information regarding their diagnosis, prognosis, and treatment alternatives. Their vulnerability is often exacerbated, especially in the context of obstetrics and gynecology, by their disclosure of personal, intimate information about themselves with no corresponding disclosures on the part of the practitioner. This one-sided dependence or vulnerability of patients is unavoidable in many respects and not necessarily conducive to a bad outcome;

nonetheless, it confirms and sometimes heightens the privileged status of the doctor vis-à-vis the patient. The legal and moral requirement of informed consent imputes privilege to the patient's decision but does not eliminate the power discrepancy between the two. In fact, the language of "informed *consent*" suggests dominance on the part of the one who defines the parameters and chooses the context in which consent is requested. Language involving "choice" rather than "consent" would impute greater autonomy to the patient's decision.[72] So routinely is the language of "informed consent" used in the clinical setting, however, that efforts to replace it with "informed choice" are unlikely to be successful.

To the extent that privilege connotes power, men in general occupy privileged positions vis-à-vis women in general because they predominate in positions of power and policy-making. Laws and educational practices have in many cases reduced this overall discrepancy, in some cases by imputing privileged status to women through policies of affirmative action. In many countries, women occupy more positions of leadership or privilege than in the past, but they are far from predominant vis-à-vis their male counterparts. The number of women entering medical school is in some instances greater than the number of men, and residencies and fellowships, especially those devoted to women's health care, have been increasingly comprised mainly if not entirely of women. Eventually, women may predominate in dominant positions, but that day is far from here as yet, especially in the more prestigious or remunerative professions.

A profession is an occupation through which individuals are equipped through their education and training to exercise specific power or expertise in behalf of those who lack such power or expertise. However, the goal or end of a profession is to empower the other, whether client or student or patient, so that he or she no longer needs the services of the professional.[73] To the extent that the professional seeks to maintain or increase her own power vis-à-vis the other, this goal is betrayed. Standpoint theory suggests a means by which the end of the profession may be effectively pursued—by empowering the disempowered.

Admittedly, empowering patients and women so that equality between them and their counterparts is fully achieved is an ideal that may be critiqued as utopian. Nonetheless, the ideal (discussed further in chapter 14) can be approximated through applications of standpoint theory to the clinical setting. A recent example of how this might be done in research settings was the practice of inclusion of "consumers" in evaluation of research proposals by the U. S. Department of Defense Breast Cancer Research Integration Panel.[74] Consumers were defined as survivors of breast cancer and their family members. Following a recommendation from the Institute of Medicine, patients with breast cancer were invited to serve on the review panel, along with the scientists, to review proposals and participate in decisions about funding. Appointment to such panels is commonly construed as a sign that the appointee enjoys a dominant position in the field.

In questionnaires completed by scientists and consumers subsequent to the review process, the majority of both groups felt that inclusion of consumers had enhanced the process. Given that the consumers as such lacked scientific expertise, their input could not have improved the quality of the science in the submitted proposals. Nonetheless, the scientists as well as the consumers who had participated felt that inclusion of nonscientists who had experienced breast cancer improved the quality of the review process and provided input critical to determination of whether scientifically meritorious proposals fit programmatic goals. Positive assessment of this application of standpoint theory was demonstrated most convincingly through affirmative answers to the question of whether a policy of inclusion should be continued.

Increasingly, policy-making groups recognize the ethical and epistemological merit of involvement by nondominant, affected individuals in their deliberations. In clinical settings also, the appropriateness of such involvement is increasingly recognized. Hospital lawyers tend to assign privileged status to the decisions of competent, informed patients; legal statutes and court decisions generally support this. Nonetheless, input from patients is less likely to be given privileged status when they belong to nondominant groups, such as those who are economically or educationally disadvantaged, those who do not speak the same language as their caregivers, the very old or very young, people with disabilities, and those from different cultural, racial, or religious backgrounds. Studies also suggest that the input of women is less likely to be accorded privileged status.[75] The unfortunate result is that decisions are less informed and ethically justified than they might be.

This book attempts to accord privileged status to the input of women through persistent recognition that they are the ones most affected by decisions about their health and less likely than men to be accorded that status. Because women in health care as in other areas of life are seldom accorded that status, this is a remedial effort. Admittedly, this attempted remediation is but partial because, while my standpoint matches that of other women in many ways, it cannot wholly capture the uniqueness of each woman's standpoint. Neither do I consider my egalitarian and standpoint-based approach theoretically or practically adequate to the end of justice in health care. I simply offer a deliberate effort to be as inclusive as I can of women's views about our care and its impact on us. With Donna Haraway, I want to avoid the pretense of objectivity of those who purport to articulate universal truths, because I believe the best approximation of objectivity occurs by establishing "webs of connection" through shared conversations about the "situated knowledges" of different individuals and groups.[76]

If the principle of justice is crucial to resolution of ethical conflicts and if gender justice is a necessary subset of justice, issues involving women's health care must be examined from the standpoint of women themselves. This standpoint is particularly important for clinicians who care for women because our status as patients exacerbates the risks posed by gender-based nondominance. Race, ethnicity, religion, class, ability, age, and sexual orientation are other ethically relevant differences that need to be identified and examined from the perspective of justice. Men as well as women in any of these groups are treated unjustly if their differences become grounds by which they are valued less than others. While focusing on justice toward women, therefore, I necessarily address concerns about injustice toward nondominant groups to which men belong.

Some nondominant individuals whose standpoint deserves privileged status are unable to understand, anticipate, or articulate how decisions formulated by others will affect them. Children and adults with cognitive impairment belong in this group; if moral status is imputed to them, embryos and fetuses belong there as well. If women are in dominant positions vis-à-vis other persons because of factors such as age or class or ability, we too should impute privileged status to our nondominant counterparts.

As we have seen, the verity of justice, like respect for autonomy, beneficence, and nonmaleficence, is subject to different interpretations and justifications, as are the different ethical and political theories with which they are associated. Any of these terms or theories could be the subject of an entire volume, or multiple volumes of refutations, interpretations, and justifications articulating different views. My aim is philosophically more modest and practical. I simply intend to consider a range of cases and issues that arise in caring for the health of women across the life span, pointing out how different principles or verities are applicable to some of the variables that inevitably arise. Some practitioners and patients may find these considerations helpful to their own examination of ethical quandaries. Others may interpret the verities and variables differently, and they may articulate or defend other prioritizing maxims to apply to complex cases. Both kinds of response are welcome.

In sum, the egalitarian perspective of this book identifies relevant variables and considers these in light of well-established ethical verities and maxims. The particulars of cases help to clarify the ambiguity of the verities. Justice, which necessarily involves equality (but not sameness) of care, serves a mediating function in situations of conflict; it also serves as an ideal to be approximated as fully as possible. The concept of equality that underlies this perspective is one that imputes the same value to everyone, regardless of differences among them. It requires attention to differences so that inequalities associated with them may be reduced. The standpoints of nondominant groups are crucial to identification of these differences; these provide a means by which the nearsightedness of the dominant decision-making group can be alleviated. Because women are the nondominant group on whom this book focuses, gender justice is central to consideration of the issues. As the next chapter illustrates, many features of women's health care pose significantly different challenges than those addressed in other areas of health care.

2

Distinguishing Features of Women's Health Care

As discussed in chapter 1, identification of differences is the first step required for an egalitarian approach to ethical issues, and standpoint theory provides a strategy for recognizing these differences. The second step is to determine the extent if any to which the identified differences are associated with inequality—that is, disadvantage or disempowerment. The third step is to find ways by which to reduce the associated inequality, and the fourth step is to implement these measures. Some differences associated with inequality between patients and practitioners or between women and men are not changeable (e.g., only women can be pregnant); others, such as those that arise from social, economic, and cultural practices, are changeable. In either case, an egalitarian perspective calls for efforts to reduce the inequality associated with differences based on gender or on any other feature irrelevant to the value that ought to be attributed to every person.

To implement an egalitarian perspective in the context of health care requires attention not only to differences based on variables such as gender, race, and class but also to more specific differences such as the medical prognosis, the risks and benefits of interventions, and the relationships between patients, clinicians, and family members. It also requires clarification of the concepts of respect for autonomy, beneficence, and nonmaleficence in light of the relevant variables, as well as efforts to maximize the implementation of these principles with regard to those affected through use of prioritizing maxims. Although justice is rarely mentioned in some accounts of bioethical issues that concern women, it is central not only to resolution of conflicts raised by particular cases but also to assessment of different models of the practitioner-patient relationship and to regulation of health care by professional societies and governmental bodies.

Many ethically relevant variables in health care apply to men, women, and children alike. Some, however, apply exclusively to one group because its members are distinguishable in ethically relevant ways. This chapter is intended to facilitate understanding and application of an egalitarian perspective by identifying ways in which women's health care is different from other areas of clinical practice. In light of these features, I critique models of the practitioner-patient relationship that, while developed for physicians, are applicable to anyone engaged in clinical encounters with women. I also consider how the casuistic and principlist methods discussed in chapter 1 may be amended to account for a unique feature of women's health care: the possibility of initiating, prolonging, or terminating the life of an embryo or fetus within them. In this context, I examine and critique the tendency to treat the fetus as a second patient. Finally, I briefly consider differences between professional guidelines and government regulations as mechanisms by which ethical decisions in health care may be promoted for women and other nondominant members of society. These differences also deserve critique from an egalitarian perspective.

Some sex and gender differences

The terms "sex" and "gender" have sometimes been distinguished from each other on grounds of biological versus social influences on human behavior. In fact, these influences often intertwine, and both affect women's health. Nonetheless, most of the distinguishing features of women's health care are mainly biological or mainly social. The biological differences are generally unchangeable, but this is not necessarily the case for social attitudes and practices—even if they are triggered by the biological differences, and even though social change often seems more difficult to effect than biological change. Gender-based features of women's health care are often more numerous and complicated than those based solely on biological sex.

The most salient distinguishing feature of women's health care is the fact that most women are capable during a considerable portion of their lives of conceiving and bearing children. Although this sex-based characteristic is often relevant to treatment of women, it also has many gender-based or social implications. Ethically relevant variables that arise from these implications include (but are not limited to) the circumstances in which a pregnancy is initiated, continued, or terminated; the costs and availability of medical assistance during pregnancy; the impact of pregnancy on women's lifestyles; societal supports (or lack of support) for pregnant women; and social attitudes and laws about decisions to continue or terminate pregnancy. In addition, the ethical complexity of health care of pregnant women and research involving women of reproductive age is inseparable from diverse positions about the moral status of the fetus.

As indicated in chapter 1, another distinguishing feature of women's health care is that their encounters with clinicians are often initiated not by illness or disability but by a normal and health-affirming event in their life cycle (pregnancy or menopause) or by the fact that they are the principal caregivers of others for whom they seek care. Although elderly women obtain health care more often than elderly men, this is mainly due to the fact that their life span is longer than men's. If an extended life span is a mark of health, most women are healthier than most men; this difference is probably due to social or gender-based factors as well as biology.

From an egalitarian perspective, the fact that patients are women presents a challenge to practitioners to avoid reinforcement of harmful gender stereotypes. A stereotypic construal of women as vulnerable, dependent, passive, emotional, and less informed or rational in comparison with men coincides with a construal of patients as vulnerable, dependent, passive, emotional, and less informed or rational than their doctors. Sick people sometimes match these stereotypes, but men are as likely as women to match them. In normal pregnancy and during menopause, the major responsibility of the practitioner is to help the woman maintain her health through the duration of the experience; a concomitant challenge is to facilitate her recognition that her condition is not a sign of ill health.

Unfortunately, the medicalization of normal events in women's lives gives some women the sense that these conditions constitute illnesses. The power discrepancy that usually prevails between patients and doctors may lend credence to this false impression. Good care of healthy women is not unlike routine practices of preventive care in other settings. To the extent that such care is distributed across income levels, these practices facilitate more equitable care. While encouraging women to view pregnancy or menopause as normal events in the life cycle, clinicians also need to ensure that medical assistance is available to women for health needs that may or may not be related to these conditions.

Another gender-based feature of women's health care occurs throughout the life span and throughout the world; this is what Diana Pearce dubbed "the feminization of poverty."[1] The term "juvenilization of poverty" could also be introduced to describe the impact of poverty on the children of poor women.[2] Although many poor families receive government support for their children, support for pregnant women's health care often focuses exclusively on concerns about the fetus, treating the woman as if her sole importance stems from her pregnant status.

The correlation between poverty and quality of health care has been well documented: the greater the income, the more people can afford a healthy life style and the greater the likelihood that if and when they become ill they will be treated optimally.[3] Expensive, elective treatments such as reproductive technologies and cosmetic surgery are typically available to the affluent but not to the poor. Ironically, the availability of some of these treatment modalities may be more burdensome than beneficial to affluent women who are driven to seek the interventions by social or family pressures, despite risks to themselves that their male counterparts avoid. Gender stereotypes about a feminine appearance exacerbate the burden of treatment involving mastectomy or hair loss for women; and distorted, media-propelled images of feminine beauty lead some women to adopt health-threatening behaviors to achieve conformity with these images. A stereotypic image of men as naturally prone to violence or sexual aggression poses another gender-based health threat to women—as victims of domestic abuse.

Some distinctive features of women's health care, such as the fact that many "patients" are not ill, are applicable to any specialty that offers preventive services. When the patient is pregnant, however, the clinical situation is unique in that the interests of a potential child may be affected. Research on pregnant women is also problematic because of this possibility. Transplantation of organs or tissue from living donors involves direct treatment of two patients who are unquestionably persons. In contrast, treatment of pregnant women involves direct treatment of two patients only if the fetus or embryo is in fact a second patient. Similarly, research on a pregnant woman means research on two distinct subjects if the fetus is considered apart from the pregnant woman. (Whether the fetus is a person is a related but different issue, examined in chapter 3.)

Obstetrics is a specialty that prevalently leads to happy, healthy outcomes. When the outcome is otherwise, the distress that follows tends to be more intense than in situations in which those involved are not as confident of good outcomes. Two factors make the distress worse for patients or family members than for practitioners: bad outcomes are a recurrent, even if unusual, event for practitioners, and they, unlike patients or family members, do not live intimately and lastingly with the consequences of the bad outcome. For example, the obstetrician who assists in the birth of an infant who is neurologically devastated, say, through cord prolapse, will not take the child home or be responsible for her lifelong care. Admittedly, cases in which the bad outcome arises from medical mistakes or neglect can and should cause greater distress for the practitioner than those in which the bad outcome was unavoidable. Nonetheless, the standpoint of the one who is most burdened by decisions made in this context, surely deserves a more privileged status than that of others.

Some of the distinctive features of women's health care make this area of clinical practice more attractive than others to aspiring clinicians. For others, the opposite is the case. Debts incurred in the course of training and income or lifestyle goals influence the choice of clinical specialties and practice settings for many individuals. When obstetrics is considered, other factors influence these choices, especially for women. Because normal births as well as difficult births and complications of pregnancy can occur at any time, obstetricians are on call at any hour of day or night throughout the year. Many women seek predictable or reduced work schedules to accommodate their personal reproductive plans and responsibilities for children. Team practices allow many obstetricians to adjust their work schedules to accommodate other responsibilities or personal goals, at least after the completion of residency training. From the patient's standpoint, however, team practices may limit her ability to ensure that a particular clinician assists in her care or delivery.

When women have the option, many prefer women as their doctors. Some are required by their cultures to be examined only by women. To satisfy the increasing number of requests for female practitioners, many team practices have been eager to recruit women for their staffs. Their efforts are much more likely to be successful than in the past because the number of women in medicine is considerably greater, especially in obstetrics and gynecology. A commitment to women's health has encouraged many women to join this specialty or to focus on women's health in other specialties. Provocatively, one experienced (male) practitioner has even proposed that only women should be obstetrician/gynecologists.[4] Respect for autonomy argues against this suggestion because its implementation would not only reduce the practice options of male doctors but also eliminate the option of a male doctor for women who prefer this. Standpoint theory suggests that female practitioners are more likely to be aware of some of the complex issues faced by women as women, but other prevalent differences between clinicians and their nondominant patients (e.g., class, sexuality, ability, ethnicity) still argue for privileging the standpoint of patients, both male and female, in the clinical setting.

Reproductive and gynecological care deals more than other specialties with intimate sexual histories and lifestyles that practitioners may personally find morally objectionable or psychologically disturbing. Some clinicians are prone to judge the moral practices or values of patients, but this is not the role or right of the health professional as such. Occasionally, practitioners are tempted to talk about personal disclosures of patients to their colleagues or others. Duties of confidentiality and respect for privacy, both required by respect for patient autonomy, call for resistance to this temptation, no matter how titillating or intriguing the information imparted. Moreover, because the profession of health care permits practitioners to have access to patients' bodies and to intimate details of their lives, an inadvertent voyeurism may influence the behavior of clinicians. This possibility is exacerbated in reproductive and gynecological care because the power discrepancy that usually prevails between patients and clinicians offers a potential not present in other settings for sexual abuse of women. From an egalitarian perspective a challenge this poses for institutions is not only to have policies in place that identify and punish offenders but also to minimize the power discrepancy that enables abuses to occur.

Because their patients may be minors or adults, obstetrician-gynecologists and family practitioners grapple more frequently than colleagues in pediatrics and medicine with moral and legal questions about competence for consent to treatment. With some exceptions (such as emancipated minor statutes), laws in most jurisdictions tend to assume that decisions by adults are autonomous and those by children are not. Ethically, this distinction is inadequate if respect for autonomy as well as nonmaleficence and beneficence are maximally upheld, and if the standpoint of patients is to be respected regardless of their age. But autonomy is lacking or deficient in some healthy, able adults and present in varying degrees in many older children and adolescents. The moral challenge to the practitioner, therefore, is to determine the extent of the patient's capacity for decision-making and attempt to respect her autonomy in light of that determination.

Although patients and doctors sometimes develop close personal as well as professional ties to one another, neither party relates to the other as a lone individual. This is especially true in obstetrics, where many women see several doctors through the course of their prenatal care, and which physician will be available during delivery is often beyond their control. On their clinical visits, patients are often accompanied by their partners, relatives, or friends; those who come alone are also, inevitably, enmeshed in and influenced by those relationships. Consequently, to think or speak of "the doctor-patient relationship" without acknowledging the multiple, rich, and complicated relationships in which both individuals are simultaneously and unalterably embedded exemplifies the fallacy of abstraction—that is, using a term whose meaning is inseparable from that of another term without reference to the other term. An egalitarian account of relationships between physicians and patients would acknowledge the plurality of relationships that occur in interactions among patients, their family members and friends, and all of the clinicians involved in their treatment. In the next section, I examine prevalent models of "the doctor-patient relationship" in light of that account.

Models of the practitioner-patient relationship

Most models of the physician-patient relationship focus on the tie between an individual doctor and a specific patient, thereby tending to minimize or ignore the centrality of justice in health care and gender justice in women's health care. The prevalent models emphasize the obligations of clinicians to respect and promote the best interests of the patient but give different weight to different interests. These interests include not only the patient's health and well-being but also her choices regarding treatment or nontreatment. Linda and Ezekiel Emanuel have identified four models that they consider applicable to different circumstances: paternalistic, informative, interpretive, and deliberative. The American College of Obstetrics and Gynecology has endorsed this account in their recommendations to physicians regarding appropriate treatment of women.[5]

In most cases, the first two models are at odds with an egalitarian approach to health care. In the paternalistic model, the physician attempts to promote the patient's health or welfare without regard for her autonomy. This implies that her health interests override her autonomy interests. For patients who are not autonomous, a paternalistic model is inapplicable because their health interests can be promoted without either disregarding or overriding their autonomy. It is not paternalistic, for example, to provide urgent necessary treatment to an unconscious patient, unless she has previously indicated her objection to it or a proxy indicates that the patient would not consent to it. As maxim 3 indicates, autonomy may occasionally be overridden on grounds of others' welfare, but coercive treatment of a competent, adequately informed patient cannot be justified solely on grounds of the practitioner's desire to promote her health. Accordingly, this model is inconsistent with widespread acceptance of the priority of patient autonomy and with recognition of the patient's privileged standpoint.

In the informative model the practitioner is "a provider of objective and technical information regarding the patient's medical problem and its potential therapeutic solutions," and the patient "has complete control over" clinical decisions.[6] The physician's role is purely instrumental: she simply implements the patient's informed choice. Ignored here is the fact that many patients are not autonomous, some are only partially autonomous, and some autonomous patients want direction or guidance as well as information or prefer to have their practitioners or others make decisions regarding their care.[7] A further flaw of the informative model is its implication that the physician is not responsible for what she does or doesn't do. The practitioner who defines her role solely as a provider of information and the patient as the sole determiner of clinical decisions fails to fulfill her own responsibility as a moral agent, who, as such, may be obliged to advise the patient against a course that is medically contraindicated or morally unjustified. Worse, perhaps, the informative model suggests that the clinician doesn't care what the patient chooses but only about implementing her choice, even if this is highly likely to have dastardly consequences. The patient's autonomy is thus the only interest to be promoted.

A paternalistic model of the physician-patient relationship still prevails in many clinical encounters, but many clinicians who treat women of reproductive age are more attracted to the informative model. The attraction arises from an understandable desire to bypass the myriad ethical controversies and emotionally charged issues that arise in reproduction—by simply acting as instruments of the patient's will. The physician thus sees herself as ethically neutral or, better, as exercising a morally appropriate nonjudgmental attitude toward the patient. In some cases, ethical neutrality is possible and morally justifiable. In other cases, however, it is morally irresponsible. Maxim 1, which in most cases gives priority to respect for patient autonomy, is a crucial guideline, but it does not imply that the moral obligations of physicians as such are satisfied by uncritical fulfillment of patients' requests. An egalitarian model of the practitioner-patient relationship demands regard for the moral integrity of both clinicians and patients.

Although the autonomy of competent patients is accorded unquestioned priority in the informative model, philosophers have increasingly questioned simplistic interpretations of autonomy, and bioethicists and clinicians alike have argued against its primacy in clinical decision-making. Relationships to others inevitably and appropriately influence the choices we make. Models of "*the* doctor-patient relationship" seem to ignore these ongoing ties by suggesting that only two parties are involved. Nor is autonomy an all or nothing capability; adults as well as older children and adolescents may be partially autonomous. Addiction, mental illness, cognitive impairment, and intense pain—all of these may reduce but not eliminate the autonomy of patients. In an informative model, deficiencies in autonomy are apparently not taken into account; in a paternalistic model, whatever autonomy is present in patients is ignored or overridden.

The interpretive model recognizes that the autonomous decisions of each patient are enmeshed in a personal value system to which the clinician may lack access. As described by the American College of Obstetrics and Gynecologists, this model is comparable to the nondirective model of genetic counseling: the practitioner's role is to help the patient "clarify and integrate her values into the decision-making process, while acting as an information source regarding the technical aspects of any given medical procedure."[8] Although this approach is ethically appropriate in some situations, a crucial flaw arises from the fact that practitioners at times have values that are at odds with those of their patients. If they are faithful to their own moral values, they may not in those instances facilitate decisions they consider morally objectionable. Like the informative model, this model gives priority to the patient's autonomy without acknowledging that the practitioner still shares in responsibility for the patient's treatment. While both models impute privileged status to the patient's standpoint, they are inadequate in that they fail to impute any moral relevance to the clinician's standpoint.

In contrast to the preceding models, the deliberative model attempts to incorporate the standpoints of both physician and patient. This model is egalitarian in that it takes account of "the potential for an unequal balance of power to the physician-patient relationship."[9] In practice, however, the relationship between physician and patient is not dyadic, although other models construe it that way. An egalitarian model takes account of power differences not only between an individual doctor and patient but also of power differences across the spectrum of interactions among people involved in, or affected by, health care decisions, including those between doctors and nurses or other clinicians and in relationships with family members as well as patients.

Although an egalitarian model cannot settle the question of whether human fetuses have the same value as humans already born, it does suggest that different standpoints on this question should be considered when decisions are made about treatment of pregnant women. Unfortunately, the casuistic and principlist methods discussed in chapter 1 shed no light on how to incorporate such considerations into an analysis of cases or issues. In the next section, therefore, I explore ways of amending the reigning formulations of these methods so that they take account of pregnant women as well as other patients.

Possible modifications of principlist and casuistic methods

All of the distinguishing features of women's health care are ethically relevant in many cases, but one that is both unique and uniquely troubling is that some patients are pregnant. Proponents of principlism and casuistry do not adequately address issues involving pregnant women because they neither identify nor defend a position on the moral status of the fetus, which inevitably affects decisions on these issues. The most recent edition of *Clinical Ethics*, for example, fails even to consider pregnancy, abortion, or infertility treatment as topics relevant to the field.[10] This omission virtually excludes pregnant women from the domain of clinical ethics, violating the authors' own version of casuistry, which calls for attention to the particularities of cases.

A schematic by which to incorporate concerns about the fetus into their interpretation of the principles of Beauchamp and Childress was proposed by Frank Chervenak, an obstetrician and gynecologist, and Laurence McCullough, a philosopher, in 1985. Presumably assuming that beneficence encompasses nonmaleficence, their modification of the Georgetown mantra is the following:[11]

Best Interests of Mother		*Best Interests of Fetus*	
Maternal autonomy-based obligations of physician	Maternal beneficence-based obligations of physician	Fetal beneficence-based obligations of mother	Fetal beneficence-based obligations of physician

Although the authors thus identify obligations applicable to physicians who care for pregnant women, their schematic offers no clues on how to prioritize these obligations in cases of conflict. In their arguments for specific positions, however, they implicitly invoke justice as a relevant principle for cases of conflict by arguing that one set of interests outweighs the other. This accords with the balancing function that Beauchamp and Childress propose as a means of settling conflicts that arise in applications of their principles. On the issue of coercive treatment of pregnant women, for example, Chervenak and McCullough weigh "fetal beneficence-based obligations" and "maternal beneficence-based obligations" against "maternal autonomy-based obligations" and conclude that the former outweigh the latter. Their positions on different ethical issues faced by pregnant women rely on their consideration of women and their fetuses as separate or separable patients.

By distinguishing between the interests of the woman and her fetus, Chervenak and McCullough apply the principle of beneficence differently to each; the autonomy-based obligations are obviously only applicable to the woman. The authors' consideration of the fetus as if it is separable from the pregnant woman is another illustration of the fallacy of abstraction. Neither conceptually nor practically is it true that fetuses as such are separable from pregnant women. Embryos are occasionally separate or separable from women (e.g., when they are formed through in vitro fertilization or flushed from the woman's body after in vivo fertilization), but fetuses, once separated from women, are no longer fetuses but newborns or abortuses or stillborns. Scholars taking different positions on "maternal-fetal conflict" seem to ignore this inseparability when they argue for the priority of either the fetus's or the woman's interests.

As already indicated, the casuistic framework of Jonsen, Siegler, and Winslade fails to take account of the uniqueness of pregnant patients. If they were to amend their method so that it incorporates recognition of the fact that some patients are pregnant, two of their topics, medical indications and quality of life, would need to be subdivided into those applicable to the fetus and those applicable to the woman. However, this modification would again exemplify the prevalent but misguided tendency to construe the fetus and the pregnant woman as separate or separable, and it offers no guidance on how to prioritize fetal and maternal interests.

The topic of "contextual factors" in the casuistic method allows inclusion of others' interests, including those of the potential father, as morally relevant, whereas the framework proposed by Chervenak and McCullough only identifies "maternal interests" and "fetal interests" as morally relevant.[12] However, their method as well as an amended method of casuistry are both preferable to methods of analyses that totally ignore the unique status of pregnant patients, and the prioritizing guidelines or maxims proposed earlier may be used to resolve or reduce conflicts that arise between the interests of fetus and pregnant woman if these are treated as if they were separate. The application of the proposed maxims to specific cases depends crucially on the extent, if any, to which embryos or fetuses[13] are regarded as separate patients.

Through different approaches to the relevant issues, John Robertson and Carson Strong address the unique status of pregnant patients. These authors posit an essential tie between pregnant women and the developing fetus. For them, the question of whether the fetus is a separate or separable patient depends on whether, when, and to what extent (if any) it has moral status. The starting point of the arguments through which each defends positions on ethical issues involving pregnant women is their answer to this question, which is addressed more fully in chapter 3.

Robertson's methodology has an additional starting point, one that suggests a form of principlism because it affirms as paramount the principle of "procreative liberty." This liberty, he says, is "the freedom to reproduce or not to reproduce in the genetic sense, which may also include rearing or not, as intended by the parties."[14] It includes the right of a man or woman to provide gametes to another, as well as the right of a woman to gestate and give birth to the genetic offspring of another woman. The "individual's procreative liberty should rule," he says, "unless there are compelling reasons to the contrary."[15] Although he mainly affirms the rights of couples rather than those of women as individuals, his methodology generally exemplifies a libertarian-oriented version of liberal theory.

For Robertson, procreative liberty is a negative rather than a positive right. This means that the state may not interfere with anyone's choice about procreation but also is not obliged to facilitate its exercise through funding of reproductive services. Whether the state should alleviate conditions that constrain the exercise of procreative liberty is "a separate issue of social justice" which Robertson does not intend to address.[16] Nonetheless, his claim that "reasons to the contrary" may at least occasionally outweigh procreative liberty implies recognition of a need for some form of balancing, as recommended by Beauchamp and Childress.

Strong also defends procreative freedom as a fundamental negative right of individuals or couples. Although he grounds this right in the principle of "respect for persons," he calls his methodology a "modified casuistry" rather than a form of principlism.[17] In effect, though, his approach combines elements of both. Using the term "values" to include principles as well as rules or guidelines, he argues that priorities regarding these values may be different for individual cases than they are for "types of cases."[18] Strong's delineation of values central to reproduction and perinatology includes reproductive freedom, the well-being of procreators, potential procreators, and potential offspring; respect for life; and the well-being of society in the immediate as well as distant future. These may be construed as specifications of the principles of Beauchamp and Childress, but greater specification is obviously both possible and necessary.

The greater specification Strong proposes for fetuses is based on the degree of similarity between the developing organism and "descriptive persons," that is, individuals who possess self-consciousness.[19] According to this paradigm, "the moral standing of the fetus becomes progressively stronger as fetal development proceeds."[20] Since fetuses never match the paradigm of descriptive personhood achieved by women, there should always be "a presumption in favor of the woman's interests when conflicts arise."[21] Strong imputes a basic right to procreation to men as well as women and maintains that "the strength of *parental* obligations can be affected by the fetus's moral standing."[22] On various issues, however, he acknowledges that the risks and burdens of reproduction fall more heavily on women than on men. He is thus more open to an egalitarian account, one that privileges the standpoint of women, than are other authors.

An obvious weakness of Jonsen and Toulmin's and Strong's casuistry relates to the selection of paradigmatic cases. Descriptive personhood, for example, serves as a relevant paradigm for those who believe that its achievement entails obligations that lack of it do not entail. Those for whom genetic humanity alone entails equal obligations toward all who possess it, regardless of their developmental stage, embrace a different paradigm. Because of their different views about the moral status of the fetus, practitioners and patients alike may utilize different paradigms on issues involving pregnancy. An egalitarian approach recognizes the relevance of different paradigms for different people. It does not imply, however, that any paradigm is acceptable; acceptable paradigms must meet a minimal standard of egalitarian justice by requiring respect for individuals who hold positions that are at odds with each other but consistent with defensible starting points.

Another weakness of casuistry, even when it is modified as Strong suggests, is that it fails to provide adequate guidance for prioritizing the values or principles at stake. While Strong proposes a means of "assigning priorities" by applying paradigmatic cases to new ones, he assigns "prima facie" status to values such as "the moral right to noninterference with freedom to procreate," without explaining how this value may be overridden in some circumstances.[23] He simply asserts "a presumption that the prioritizing should take place in the context of individual cases" and "be supported by an argument."[24] Although he doesn't acknowledge the need for prioritizing maxims as such, the arguments that he subsequently develops for particular cases are consistent with the maxims sketched in chapter 2.

Many scholars who write about issues involving pregnant woman attempt to bypass the question of fetal moral status because they consider the abortion issue, to which it is obviously related, interminably controversial and irresolvable. Chervenak and McCullough attempt to avoid the issue by distinguishing between concepts of patienthood and personhood, and they are hardly alone in considering pregnant women as two patients rather than one.[25] In the literature of obstetrics, for example, fetuses are described as "a whole new patient population," and books such as *Fetology* and *The Unborn Patient* have become commonplace in the libraries of physicians who treat pregnant women.[26] But treating a gestating woman as two patients suggests what is impossible: that she and the fetus exist or are able to exist apart from each other. As Margaret Little puts it, the *essential* tie between them is "left out of the conceptual paradigm."[27] In the next section, I explain more fully why this omission is both conceptually and practically problematic.

Who is the patient?

The question "Who is the patient?" is relevant not only to pregnant women and the practitioners who treat them but also to infertility specialists and their patients, including fertile partners of infertile patients and those who may provide gametes or agree to gestate a child for another. Note, however, that the term "patient" does not apply exclusively to persons or potential persons: veterinarians treat patients that fit neither characterization. Attribution of moral status is thus a separable question from determination of patienthood. Some practitioners who treat human patients view those in persistent vegetative state as patients but not persons, despite the fact that they are legally persons.[28] It is plausible, therefore, to consider fetuses patients even if they are not persons, as Chervenak and McCullough propose.

Competent adults choose to be patients by seeking or consenting to diagnosis or treatment for themselves; those who choose otherwise—for example, by leaving the hospital against medical advice—are no longer patients, even though they may have conditions that deserve treatment. Those who refuse life-saving treatment while remaining in the hospital are no longer patients with regard to their life-threatening condition; they may then become patients as recipients of palliative care to ease their dying. Similarly, women who leave the hospital after free and informed refusal of medically recommended surgical delivery are no longer patients. If they remain in the hospital, however, they may then become patients as recipients of comfort care or measures that facilitate vaginal delivery.[29]

Choosing to be patients is obviously not possible for those who are decisionally incapacitated; their patienthood status is necessarily determined by others. Infants and profoundly impaired adults, for example, become patients when parents or guardians seek treatment in their behalf. If fetuses are considered patients, they can only become so by being presented for care by others. Individuals unrelated to fetuses may attempt to secure care for them, but the only person who is indispensable to presentation of a particular fetus as patient is the pregnant woman herself. Regardless of who seeks treatment on its behalf, the patienthood of the fetus is thus dependent on others and on the patienthood status of the pregnant woman.

As already indicated, Chervenak and McCullough consider the controversy regarding personhood (or lack thereof) in fetuses avoidable through their focus on the fetus as a patient.[30] Determining whether the fetus is a patient, they claim, allows practitioners to treat it as such, even, at times, over the objection of the pregnant woman.[31] Accordingly, they identify variables by which clinicians may make this determination. The criteria they propose are morally relevant but inadequate for determination of patienthood if the woman decides not to present her fetus for care. Even if some fetuses are patients, this does not imply that they are separate or separable patients. Perhaps the most compelling support for the view that fetuses are separable or separate patients occurs in the context of maternal-fetal surgery, when the woman's uterus is opened and the fetus is removed from it for treatment. But the fetus is still not a separate or separable patient because its physical connection to the pregnant woman is maintained through the umbilical cord. As long as this connection remains, even if the fetus is considered a person, it is never treatable as a patient without the pregnant woman being treated as a patient. This inseparable entwinement cannot justifiably be ignored.[32]

Determining whether the fetus is a patient does not settle moral questions regarding its treatment because answers may still differ on grounds of whether the fetus is or is not a person. If there are two patients with conflicting interests, and one is a person but the other is not, the interests of the patient who is clearly a person may trump those of the patient who is not a person. Persons as such have a legal and moral right to life, which may not be claimed for nonpersons to whom lesser, or no, moral status is imputed. With regard to other rights or goods, the verities apply more compellingly to patients who are uncontroversially persons than to those whose personhood is disputed or denied. Regardless of whether agreement can be reached on whether fetuses are persons, then, the issue is not ultimately separable from that of patienthood. The moral status of the fetus remains an unavoidable and crucial variable in addressing ethical questions involving pregnant women. Chervenak and McCullough implicitly acknowledge this when they attribute "dependent moral status" to some fetuses.[33]

Beyond moral status, another variable with regard to fetuses is that they cannot all be considered patients even if, for the sake of argument, patienthood is imputed to them. Most patients seek medical assistance because they need it, but some seek it for nonmedical reasons, and physicians would be remiss if they treated these individuals as patients by providing medically unnecessary treatment solely on grounds of their requests. When physicians provide unnecessary treatment such as cosmetic surgery for enhancement of appearance or infertility treatment for healthy postmenopausal women, they still must weigh the hazards of the treatment against the expected (nonmedical) benefit to the patient, and they must decline to provide it if the medical risks are high. Pregnant women are encouraged to seek prenatal care on the grounds that this will promote their health and that of their potential children. Whether all pregnant women need or benefit by the care of physicians has nonetheless been questioned. One high-risk obstetrician, for example, has argued that healthy pregnant women do not need obstetricians because prenatal care and assistance in childbirth by physicians does not generally improve the outcome for the woman or the newborn.[34] According to studies he cites, pregnant women are not only well cared for but also tend to be more satisfied with the care they receive from nonphysicians such as midwives than with the care they receive from obstetricians.

On Chervenak and McCullough's understanding of "patient," a fetus may become one when it needs medical assistance and the pregnant woman seeks such assistance on its behalf. The analogy that supports this view is that of an adult who brings a minor for needed health care; the minor thus becomes a patient. If parents of children or guardians of decisionally incapacitated individuals fail to present them for necessary care, they may be accused (and convicted) of neglect; others in society will then be required to assume this responsibility, through either court-ordered hospitalization or treatment. The requirement that anyone in need of medical assistance *should* be considered a patient implies that such an individual has an independent claim or positive right to care. Such individuals are thus regarded not only as patients but also as persons who, as such, have independent, not dependent, moral status. In contrast, nonpersons, such as pets, may not become patients when they need care. Whether they become patients depends on their being presented for care by those responsible for them or others who choose, but are not obliged, to fill that role (e.g., members of an animal humane society).

Admittedly, an ethically relevant difference between human fetuses and nonhumans whose patienthood status depends on others is that the former are uncontroversially regarded as having at least the potential for independent and full moral status or personhood. Arguments based on potential personhood are unnecessary to those whose starting premise is that (actual) personhood begins with human fertilization. To others, the status of potential personhood is legally and morally significant and, in some cases, compelling. If the interests being compared are proportionate, however, the interests of potential persons cannot override those of actual persons. Indeed, it may be argued that the interests of potential beings can never override those of actual beings of any kind.

A child or pet in need of care may be physically presented to a physician or veterinarian by someone other than a parent or owner. Regardless of who "presents" an individual in need of care, however, the patient is then left in the hands of the appropriate practitioner, and the "presenter" may then turn to other tasks or interests. In contrast, when fetuses are "presented" for care, the crucial "presenter" cannot leave the facility to resume other activities. More significantly, she cannot consent to testing or treatment of the fetus apart from herself. Any intervention on behalf of the fetus can only be provided through her body, often with risks or harms to her. Empirically, then, the pregnant woman is the only presenting patient when care of a fetus is contemplated or undertaken. As *pregnant* woman, she is one patient, not two, albeit one whose choices and welfare importantly and inevitably affect her potential offspring even as they may also affect the choices or welfare of those already born.

Chervenak and McCullough consider the pregnant woman as more than one patient, but not in all situations. An individual is a patient, they maintain, "when the *individual* is (1) presented to a physician (2) for the purpose of applying clinical interventions that are reliably expected to protect and promote the interests of that individual."[35] In light of the fact that some women present their fetuses for abortion, the second requirement is crucial. With regard to the first requirement, the term "individual" is problematic. Webster's dictionary defines "individual" as "separate and distinct from others of the same kind."[36] Because of the essential physical connection between fetuses and the women in whom they develop, fetuses do not fit this understanding of the term. As already mentioned, the meaning and reality of a human fetus is accurately understood as contained within the meaning and reality of any pregnant woman. Recognizing the genetic distinctness and potential for personhood of the fetus is entirely compatible with this position.

Just as fetuses cannot be presented for treatment as individuals apart from pregnant women, neither can conjoint twins, who at birth are legally and morally distinct persons despite their physical dependence on each other. At least in some cases, however, conjoint twins are separable without changing the fact that each is an individual person. Fetuses, once separated from pregnant women, are no longer fetuses. The situations are analogous in that treatment of the pregnant woman may affect the fetus, and treatment of one conjoint twin may affect the other. They are disanalogous, however, in that treatment of the fetus always affects the pregnant woman, whereas treatment of one conjoint twin does not always affect the other. The pregnant woman and both conjoint twins may be separate or separable patients because each is treatable without affecting the other to whom they are attached; fetuses cannot be separate patients because they are not treatable without affecting those to whom they are attached.

An interesting contrast to the view that fetus and pregnant woman are two distinct patients is the tendency of infertility practitioners to view couples as a single unit rather than two distinct patients. Here, however, the couple as patient is comprised of physically separate persons, only one of whom, usually the woman, may require treatment. Regardless of whether infertility is due to the male partner or the couple together, both partners are patients because treatment of the male partner always occurs through the woman's body. Healthy individuals who undergo treatment on behalf of others—for example, by providing gametes, gestation, organs, or tissue for others—are also patients as well as persons. If the presenting condition is female infertility, the woman alone may be considered the patient because she is the only one treated for a condition that she alone has.

Pregnant women occasionally present themselves as patients for care of conditions unrelated to their fetuses or potential children. Even then, they necessarily present the fetuses within them. Except when abortion is desired, women usually want and expect the clinician to do what is medically best not only for themselves but also for their potential children. Arguments for treating fetuses as distinct patients are consistent with the latter goal insofar as fetuses are destined or intended to become indisputably persons after birth. However, this rationale is based on the potential rather than the actual status of an existing being. In situations of conflict, proportionate obligations to existing persons generally override obligations to possible or potential persons. Because decisions intended to benefit the potential child can only be implemented through the woman, fetuses are not patients in their own right—that is, apart from the patients on whom they depend for survival or treatment—unless their status as patients is determined on grounds that they are already persons.

The variables that Chervenak and McCullough propose for determining whether fetuses are patients (regardless of whether they are persons) are based on two distinctions, one biological and the other psychological. The first distinction is between viable and previable fetuses; the second, which applies only to previable fetuses, distinguishes between those that the pregnant woman has decided to abort and those she has chosen to carry to viability or term.[37] On grounds of these distinctions, they argue that either of two criteria identifies a fetus as a patient: its viability, or the decision of the woman to continue her pregnancy. For these authors, a fetus that satisfies either criterion is a patient, that is, an individual "presented to a physician for the purpose of applying clinical interventions, etc." By becoming a patient, they argue, the fetus acquires "dependent moral status." As discussed in the next section, this view is at odds with their attempt to bypass the moral controversiality of abortion.

Patients and "dependent moral status"

While acknowledging that persons as such have "independent moral status," Chervenak and McCullough attribute "dependent moral status" to all viable fetuses and some previable fetuses on grounds that they are patients. A viable fetus, they argue, has dependent moral status because its ongoing development is "reliably linked to later achievement of independent moral status."[38] A previable fetus, however, has dependent moral status if and only if the pregnant woman "presents the previable fetus to the physician, that is, when she elects to continue her pregnancy to viability."[39] The latter criterion seems to ignore the fact that a fetus as such is not presented to the physician; instead, a woman presents herself as a pregnant person who in many but not all cases desires care for herself and her potential child. It also ignores the fact that a woman's decision to continue her pregnancy is not necessarily accompanied by presentation of herself to a physician. By Chervenak and McCullough's account, some fetuses that women have elected to carry to term are not patients until and unless they become viable. At that point, the authors apparently consider them patients even if the pregnant woman does not seek health care.

Although dependent persons (e.g., children) as well as nonpersons (e.g., pets) become patients when presented to practitioners for diagnosis or treatment, this does not imply that they thereby acquire "dependent moral status." Children and incompetent adults have independent moral status despite their dependence on others; they thus have a right to life and health care, and practitioners have duties to them as patients independently of their parents or others on whom they depend for care. By arguing that physicians have similar duties to fetuses that meet their criteria for patienthood, Chervenak and McCullough in effect regard these fetuses as having the same moral status as children and incompetent adults who have independent moral status.

The difference between the criteria for patienthood that Chervenak and McCullough propose for viable versus previable fetuses is morally significant in its own right. For viable fetuses, moral status depends on achievement of a specific developmental milestone; for previable fetuses, it depends on the subjective decision of the pregnant woman, which may be made at any point after the woman knows she is pregnant, until the viability criterion is applicable. Although the authors deny that fetuses in either category have "independent moral status," they argue that the pregnant woman's wishes may be overridden for the sake of the viable fetus if her refusal is likely to harm her and her fetus, or when the apparent urgency of the situation prevents recourse to the courts.[40] In these cases at least, the moral status of the fetus is obviously not dependent on the autonomy of the pregnant woman, who is indisputably a person with independent moral status.

As is the case with infants for whom parents are unable or unwilling to care, it may be argued that others are obliged to present viable fetuses for care if the pregnant woman does not do so. This implies that the pregnant woman herself may be coercively presented and treated involuntarily for the sake of the fetus. Chervenak and McCullough do not argue in favor of such coercion outside of the health care setting, but their position supports this conclusion. If the decision of a pregnant patient is overridable by the interests of the fetus-as-patient, the alleged moral status of the fetus is obviously not dependent on the woman's. In effect, the right of the fetus to treatment is as independently established as is that of any child or adult.

With regard to previable fetuses, Chervenak and McCullough acknowledge that the legal option of abortion constitutes an impediment to their being patients. They claim, however, that women who reach a "settled" decision to continue their pregnancies are obliged to present their previable fetuses to the physician, and once they do that, the physician is morally obliged to treat the fetus as a patient whose interests may be at odds with hers. In other words, a woman's decision to continue her pregnancy commits her to accept what others decide on behalf of her fetus. As with viable fetuses, however, Chervenak and McCullough still maintain that previable fetuses have dependent rather than independent moral status.

From the standpoint of those who impute full moral status to embryos or fetuses, Chervenak and McCullough are correct that fetuses are patients in their own right. Had these authors supported that starting position, however, they would have no need to argue for either viability or the woman's decision to continue her pregnancy as determinative of patienthood. Rather, all fetuses would then be considered patients precisely because they are persons. From that standpoint, viability suggests an analogy with patients who are indisputably persons, such as children and individuals dependent on life support, whose survival or viability is not simply a matter of developmental level or decisional capacity but also, and sometimes only, a function of whether others are willing and able to treat them. The woman's decision to continue her pregnancy is simply irrelevant to determination of whether human embryos or fetuses have rights and responsibilities that are objectively and independently attributable to them as persons—that is, as individuals with full moral status. Fetal personhood thus implies fetal patienthood, regardless of whether pregnant women themselves make that determination.

As discussed in chapter 3, full moral status is generally attributed to persons as such, and partial moral status is attributed to individuals who are not persons but who have some moral status or standing of their own, regardless of whether it is attributed to them by others.[41] For those who impute partial moral status to fetuses, obligations to people already born are clearly more compelling than those that apply to persons who are born. But Chervenak and McCullough's distinction between dependent and independent moral status is unrelated to the important difference between partial and full moral status. Instead, their position is that fetuses either have it or don't have it. Once fetuses meet either of their criteria for patienthood, their interests may be as compelling as, or even override, those of the pregnant woman. The dependent moral status they attribute to some fetuses is thus equivalent to full moral status or personhood.

Because some practitioners believe that fetuses are patients with moral status of their own, but others do not, clinical practice varies with regard to ethical issues involving reproduction. Some physicians, for example, perform abortions only for compelling medical reasons; some never perform them, and others perform them routinely if the woman wishes to terminate her pregnancy. Some practitioners support coercive treatment for the sake of the fetus after viability (e.g., Chervenak), while others oppose coercive treatment of pregnant women for any reason. In light of these differences among their members, professional health care organizations usually provide guidance that respects their different moral standpoints as well as the different standpoints of researchers and study subjects. Similarly, federal regulations and state statutes attempt to articulate requirements applicable to all citizens, whose moral positions on key issues differ considerably. In the next section, I briefly consider some of these mechanisms for ethical guidance of clinical practice and research. To be just in their provisions about women, laws and policies must take account of the distinguishing features of women's health care, as well as the variable standpoints of those who provide treatment or conduct research.

Guidelines and regulations

Practitioners and patients alike have long grappled with ethical questions that are especially complicated, emotionally charged, and controversial in women's health care. As in other areas of life, many people look to personal or religious guidelines to facilitate resolution of these questions. For example, the "golden rule," consideration of what one would do in circumstances resembling those faced by another, often serves as a personal guide for clinicians, patients, and family members.[42] Specific religious teachings often provide more specific guidance. However, the personal ethical codes of individual practitioners don't necessarily mesh with the values of all of their colleagues and patients, and vice versa. Accordingly, professional guidelines for clinicians are generally worded broadly enough to accommodate diverse standpoints, some of which may arise from incompatible starting points. To allow practitioners to consider a wide range of clinical and ethical variables as they see fit, these guidelines usually serve an advisory rather than regulatory function with regard to clinical practice.

Unlike professional guidelines (which are often issued in the form of committee opinions), government regulation, or laws, articulate duties rather than recommendations and tend to be stipulative and definitive rather than flexible and advisory. Failure to observe guidelines may incur professional criticism and may be invoked in courts of law to demonstrate to judges or juries how practitioners are advised to act or not act in accordance with the mores of their professions. Failure to observe government regulation risks harsher civil or even criminal penalties. Professional guidelines are developed mainly by the professionals to whom they apply, whereas regulations are usually determined by legislators who are not directly affected by them. The ethical priority of legislators is, or ought to be, the common good, whereas professional guidelines generally focus on the interests of individuals directly affected by the professional practice under consideration.

While addressing the practices of specific professions, professional guidelines are primarily concerned with maximization of respect for the autonomy of the professionals to whom they apply, so that these individuals can adequately address the nuances of cases whose complexity cannot be fully anticipated in regulatory formulations. Not following guidelines in specific cases may thus be defensible to others in the profession through appeal to verities that apply to patients in very different circumstances. Because of their generality, however, professional guidelines are inadequate guides to moral decision-making on the part of individuals who address issues from different, and sometimes incompatible, moral standpoints. An egalitarian perspective, I believe, is more likely to provide such guidance.

Various professional societies of health caregivers have developed guidelines for their members, whether physicians, researchers, nurses, social workers, therapists, subspecialists within these groups, or other health care workers. Typically, the guidelines are formulated in conformity with existing laws by a select committee of members, some of whom may have training in law or ethics as well. Outside experts and input from patients or research subjects is sometimes sought to facilitate the development of the guidelines, which are made available to members after approval by the organization's leadership. As new issues unfold, old guidelines are sometimes amended or new ones are developed.

Guidelines that specifically target physicians who treat women include those developed by the American College of Obstetrics and Gynecology, the American Society for Reproductive Medicine, and the International Federation of Gynecology and Obstetrics, but guidelines developed by most health care specialties and disciplines are also applicable to treatment of women. Many of these organizations invoke the principles or verities developed by Beauchamp and Childress in support of their recommendations. Most oppose exclusively paternalistic or informative models of "the practitioner-patient relationship," affirming instead the importance of interpretive and deliberative ties between the two. Few guidelines, however, extend the domain of their ethical concerns beyond the individual practitioner and her patient to consider issues from a fully egalitarian perspective—one that acknowledges and addresses the injustice toward others that may arise from decisions made by or on behalf of individuals.

Hospitals usually develop their own ethics policies or guidelines for clinical care and the conduct of research. In the United States, programs that pursue research with human subjects are federally mandated to examine research proposals to ensure that they conform to specific ethical criteria. Throughout the world, bioethics commissions or councils are often appointed to advise government officials about regulations that they may enact. The regulations articulated by the governing authorities are applicable to different jurisdictions: statewide, citywide, provincewide, or nationwide. The range of regulation to which this leads makes it difficult sometimes for clinicians to know which set of rules is applicable to a particular practice setting or patient. It also spurs some patients to look for care in a jurisdiction other than their own. Reproductive laws and euthanasia laws, for example, vary from country to country and from state to state.

Regulations differ from guidelines in that they are primarily concerned with avoidance of harms that could occur if clinicians and clinical practice were not subject to scrutiny by the law. A common example of government regulation of medical practice is the credentialing requirements of physicians. Because laws are mainly intended to promote the common good rather than the particular goods of individuals, justice is paramount; this necessarily entails curtailment of autonomy in some cases or for some people. The conception of justice generally invoked to support regulation of health care is one that permits some inequality so that individual liberty will be constrained as little as possible. This is essentially a Rawlsian conception of justice rather than an egalitarian conception.

As discussed in chapter 14, justice is not only a principle by which social conflicts may be resolved and priorities among moral obligations may be determined. Justice is also an ideal that provides moral guidance to those whose sense of morality involves more than fulfillment of obligations. The ideal of justice toward which an egalitarian perspective points is one in which every person is enabled to flourish optimally through development of her different capacities. Through emphases on different verities, professional guidelines and government regulations can facilitate, but not ensure, achievement of this ideal.

Some practitioners and libertarian-minded patients would probably prefer total lack of government regulation of clinical practice. To maximize respect for the autonomy of clinicians as well as patients, regulation should be minimal and guidelines should provide helpful advice in situations of ethical complexity. However, to distribute potential harms and benefits fairly so that justice is maximized, some measure of government regulation is necessary. In other words, in situations of conflict, whether these arise for individuals or for policy makers, justice is, or should be, the final arbiter.

From the standpoint of individuals, who are ultimately responsible for their own moral decisions, guidelines and regulations are ethically relevant in their own right and helpful also in informing them about factors to consider in making their decisions. However, the very generality of these mechanisms means that they are unable, by themselves, to provide the individual with solutions to dilemmas that are consistent with starting points that the guidelines and regulations don't address. For a particular woman facing an unwanted pregnancy, for example, the fact that the legal availability of abortion is supported by most medical organizations doesn't settle the question of whether her decision on the matter is morally justified. Neither does it settle the question of whether she is acting in conformity with her own beliefs or her responsibilities to others already born. From an egalitarian perspective, the woman's standpoint is not only unique but uniquely relevant to all of those affected by her decision. Its privileged status, however, does not preclude assessment of the starting point and end point that determine the direction of her standpoint.

3

Different Starting Points, Standpoints, End Points

The majority of questions addressed in contemporary bioethics involve the beginning and end of human life. These thresholds define the span of time in which decisions can and must be made by and on behalf of individuals who are persons. Persons as such have standpoints that are morally relevant to decisions affecting them; in clinical settings, they are universally acknowledged to have a right to life and health that other persons are morally obliged to respect to the extent that they have the capability for doing so. Moral obligations may also be due to nonpersons or potential persons, but these are ordinarily less compelling than those toward persons. From an egalitarian perspective, all persons have the same value, but nonpersons and potential persons do not have the same value as persons.

Ongoing controversy about the morality of abortion usually hinges on the question of whether fetuses are persons. Questions about personhood also emerge with regard to born individuals who lack brain development (anencephalic infants) or higher brain activity (irreversibly comatose individuals). Regardless of whether individuals are persons, concerns about whether treatment might benefit them and whether they would choose treatment if they had decision-making capacity may arise. Standpoints and moral status may be imputed to fetuses and individuals who lack brain function even if they are not persons.

Birth and death are often seen as the beginning and end of life, but different construals of both terms are defensible. Women who have given birth typically recognize that their newborns were alive before they emerged from womb to world. Clinicians who assist women in maintaining or terminating their pregnancies are aware that when fetal demise occurs, fetal life has ended. The factors known to precipitate birth are limited, but its timing is relatively predictable. When a human life begins, however, is disputed, as is its ending—despite legal and clinical criteria for determining death.

Questions about life and death are usually more troubling and ethically perplexing than other questions. Unfortunately, however, discussion of these topics is prevalently beset by the ambiguity or inaccuracy of key terms. Disagreement may be masked through use of the same term for different meanings, and agreement may be unrecognized because different terms are used for meanings that are the same. In what follows, therefore, I begin by examining terms commonly used in discussions about the beginning and end of life. Unnecessary disagreement and unwarranted agreement is avoided through agreed-upon usage. However, this doesn't necessarily lead to understanding or appreciation of the different standpoints of those who use the agreed-upon terms. For most people, the starting point and end point that determine their standpoint on ethical questions involve not only their conceptions of life and death but also their conceptions of other values, including those identified through the ethical verities or principles.

To facilitate understanding and critique of arguments developed from different standpoints, I also explore the meaning of terms mainly used by bioethicists and philosophers: "moral status," "moral agency," and "personhood." These usually occur in discussions of possible criteria for determining what constitutes a person who as such has full moral status and the rights that accrue to one who has that status. I consider a range of positions on the moral status of human beings because these may lead to different conclusions about what should or should not be done in health care. These different positions have implications applicable mainly to women when they arise at the beginning of life; at the end of life, the implications apply to men also.

Key terms

Language expresses concepts, and concepts are generalizations based on particular experiences.[1] Because all of our experiences are unique, concepts inevitably fail to wholly capture their meaning. Similarly, language cannot fully express the concepts it is intended to convey. Clinicians are reminded of the gaps between language and concepts when they discover that patients or family members have a different understanding of a term they use, and when the outcome or experience of a treatment is at odds with what they thought would happen. Patients and family members are reminded of gaps in communication when they find that the physician's interpretation of risks and benefits of treatment are different from their own. Miscommunication in clinical encounters is reducible through attempts to see the world from the standpoints of others, especially those whose standpoints tend to be forgotten or ignored because they are nondominant.

The terms "life," "death," "human being," and "person" are routinely used without questioning their meanings. In fact, however, each of these may have different meanings for the parties involved. Life, for example, is prevalently recognized as a biological process that begins and ends in organisms, but some scientists believe it neither begins nor ends because all of life is continuous.[2] Even if everyone agreed that life has a beginning and end, questions would persist about when it starts, what it entails, and when it ends. Different rights and responsibilities are associated with these different meanings.

Although separate cells and tissue, as well as whole organisms, may be "living," the term "life" is usually reserved for distinct organisms whose parts work together to sustain its functions. When the organism is no longer capable of sustaining these functions, it is "dead"; when it, while still living, is thought to be close to death, it is "dying." What functions must be maintained or lost to indicate that an organism is alive or dead is critical to determination of either characterization. Accordingly, the criteria for determination as well as definitions of life and death are debatable. The meaning of either term is indicative of the other's meaning, as its opposite or antonym.

The difference between life and death in human beings is clear if we envision a first-year medical student in an anatomy course, examining the body of someone who has bequeathed her body to science for research or education purposes. The medical student is obviously living a life, and the cadaver is obviously a dead human being. But the difference between life and death is not so clear if instead we imagine two individuals in adjacent surgical suites. One no longer has any detectable brain activity and her other vital functions are being maintained through mechanical support so that her heart may be transferred to the patient in the other suite who is awaiting transplant. No one disputes that the potential recipient is someone in whom human life is present, but the potential donor may or may not be considered dead.

Laws in many jurisdictions define death as the complete cessation of brain function and life, correspondingly, as maintenance of whole brain function. Some scholars agree with these criteria; others, however, argue that human life ends, or death occurs, when cerebral function is lost but brain stem function remains.[3] By the latter account, some patients who require constant medical support (e.g., artificial feeding) to maintain their cardiac and respiratory function are already dead; the corresponding definition of life is maintenance of higher brain function or cerebral activity.

The preceding definitions of human life and death are inapplicable to early fetuses or embryos, but this doesn't mean that other definitions are not applicable to them also. One traditional definition of death is applicable to any living organism: separation of soul and body. Contemporarily, the term "soul" is seldom used by philosophers, but religious ethicists and members of the public sometimes use the term for that which is essential to human life or personhood.[4] Different conceptions of the body/soul relationship influence the priorities of patients, family members, and practitioners. The body, which is empirically discernible, is typically construed as subject to the soul, which in living humans may be equated with mind, a nonempirical principle, or power. On grounds of this distinction, loss of mental function is prevalently considered worse than loss of physical function.

Despite their ancient origins, the views of Plato and Aristotle about the body/soul or body/mind relationship are still operable in decisions about the beginning and end of life. Plato's position is implicitly endorsed by those who give such weight to cognitive capability that mere bodily function counts for little or nothing. The soul or mind, for Plato, is all that is essential for a human being as such. Body and soul are an aggregate union, and separation of one from the other is desirable because the body is an impediment to the fullness of a human life.[5] From a Platonic standpoint, therefore, death is not tragic but liberating. Religious traditions that subscribe to belief in the immortality of the soul and disparage the pursuit of bodily pleasures are well-supported by this view of the body/soul relationship.

Aristotle describes all living human and nonhuman organisms as essentially comprised of body and soul.[6] As form is to matter, so soul is to body: an essential union. Different types of soul—vegetative, sentient, and rational—inform the bodies of plants, animals, and humans, respectively, as long as they are living. For Aristotle, the three types of soul form a hierarchy through which functions that define a lower type (e.g., vegetative or sentient vis-à-vis rational) are also present in the higher type. The soul itself is not empirically ascertainable, but its presence is revealed through operations or functions specific to the kind of being it is: growth and reproduction for plants, mobility and sentiency for nonhuman animals, reason and autonomy for human beings. Characterizing the condition of individuals that grow and reproduce but lack the ability to feel pain or function cognitively as "persistent vegetative state" is consistent with this account. Although such individuals still have a soul, the soul is vegetative rather than rational. Living individuals may be human in appearance, but if they never express the capacity for reason or autonomy, they lack what Aristotle considers essential to human life as such.

Drawing on Aristotle's account, Aquinas identifies the point at which God infuses a soul into a developing human organism as the beginning of a new human life.[7] An empirical way of putting this with regard to embryos or fetuses is to define their death as the cessation of their ability to continue development. A fetus developing within a woman's body is clearly living, and its parts work together to sustain the functions of which it is capable. But the fetus is not capable of sustaining these functions apart from the woman until viability. In a sense, the life of the fetus as such ends at birth, when it is no longer a fetus but a newborn. Nonetheless, on grounds of two analogies, the developing fetus may still be considered *a* life: congenital twins who are unable to maintain essential life functions apart from each other, and patients who are dependent on life support. Despite their dependence on others for survival, each congenital twin and each patient on life support is regarded as *a* human life. Even if the fetus is nonviable or previable, it is, arguably, *a* life because it is alive while dying, and dying is a stage in the process of life. Accordingly, a "stillborn" infant should not be referred to as "nonviable" but as dead—that is, no longer alive. In other words, death, as already mentioned, is the end of the process called life.

"Human," "human being," "human life," and "person" are used synonymously in common parlance and by some bioethicists and philosophers.[8] Whether the meanings of these terms are interchangeable may not even be considered in the relevant discussions. However, the meanings assumed or attributed may actually be the same, overlapping, or different, regardless of whether this possibility is recognized. The term "human," for example, may refer to organisms or only to parts of them. In either case, "human" identifies the entity as biologically distinguishable from others. The ways in which human organisms differ from others may be disputed, but some characteristics that are only present in humans are not present in all humans.

As an adjective, the term "human" refers to any tissue or organism whose DNA shows that it belongs to the species *Homo sapiens*; as such, it is genetically human. A human hair follicle is human in this sense, but acknowledging this is not equivalent to considering it *a* human. Moreover, at the early embryonic (blastocyst) stage, the developing entity is potentially more than *a* living organism because it may become more than one individual. In other words, "it" is potentially "them."

As a noun, "human" is frequently used interchangeably with "human being" to refer to an individual member of the species. Although both terms are usually used for living organisms, "human" may also be used for organisms that are no longer living, such as human cadavers. A human newborn or fetus is a human or a human being, whereas separated human gametes or blood cells are human only in the adjectival or genetic sense.[9] To some, "being" means "living"; "human being" then applies (obviously) only to living human organisms. "Being" may also be used more extensively as a synonym for "existing," which is applicable to nonliving or inanimate entities (e.g., a painting) and even to ideas that exist only in someone's mind (e.g., a conception of the painting).

Unlike terms that are biologically meaningful (e.g., "human" and "life"), "person" is a philosophical, moral, or legal designation. However, the biologically meaningful terms are based on descriptive criteria that identify individuals to whom they apply. Different positions on personhood are based on different criteria, and full moral status is attributed to those who fit the criteria. Nonpersons and potential persons may also have moral status, but this may be overridden by the moral status of persons. In other words, moral status may entail a range of stringency in the obligations it imposes on others. From an egalitarian perspective, all persons have the same value or moral status, regardless of their age or condition. Using the terms "human being," "human life," and "person" synonymously thus carries significant moral weight.

Meaning and significance of moral status

What is "moral status" and why is it such a significant moral variable? Basically, the term refers to the value an entity possesses independently of other entities.[10] Its inherent value renders the entity deserving of certain behaviors or attitudes on the part of others; these are their moral obligations to the entity. An entity with moral status deserves these behaviors or attitudes regardless of whether they are forthcoming, and regardless of whether it has comparable obligations toward others. The specific content of these obligations and who is specifically obligated to fulfill them are questions whose answers depend on the circumstances (variables) of the case. People who are ill, for example, deserve health care from knowledgeable practitioners, but not from those incapable of providing the care they need.

Ascriptions of moral status are generally based on characteristics or properties present in most members of a group; the ascriptions apply to all members of the group even though some may lack these characteristics. Full moral status may therefore be attributed to all human beings, including those who are profoundly impaired, because most humans possess valued capabilities such as cognition, speech, and autonomy. Some scholars define the group of humans who have full moral status more narrowly—for example, as comprised only of those who possess the valued capabilities. Humans who are profoundly impaired are then imputed to have less moral status than those who do. Accordingly, moral status may be construed as full or partial. Partial moral status covers a wide range of possibilities, depending on the criteria by which membership in the group is defined. Multiple criteria may be required for full moral status and fewer criteria for partial moral status.[11]

Attribution of any degree of moral status implies a duty to respect individuals to whom this status is imputed.[12] Respect entails recognition of the individual's worth as a member of the group; how it should be expressed varies according to the values on which it is based and the capabilities of those who are obliged to render the respect. For Kant, respect for the moral status of persons means that each should be treated by other persons as an end in herself (or himself) and never only as means to others' ends. The essential attribute on which he bases this claim is autonomy. Individuals incapable of autonomy are not owed the respect due to persons.

Some scholars argue that the same respect that autonomous humans merit is also due to nonautonomous humans, such as fetuses and infants. Those who consider abortion murder hold this view. If fetuses or newborns are members of distinct groups of humans whose characteristics are not deserving of the respect attributed to the group of humans who have cognitive capacity, they may deserve less respect due to less moral status. If they are seen as members of the group that generally possesses this capacity, they deserve the same respect.

Other scholars attribute partial moral status to some humans and nonhumans, either as gradually increasing during the course of prenatal development or as acquired at some threshold of development. Depending on the criteria that determine full moral status, individuals to whom it is attributed don't necessarily retain it throughout their lifetime; the moral status of those who meet the criteria early in their lives may be lessened or lost if they subsequently fail to meet these criteria. A patient who lapses into "persistent vegetative state," for example, may no longer have the moral status she had achieved before she lost her ability to respond meaningfully to external stimuli.

Because moral status means that an individual is independently deserving of respect, it implies that she has rights, both positive and negative. Persons as such are generally accorded a positive right to life and basic health care on grounds of their full moral status. As discussed in chapter 1, negative rights are more compelling than positive rights; in the language of the verities, this means that nonmaleficence trumps beneficence (maxim 4). Fetuses and individuals who are permanently comatose or "vegetative" may or may not have rights of either kind, depending on what moral status, if any, is attributed to them.[13] Nonhuman animals may be accorded rights at a lesser level than that accorded to born human beings with cognitive capacity. On grounds of this rationale, for example, it is always wrong to inflict pain on an animal needlessly, but it is not necessarily wrong to kill the animal painlessly.

Debates about abortion as well as debates about termination of life-sustaining treatment after birth prevalently involve the use of rights language. The pivotal rights upheld by opposing sides in debates about abortion are the right to life of the fetus and the right to choose of the pregnant woman. If the same moral status is imputed to both, the fetus' right to life may override the woman's right to choose. If the fetus has partial moral status, the woman's right to choose may prevail because she has full moral status.

The pivotal rights asserted in debates about whether to withdraw or forego life-sustaining treatment after birth are the individual's right to survive through mechanical support, the right to have currently or previously expressed wishes honored, and the right not to be continually subjected to invasive medical interventions that can only sustain a minimal level of function. Two different and competing notions of human life are at stake here: one reliant on a level of functioning that characterizes living nonhumans, the other reliant on a level that only characterizes living human beings. In either case, full moral status may be imputed to the individual if she is seen as a member of a group whose attributes typically merit this evaluation.

Moral relevance of the gestational tie and other relationships

Obligations of human beings toward others are not based solely on moral status. Most if not all moral obligations are inseparable from relationships to others who may or may not be persons. On a broader social level, duties of promise keeping, truth telling, gratitude, and restitution also arise from relationships between persons. As discussed in chapter 2, relationships between practitioners and patients are particularly important in clinical settings. Occasionally, these relationships entail obligations for the clinician but not the patient because the patient is incapable of autonomous decision-making. For most people, however, whether or not they are involved in health care, fulfillment of duties based on one relationship are sometimes at odds with fulfillment of duties based on another. In the context of health care, women tend to experience these conflicts when they find themselves unable to fulfill their obligations as patients while also fulfilling their obligations as mothers, spouses, or daughters.

Arguably, obligations also arise from relationships to entities that have the potentiality to become indisputably persons. These relationships inevitably raise questions about moral status, as consideration of the gestational tie makes clear. However, the relationship may be different no matter what moral status is imputed, depending on whether an embryo is developing within the woman's body (in vivo) or outside of her body (in vitro).[14] The physiological relationship between the woman and the developing organism is obviously different in these situations, and the emotional relationship is likely to be different also. Because of their different relationships to their embryos, the standpoint of women who are not pregnant is different not only from that of their male partners but also from that of women in whom pregnancy is already established.

No matter how pregnancy is established, whether through sexual intercourse or transfer of an embryo formed in vitro, the tie between a woman and her developing fetus is unique among other human relationships. Unfortunately, although this intimate connection is a morally significant variable in any decision involving pregnant women, it is often neglected in debates about abortion. Instead, the debates tend to focus exclusively on the moral status of the fetus, one side claiming that abortion is wrong because the fetus is a person, the other that abortion is permissible because the fetus is not a person. As discussed in chapter 9, neither side presents an adequate argument through this focus.

An early and significant exception to the tendency to ignore the uniqueness of the gestational relationship is an article by Judith Jarvis Thomson, in which she argued that even if the fetus is a person, no woman should be forced to maintain a constant biological connection to another person for nine months, even if this is the only means by which the life of the other person can be sustained. The analogy used in support of her position was the following: "You wake up in the morning and find yourself back to back in bed with an unconscious violinist. A famous unconscious violinist. He has been found to have a fatal kidney ailment, and . . . you alone have the right blood type to help."[15] Thomson went on to explain that the Society of Music Lovers had kidnapped you and arranged for your circulatory system to be connected to that of the violinist for the nine months necessary for his cure. To disconnect the two of you now would be to kill him.

By employing this preposterous analogy, Thomson provided a corrective to the nearsightedness of her contemporaries who had argued for or against abortion solely on grounds of the moral status of the fetus. No actual relationship between persons, including that of congenital twins, adequately demonstrates the uniqueness of the tie that must be severed if the life of a fetus is to be terminated.[16]

Thomson's recognition that abortion cannot be adequately refuted or defended through exclusive focus on the moral status of the fetus may well have been influenced by the fact that her standpoint was that of a woman: that is, someone whose body might be personally affected by this relationship. Most of the philosophical arguments developed at the time were written by those who lacked this relevant perspective. Admittedly, if the tie on which she focused, while assuming that the fetus has as compelling a right to life as an unconscious violinist, could be severed without terminating the life of the fetus, Thomson's argument would not necessarily lead to the same conclusion. At that point, arguments on both sides could be legitimately mounted on grounds that the fetus is or is not a person. Other relationships, including the relationship between the potential father and the fetus would then assume a more persuasive relevance.

As discussed in chapter 2, some authors who address reproductive issues try to bypass the abortion controversy by focusing on the fetus as a patient or potential person rather than as an actual person. In doing so they are prone to ignore the physical connectedness that makes this experience unique for the gestating woman, not only physiologically but also emotionally and socially. Scholars who emphasize the autonomy of the pregnant woman may also fail to appreciate the moral relevance of this relationship. Here, as in other contexts, the autonomy of the individual is inseparable from relationships that are indiscernible to others.

Women who have been pregnant are less likely to ignore the significance of the intimate tie between women and their fetuses than those who have not had this experience. And women who have not been pregnant are more likely than men to appreciate this relationship as a desired or undesired experience for them personally. As many women recognize, however, each one's experience of pregnancy and of individual pregnancies is different. Although the standpoint of the pregnant patient should be given privileged status when she is most affected by health care decisions, this does not imply that those who have not been (or cannot be) pregnant lack relevant insights or understanding regarding the experience. Foremost among those whose standpoints may be relevant but less privileged than that of the pregnant woman is the potential father. To the extent that he acknowledges his genetic tie to the fetus and his responsibility for the life of a potential offspring, his standpoint is more compelling than that of those who are not personally affected by the pregnancy.

Even those who are not permanently or personally affected by pregnancy may have relevant insights or understanding regarding the experience. Just as the oncologist who has never had cancer but has treated thousands of cancer patients over the years acquires helpful information or suggestions for new patients, so the obstetrician who has cared for thousands of pregnant patients often has useful advice for pregnant women. The practitioner's experience is indirect but (usually) extensive; the patient's experience is direct but limited. Both patients and practitioners, therefore, have standpoints that are ethically and epistemologically relevant to clinical decision-making.

Practitioners who recognize that the standpoint of patients deserves privileged status in decisions affecting them may have a better knowledge base from which to make their clinical decisions than those who deny this. Nonetheless, no practitioner who cares for pregnant women can avoid the complicated question of the moral status of the fetus simply by eliciting their input and granting it privileged status. Unquestioning compliance with another's decision is never an adequate justification for one's own decision. Tempting though it may be, such compliance, while consistent with the informative model of the physician-patient relationship, entails at least partial responsibility for the decisions of another.

Like the general public, clinicians embrace a wide range of positions about fetuses, and these form the starting points from which other views follow, including those involving patients whose moral status is disputed because they lack abilities considered central to persons as such. In light of the interminable controversy about moral obligations (if any) to the fetus, as well as controversies about treatment or nontreatment of patients who are permanently comatose, it is doubtful that there will ever be consensus on the matter. By examining a range of positions, however, individuals can clarify their own views and develop more informed and respectful attitudes toward those of others.

Personhood and potential for personhood

Full moral status is usually attributed to persons regardless of whether they have moral agency—that is, the ability to make moral decisions. But the term "person," as already suggested, is also used for human beings that are not currently or will never be capable of moral agency. In other words, all moral agents are persons who as such have full moral status, but personhood and full moral status do not necessarily entail moral agency. Although attributions of personhood have momentous implications for decisions made at the beginning and end of life, disputes about the criteria for personhood are persistent. Different standpoints on issues in bioethics develop from whatever criteria are embraced, either implicitly or explicitly, for determination of personhood. Addressing the variable of different starting points about personhood is crucial to resolution of ethical issues in women's health care because some but not all of these imply that fetuses are persons whose interests are separable from or at odds with those of pregnant women.

Throughout history, "person" has been defined in a variety of ways.[17] A classical definition is that of Boethius: "an individual substance of a rational nature."[18] In a sense, this is a broader concept than "human" because it is applicable to other species and even to noncorporeal beings (e.g., God or angels) to whom a "rational nature" may be attributed. Many scholars maintain (or assume), however, that only humans are persons, even while disagreeing about when in the course of human development personhood is achieved. Some support an extremely restrictive view of human personhood, limiting it to those who currently have moral agency. Bonnie Steinbock calls this a normative view of personhood, and Mary Anne Warren calls it "a maximalist view."[19] I prefer the latter term because normative criteria may also be supported for humans who do not fulfill maximal criteria.

The maximalist position denies full moral status or personhood to human beings who have permanently lost or will never achieve higher brain function (e.g., anencephalics and those who have irreversibly lost cognitive function), as well as those who are likely to achieve personhood in time (e.g., infants). However, any of these individuals may be accorded partial moral status. Those who have lost moral agency may be considered "former persons," and those who may yet acquire it may be considered "potential persons." On a "maximalist" view of personhood, both fetuses and newborns may still be potential persons. A "minimalist" view, in contrast, attributes personhood to the developing human organism from the onset of fertilization until complete cessation of cardiovascular and brain function.

An interesting nuance regarding the minimalist position on personhood arises in conjunction with the possibility of somatic cell nuclear transplantation, also called cloning. As discussed in chapter 13, human cloning involves activation of development in a human enucleated egg to which the nucleus of an adult cell has been transferred. Some scholars support minimal criteria for a full right to life or personhood in these entities, as well as in embryos produced through fertilization. Accordingly, they argue that even if embryos are produced through cloning, which they oppose, it is better to transfer them to a woman for gestation than to destroy them for use in research.[20]

Former personhood is relevant to end-of-life decisions because former persons may have indicated their wishes about care prior to their loss of the capacity for knowledgeable and autonomous decision-making. Arguably, respect for their autonomy, as previously expressed by those who are no longer autonomous, has priority in ethical decisions made on their behalf. Potential personhood is relevant to beginning of life decisions on grounds that prevention of the birth of an already living human entity that has the capacity to become indisputably a person through moral agency, is a greater harm than preventing its life or potentiality in the first place. As Aristotle would put it, potency is not mere negation or privation; it is a positive capacity for actualization. His distinction is applicable to the difference between contraception, as thwarting fertilization, and abortion, as ending the process of development.

Scholars have argued both for and against the moral relevance of potentiality for personhood in decisions about human fetuses. Brian Johnstone, for example, distinguishes between three uses of the term "potential" and then argues that all of these are applicable to human embryos.[21] A weak sense of "potential," he says, is present when one entity can be transformed into another by any kind of cause; a strong sense is one in which something has the capacity for transformation within itself; and a statistical sense of "potential" simply means that there is "high probability" that one thing will be transformed into another. In response to those who claim that the potential of gametes is comparable to the potential of embryos, Johnstone denies that either a strong or statistical sense of potential is present in gametes. In virtue of their greater statistical potential for personhood, he believes that human embryos have a moral status somewhere between the status of gametes and the status of mature (born) human beings.

Alfonso Gomez-Lobo claims that the potentiality for personhood of the early embryo, whether in vivo or in vitro, is morally equivalent to actual personhood.[22] His argument for this position is not persuasive if the Aristotelian distinction between potentiality and actuality is maintained.[23] For Gomez-Lobo, separate gametes lack the "biological potentiality" to become undeniably persons; embryos have this potentiality because their further development can proceed without dependence on external causes. This analysis ignores the fact that neither gametes nor embryos can become indisputably persons independently of the women to whom they are biologically related through gestation. If Aristotle's account of potentiality is applied, in vitro embryos as well as gametes have a passive potency for personhood because their further development depends on external causes, but the probability of further development is greater for the embryos. In vitro embryos, however, have an active potency for personhood because they will continue their development unless it is ended through abortion.

No matter how the potential for personhood is interpreted, potential persons as well as former persons and nonpersons may have a right to life, albeit not as securely as actual personhood demands or on the same grounds. If an entity has partial moral status, the strength of its right to life depends on its degree of moral status. Characterizing a fetus as a person implies that it has a prima facie right not to be killed through abortion. A sanctity of life rationale may support this right even without affirming that the fetus is a person.

Affirming a potential for personhood in human embryos provides grounds for distinguishing between them and human tissue and organs to which no moral status is attributed. R. M. Hare fails to take into account this unique feature of embryos when he imputes the same potential for personhood to separate human gametes, ignoring the fact that ova and sperm exist in different bodies.[24] Unlike gametes, human zygotes can develop toward birth and unquestionable personhood if placed or allowed to remain in the supportive environment of a woman's uterus. Hare's thesis suggests that ova or sperm are only accidentally rather than essentially related within the developing organism.

Like Hare, Helga Kuhse and Peter Singer argue that the potentiality argument is inadequate because all that can be said about the potential of embryos can also be said about the potential of ova and sperm.[25] Consider, they suggest, a situation in which excess ova and sperm obtained for in vitro fertilization are disposed of by being flushed separately down the sink. No one, they believe, would find this action morally objectionable. But suppose that after the ova and sperm are disposed of separately, a blockage in the sink occurs, and this causes them to remain lodged together, allowing fertilization to occur. According to Kuhse and Singer, "Those who believe that the embryo has a special moral status which makes it wrong to destroy it must now believe that it would be wrong to clear the blockage; instead the egg must now be rescued from the sink, checked to see if fertilization has occurred, and if it has, efforts should presumably be made to keep it alive."[26] Assuming that reasonable people would not attempt such a rescue, they conclude that there is no morally significant difference between human embryos and human gametes.

Kuhse and Singer are probably right that most reasonable people would not attempt to rescue an egg that had been accidentally fertilized through a sink blockage. Depending on how much effort, expense, and chance of success were involved, however, some reasonable people might attempt the rescue. Those who view personhood as commensurate with fertilization might feel morally obliged to make the attempt, but they would not feel similarly obliged if it were clear that the gametes had remained separate. Moreover, some reasonable people might object on moral grounds to disposal of any human tissue, including separate gametes, by flushing it down the sink. They might insist on a more respectful mode of disposal, such as cremation or burial. Some religious traditions prohibit masturbation and the "spilling" of sperm on this basis.

Fetuses have at times been regarded as extraneous tissue, removable from women as readily and appropriately as unwanted growths or tumors. Until viability, fetuses are dependent for survival on women, and this has led some to describe their existence as parasitic. Demeaning as it is, the term "parasitic" may also be used to describe infants and older patients who depend on others for survival. For no one, however, does dependence on others imply nonpersonhood. Neither does attribution of "dependent moral status," for which Chervenak and McCullough argue, imply that the fetus is not a person who as such has an independent right to life.[27]

As already indicated, relationships between individuals are a significant empirical and moral variable in clinical decision-making. Its relevance, however, does not imply that one party in the relationship is thereby empowered to determine that the other has moral status. Although some authors allege otherwise, moral status is not conferrable by persons on nonpersons; it either is or isn't present in a subject, regardless of whether others recognize it. H. Tristram Engelhardt implicitly recognizes this in his account of personhood which, for him, requires moral agency. As moral agents, he claims, persons have no obligations to nonpersons as such, but they have prima facie obligations to respect the autonomy of persons who care for nonpersons.[28] Patienthood, in contrast, is conferrable by others—for example, by those who present dependent individuals for treatment. Among patients, independent moral status may be full or partial because some patients (e.g., competent adults) are fully and indisputably persons while others (e.g., neonates) are, arguably, not fully persons despite their independent moral status. If fetuses are merely extraneous tissue, they have neither partial nor independent moral status. If an adult lapses into a permanently comatose state, she may be similarly regarded. However, both fetuses and irreversibly unconscious adults may be accorded minimal moral status solely on grounds that they are living human organisms.

Thresholds of development and moral status

Between maximalist and minimalist criteria for personhood are thresholds of development that often have a counterpart in the traumatic loss or gradual decline of capacities that had previously been developed. Ranging from the beginning to the end of this continuum, possible criteria for imputing full moral status are the following:

Fertilization, or activation of a human egg cell (minimal criterion)

Implantation in the uterus

Individuation or development of the primitive streak

The woman's decision to continue her pregnancy

Onset of brain function

Onset and perdurance of consciousness or sentiency

Viability

Birth

Self-consciousness

Moral agency (maximal criterion)

An egalitarian perspective alone cannot resolve the question of when, if ever, human fetuses as such have the same value as born persons; neither can it resolve the question of whether born human beings who have lost or never acquired the ability to think or choose should still be considered persons. An egalitarian perspective does imply, however, that the criteria for inclusion or exclusion among those considered persons should be consistently applied to members of both groups.

Fertilization identifies the least demanding criterion for personhood. John Noonan exemplifies this position through his claim that full and independent moral status is present in the human zygote, the one-celled embryo formed when a human oocyte is activated through penetration by a human sperm.[29] At that point, Noonan argues, the embryo, whether it is formed in vitro or in vivo, has a right to life equal to that of any adult human being, including that of the pregnant woman. In other words, each genetically new human organism (even one that may yet become more than one individual) is fully a person. Noonan's position is consistent with that of Pope John Paul II: "The human being is to be respected and treated as a person from the moment of conception."[30] If this starting point regarding moral status is applied to the entire life span, human beings who are born with no higher brain function (anencephalics) and those who lose higher brain function later in life also count as persons.

Implantation of the embryo in the uterus occurs about a week after fertilization, initiating a detectable pregnancy. If abortion is defined as termination of pregnancy prior to viability, and pregnancy has not yet been established, opposition to abortion is compatible with termination of the early embryo. Individuation, that is, the determination of whether one or more embryos will develop further, is not settled until the primitive streak appears at the beginning of the third week.[31] Norman Ford considers the establishment of individuality at this juncture a necessary and sufficient condition for full moral status and a right to life equal to that of born human beings.[32]

The criterion of the woman's decision to continue gestating is obviously dependent on her knowing that she is pregnant, and this may occur considerably later than the pregnancy is clinically detectable. Women who are amenorrheic, for example, may not realize they are pregnant until well into the second trimester. An unavoidable question arises for those who impute moral status to the fetus solely on this basis: What becomes of its status if and when the woman changes her mind? Respect for autonomy demands efforts to respond to such changes. Chervenak and McCullough attempt to bypass the question by referring to the woman's decision as a "settled" one, but even "settled" decisions regarding previable fetuses are sometimes altered late in gestation (for example, after positive prenatal diagnoses of genetic or chromosomal anomalies). Once they consider fetuses to be patients, Chervenak and McCullough shift their ethical priorities from respect for the woman's autonomy to beneficence toward the fetus and toward her. At that point, however, the status they identify as "dependent" for the fetus is obviously *not* dependent on the autonomy of the woman who uncontroversially has independent moral status.

Just as the cessation of brain function has been the criterion by which death is determined, the onset of brain function has been proposed as the crucial criterion for determining whether the human fetus has full moral status or a right to life. In the developing organism, however, brain function that is detectable at about 6 weeks is considerably more rudimentary than brain function in a more developed fetus or neonate.[33] Consciousness and sentiency require different levels of brain development or activity. If sentiency is defined as the ability to experience pain or pleasure, it is distinguishable from consciousness, which may involve the ability to experience sounds or sight without sensitivity to pain or pleasure. Both are grounds by which partial moral status has been attributed to some living organisms (animals) but not others (plants). At about 8 weeks, the human fetus apparently draws back when touched with a needle; this suggests, but does not prove, that its nervous system is sufficiently developed to experience pain.[34] The criterion of sentiency is commonly invoked as grounds for a moral obligation to avoid the infliction of pain unless it appears necessary to avoid greater pain or to effect a benefit that outweighs the pain. The verity of nonmaleficence demands this.

As a correlate to the definition of death as complete cessation of brain function, Hans-Martin Sass has argued that the developing fetus acquires moral status when cortical (higher brain) function is detectable, which is about 10 weeks after fertilization.[35] Although this criterion identifies what Plato and Aristotle consider the defining function of human life as such, not everyone agrees that humans who lack higher brain function have lesser moral status than those who do. Moreover, like each of the developmental thresholds already mentioned, cortical function is not an instantly occurring achievement but a process. During the process, just when the threshold is reached is itself debatable, and detection is not always possible or accurate. This is also true when a threshold is traversed in the opposite direction—for example, when someone who has clearly demonstrated higher brain function gradually or partially loses this capacity.

Viability is another threshold that is difficult to detect. The criteria for its determination (e.g., experiencing fetal movement, or "quickening") are more subjective than the criteria for other thresholds of development. Consequently, a living organism can only be proved viable retrospectively, when its survival has already been demonstrated. The absence of viability generally means that death is imminent, no matter what is done to forestall it. In other words, the organism, while still living, is dying. Despite the uncertainties that accompany judgments about viability, the achievement of this threshold in fetal development is ethically relevant in another way: that is, the possibility of ending gestation electively without preventing live birth. This means that health care practitioners can choose a method of prenatal termination that ensures this will happen or not happen. Chervenak and McCullough are right that viability implies greater responsibility on the part of clinicians who care for pregnant women. However, their argument that this responsibility gives them the right to override the decisions of a pregnant woman about her care is not persuasive.

Birth also means that others, especially the father of the newborn, are responsible for the infant's survival and nurturance. It is a life-altering event for men as well as women because it makes them biological parents, regardless of whether they fulfill the responsibilities of parenthood thereafter. Unlike viability, birth is an empirically observable event that definitively establishes this responsibility and extends it to others. The infant no longer has physical ties to the only person who was previously physically affected by anything done or not done to the fetus. As a distinct member of society, the newborn is recognized as a person in most parts of the world; as such, full moral status and all the rights that apply to other persons are attributed to it.

In the clinical setting, the importance of birth is illustrated through the transition of care responsibilities—when the neonatologist or pediatrician assumes care of the newborn and the obstetrician continues care of the patient who is no longer pregnant. Warren maintains that "the moral significance of birth" is such that the status of a developmentally younger newborn supersedes that of an older viable fetus. She defends this position on grounds that it is impossible to treat fetuses as if they were persons without treating women as if they were something less than persons.[36] Personhood "in the full blooded sense," for Warren, requires the capacity for moral agency, but newborns and other sentient human beings who are not moral agents should be accorded full moral status as members of human social communities.[37]

Although newborns are manifestly conscious, self-consciousness or awareness of oneself as a separate being develops later in infancy. This criterion for personhood is only definitively detectible later in development. It is nonetheless a criterion that some consider sufficient to establish full moral status. Michael Tooley, for example, views self-consciousness as a necessary and sufficient condition for personhood because it indicates that the living organism has a "desire" or "interest" in survival as "a continuing subject of experiences."[38] His position undercuts the moral significance of birth by emphasizing a link between abortion and infanticide. The argument Tooley mounts in support of both practices is also applicable to human beings who have irreparably lost a sense of themselves as subjects who are consciously interested in their own survival. Peter Singer makes the connection explicit when, while endorsing Tooley's position, he contends that "only a being who is capable of conceiving herself as a distinct entity existing over time—that is, only a person—could have this desire. Therefore only a person could have the right to life."[39]

Moral agency, the maximalist criterion endorsed by Tooley, requires not only self-consciousness but also cognitive ability, recognition of the moral dimensions of decisions, and autonomy. Since this is the most demanding criterion for personhood, it is applicable to the least number of human beings. Accordingly, no one disputes that a living human being who demonstrates her capacity for moral decision-making is a person. The disputes occur either prior to the onset of moral agency or later in life, when decisional capacity may be only questionably present or manifestly absent. Also disputable is the level of cognitive ability and degree of autonomy required for an individual to act as a moral agent in specific circumstances.

Just what constitutes moral as opposed to nonmoral or amoral decision-making is even more difficult to determine. The terms "good/bad" and "right/wrong" are commonly used to describe actions (or inactions) that do not necessarily have a moral dimension. We may speak, for example, of a "good" move in chess or a "wrong" answer to a math problem. The capacity for moral agency necessarily implies that those who possess it are able to recognize a difference between acts or omissions that have a moral dimension and those that are morally neutral or amoral; it also implies the ability to distinguish between moral and immoral behavior.

The criterion of moral agency is obviously unmet by fetuses, newborns, and some adults. This capacity may also be lacking or only partially present in different circumstances, as when someone is inadequately informed or when a person's autonomy is limited by institutional or family pressures. Moreover, although moral agents have full moral status, those who lack moral agency may also have that status. Accordingly, the question of moral status remains a significant variable in positions about obligations to fetuses as well as to humans already born who have not yet achieved, have lost, or will never achieve moral agency. An important difference between fetuses and born individuals who have permanently lost or will never achieve moral agency is that, unlike early embryos, most fetuses are likely to achieve the capacity for moral agency. A similarity is that some fetuses have already lost that potential or will die before it can be actualized.

Few if any of the preceding criteria occur in a single instant; instead, some stretch of time transpires between entering and exiting the threshold, and this in itself may cause disagreement about which point must be reached for the organism crossing the threshold to become or to cease being a person. Ranging from the first moment of fertilization to the acquisition of a capacity for moral decision-making, the proposed thresholds define specific starting points or positions. As we have seen, some positions do not endorse either maximalist or minimalist criteria for personhood. These intermediate positions identify specific thresholds of development as grounds for attributing partial or full moral status. Although their proponents have applied them to fetuses, their applicability postnatally may be even more compelling.

Intermediate positions about moral status

An intermediate position widely embraced by clinicians, patients, and the public at large is that moral status is acquired or lost gradually after fertilization. Responsibilities and rights are correspondingly defined as stronger or weaker, depending on how near or far an individual is from full moral status. Norman Gillespie, for example, argues that responsibilities to prolong or protect the life of the fetus are proportionate to its degree of development.[40] Birth may then define the point at which full moral status is established. In most places, birth is also the point at which a living human being is legally a person, and death (defined as cessation of heart and lung function) is when a human being no longer satisfies the legal definition of personhood. Other scholars argue for different thresholds of development for full moral status. The President's Council on Bioethics describes the demarcation points as "meaningful discontinuities."[41] The discontinuities may also occur after birth. Supporters of intermediate and maximalist positions alike may consider those who lose decisional capacity as no longer persons who, as such, have full moral status; they may nonetheless impute partial moral status to such individuals.

Many scholars support intermediate positions that attribute some but not full moral status to human fetuses as such throughout, or during some portion of, their development.[42] Instead of viewing the fetus as gradually increasing in moral status, they identify a specific point in gestation at which the developing organism acquires a right to others' concern or care. This view is applicable to nonhumans as well as humans. The "interest view" of Steinbock, for example, identifies the onset of sentiency as the point at which moral agents have a responsibility to avoid or reduce pain in any entity capable of experiencing it. Warren agrees with Steinbock that sentiency provides grounds for attributing intermediate or partial moral status to living organisms.[43] Their positions about personhood are substantially the same also: neither believes newborn humans fulfill descriptive criteria for personhood, but both think they should be treated as if they do.

John Robertson describes his intermediate position as one of "special respect" for human embryos and fetuses, as "symbols or reminders of our membership in the human community."[44] He considers the moral demands of this respect more compelling as gestation proceeds. Prior to viability, abortion should be permitted but discouraged on grounds of respect for the pregnant woman's choice. After that,

Robertson supports legal prohibition of abortion "except where necessary to protect the life or health of the mother."[45] Viability is important not simply because it means that the fetus can survive ex utero, but also because the fetus at that point has interests—for example, in being born without disabilities. Despite the priority he imputes to procreative freedom, Robertson supports limitation of a pregnant women's right to abortion, based on the interests of the fetus or potential child. This aspect of his account accords with Chervenak and McCullough's argument that viability is a sufficient condition for treating fetuses as patients. Robertson also argues that the sentient fetus has an interest while in utero in the avoidance of pain. "Moral duties," he says, "can be owed to sentient beings" even if they are not persons.[46]

Another intermediate position is articulated by Carson Strong, who describes his approach as a modified version of casuistry.[47] Strong addresses moral status through recourse to a paradigm of personhood drawn from Steinbock's distinction between normative and descriptive persons. "Normative personhood" applies to entities that possess full moral status; "descriptive personhood" to those that possess self-consciousness.[48] Descriptive personhood implies normative personhood, but not vice versa. Individuals that are not self-conscious, for Strong, are normatively persons to the extent that moral status is conferred on them by others, based on how well they fit the descriptive paradigm. Characteristics by which the fit may be measured include use of language, capacity for rational thought and action, ability to profess values, and moral agency. The different milestones of development, including those of infants who are not as yet self-conscious, are thus grounds for "conferred moral status."[49] Strong's account of conferred moral status may be compared with Chervenak and McCullough's argument that a woman's decision to continue her pregnancy is a sufficient condition for treatment of the fetus as a patient. It is importantly different, however, in that Strong does not maintain that the pregnant woman alone confers moral status. Instead, he argues that it is conferred through social agreement, based mainly on concerns about social consequences.

Those who support intermediate positions on personhood may attribute partial moral status to all or only some fetuses, with or without specifying how close their moral status is to full or none. Others attribute the same partial moral status to fetuses throughout gestation, or only after they reach a specific threshold of development. Any of these intermediate positions implies that abortion decisions are not morally neutral if and when the fetus has moral status. More or less compelling reasons are required for moral justification of abortion when that threshold has been reached.

Support for the permissibility of abortion at any point during gestation is generally based on respect for the pregnant woman's autonomy and also, often, on beneficence or nonmaleficence toward her. With regard to autonomy, however, few authors address a crucial variable—the social conditions that often limit the autonomy of pregnant women. Robertson acknowledges that "procreative liberty may be severely constrained by social and economic circumstances," but he considers the question of whether the state should alleviate those conditions a "separate issue of social justice."[50] From an egalitarian perspective, these issues are not separable: social justice must prevail for individuals who are disempowered or disadvantaged to be as autonomous as their dominant counterparts.

If full moral status is not attributed to the fetus, the pregnant woman's right to life and, arguably, her right to choose may override its right to life because she is a person and the fetus is not. In contrast, if full moral status is imputed to the fetus at any point during development, its right to life may override her right to choose on grounds that life is the more basic or compelling right for individuals who have the same moral status.

That preservation of life is more ethically compelling than respect for autonomy is also supportable on grounds that life is not a right but a condition for all other rights. If two individuals are both persons and the life of one is threatened by that of the other, additional variables must be examined to determine the moral course of action or inaction. In this regard, an important variable to most clinicians and potential parents is the potential of a particular fetus to become a healthy newborn. The potential to be born and the potential to be born healthy are not the same, but both potentials are morally relevant to determination of what should be done or not done regarding them. In most countries, personhood is legally imputed to newborns regardless of their health status but not to fetuses even if they are healthy and viable. From an egalitarian perspective, just as people born with impairments have the same value as those born without impairments, impaired fetuses have the same value as fetuses that are not impaired.

Another variable in positions about the moral status of the fetus is a distinction between those destined to be brought to term and those destined to be aborted. This distinction is obviously related to the woman's decision to continue or terminate her pregnancy. At times, however, whether a fetus is destined to go to term depends solely on whether it has the capacity to do so. Some genetic abnormalities make this highly unlikely or impossible. As mentioned in chapter 2, Chervenak and McCullough employ the distinction between fetuses destined to go to term and those destined for abortion to support their view that some fetuses, but not all, are patients. Once a pregnant woman has declined the option of abortion, they contend that she is morally bound to make subsequent decisions that are protective of the interests of her developing fetus. This responsibility necessarily implies that some fetuses have a right to life or health independently of the woman's right to refuse treatment. The moral status thus imputed to them may be full or partial; in neither case, however, is its moral status dependent on hers, as they claim. If the fetus has partial moral status, its interests cannot trump her interests unless they are clearly less compelling (e.g., a procedure crucial to survival of a viable fetus, involving no risk or harm to the pregnant woman). If both the fetus and the woman have full moral status, the right to life of either or neither can trump the other. An ethical dilemma posed at that point could only be resolved through considerations such as respect for the woman's autonomy or beneficence and nonmaleficence toward others.

Chervenak and McCullough's argument about "dependent moral status" is philosophically problematic because it conflates what is actually the case with what someone or some group determines to be the case, regardless of the grounds for that determination. In chapter 1, standpoint theory is described as a corrective to the inevitable limitations of such determinations, especially when they are articulated by dominant individuals or groups. In effect, Chervenak and McCullough use this corrective by imputing privileged status to the decisions of the pregnant woman in determining whether the previable fetus is a patient with "dependent moral status." But reducing epistemological limitations by attending to the standpoints of those who are nondominant does not imply that the ensuing decisions match reality; it argues only that they are closer to that (objective) reality than they would be if they failed to incorporate the relevant nondominant standpoints.

Admittedly, my critique of the view that moral status of the fetus is determinable by the pregnant woman's decision is at odds with the postmodern account that reality does not exist apart from our conceptions of it.[51] It should be noted, however, that the claim or assumption that there is an objective reality not wholly or infallibly determinable by subjective decisions is supported not only by scholars who reject postmodern accounts but also by the public at large. Moreover, insistence that decisions or claims about reality do not determine reality is consistent with the view that some decisions are closer to the truth than others. I agree, therefore, that decisions about fetuses are better made by imputing privileged status to the pregnant women who carry them; I disagree that decisions made by pregnant women provide an adequate basis for declaring fetuses to have moral status.

The argument that moral status is dependent solely on the standpoint or determination of others is also problematic because it may be employed in defense of terrible injustices. History has provided atrocious examples of situations in which the personhood or independent moral status of whole categories of people was denied, allegedly justifying their being treated as nonpersons, having no independent right to life. Fetuses may or may not have a right to life, but if the verity of justice is applied to fetuses, it is logically and ethically applicable to all of those who have the same moral status, regardless of whether others recognize their status.

Although I have not articulated them at length, a wide range of positions about moral status and personhood have been well developed and critiqued by various philosophers and religious thinkers. These positions are relevant not just to scholars; they also have their counterparts in the moral reasoning of most people about decisions at the beginning and end of human life. Whether advertently or not, each position serves as a starting point from which different standpoints develop about specific issues. For men as well as women, practitioners, policy makers, and the public at large, different positions on moral status lead not only to different conclusions but also to different decisions in particular cases. When I address issues about the beginning of life in this book, therefore, my goal is to illustrate how different starting points and standpoints have different ethical implications. When I consider issues at the end of life, my goal is to illustrate how those same starting points and standpoints have ethical implications that are consistent with those made at life's beginning.

PART II

Topics, Issues, and Cases

4

Preconception and Prenatal Decisions

Providers of women's health care are usually familiar with ways by which to promote the health of potential children as well as women. The standpoint from which they counsel women in this regard is generally informed by years of experience and knowledge of preventive, diagnostic, and therapeutic alternatives. During the last half century, methods by which to predict the health and characteristics of newborns have proliferated. Since the human genome has been mapped and sequenced, the list of conditions identifiable by prenatal genetic testing has been growing. Unfortunately, however, treatment options for the identifiable conditions have not improved at the same pace. Gene therapies, for example, have been considerably less successful than had been anticipated, and most genetic disorders remain incurable. More often than not, the only way through which a woman can avoid having a child with a prenatally diagnosed abnormality is by preventing its birth through abortion.

Through preimplantation diagnosis after in vitro fertilization, a woman can avoid gestating and giving birth to a child with detectable genetic anomalies without undergoing prenatal diagnosis and termination of affected embryos. The former procedure is more expensive and, in most cases, more physically onerous than prenatal testing, but it eliminates the moral and psychological onus that testing and termination during gestation entails for many women. For some, however, the disposal of anomalous embryos, including those with lethal anomalies, is morally equivalent to abortion.

This chapter illustrates variables that are morally relevant to decisions made prenatally or prior to the initiation of a desired pregnancy. It also examines issues raised by the possibility of misattributed paternity, carrier testing, and sex selection. Cases of misattributed paternity exemplify conflicts between respect for confidentiality and disclosure of unexpected or unwanted information. Carrier testing and sex selection may be associated with discriminatory reasons for testing. As advances in genetics proliferate, prenatal tests may determine the probability of an increasing assortment of traits or behaviors deemed socially or personally desirable by potential parents for their offspring. From an egalitarian perspective, justice is the paramount principle or verity by which to settle conflicts evoked by requests for interventions that exacerbate social inequities.

Preconception counseling

Cases

1. As a newborn, Tara Gwinn was diagnosed with phenylketonuria (PKU), and placed on a diet that prevented her from developing the severe retardation associated with this disease. During late adolescence, Tara was weaned from her special diet and told that a regular diet no longer posed any risks to her health. She was also advised that if she ever got pregnant, she should return to her PKU diet to avoid the risk of maternal PKU in her offspring. Although Tara attempted to follow this advice during her first pregnancy, compliance with the recommended diet was only intermittently achieved. Despite three months of hospitalization for intravenous administration of phenylalanine-reduced nutrition, her phenylalanine levels remained high. Fortunately, however, she gave birth to a healthy daughter.

Three years later, during her second pregnancy, Tara was more faithful to the recommended diet but declined hospitalization; this time she gave birth to an affected daughter. When her second daughter was 2 years old, she told her doctor she would like to have another child. Her physician believed she should not attempt another pregnancy.[1]

2. Lily Tighe is a 36-year-old single woman who has been blind since birth. After earning her doctoral degree in sociology, she was hired to head the disabilities studies program at the state university. Although Lily attempted to adopt a child through private as well as government agencies, her efforts have been unsuccessful. She visits her physician to request artificial insemination from an anonymous donor so that she can fulfill her long-standing desire to have a child.

3. Paula Seitz is HIV positive, having been infected from her husband who died two years ago. She has no symptoms of AIDS. Now in a new relationship, she would like to have a child, but her partner and her parents are opposed to the idea. She visits the women's clinic to ask for advice on how to achieve her goal of motherhood.

4. Maggie McGee is a 23-year-old woman with cystic fibrosis (CF), married for five years to Sam, who is not a CF carrier. Her pulmonologist has warned Maggie that pregnancy would be life-threatening because her nutritional status is already so poor, and her respiratory and digestive problems are likely to be exacerbated by pregnancy. Having decided to try to become pregnant anyway, she visits her obstetrician-gynecologist to obtain preconception counseling.

Empirical considerations

In the cases described, the health risks and psychosocial risks of pregnancy vary considerably for the women involved and their potential children. In cases 2–4, the psychosocial risks to the women include the possibility that their efforts to become pregnant may not be successful, or, if they have children, their experience of motherhood brings burdens they had not anticipated. Psychosocial risks to the potential children stem from the possibility that their mothers will be unable to provide them with adequate care because of their disabilities or health problems.

The health risks of maternal PKU and of positive HIV status differ substantially in kind, severity, and probability of transmission to offspring. If HIV-positive women undergo retroviral treatment during pregnancy, they reduce the transmission risk to their fetuses by two-thirds; in those to whom the virus is transmitted, AIDS symptoms are treatable. In contrast, maternal PKU is an incurable teratogenic condition that involves 92 to 95 percent risk of severe mental retardation and 73 percent risk of microcephaly, as well as escalated risks of congenital heart disease and low birthweight.[2]

Gestation is apparently easy to achieve for Tara Gwinn (case 1), but avoidance of serious risks to her potential newborn is harder to achieve than for potential offspring in the other cases. The recommended diet for PKU consists of breads, cereals, fats, fruits, and vegetables, supplemented by a formula containing nutrients with no phenylalanine. Given these restrictions, it is sometimes impossible to provide adequate nutrition to sustain fetal development without requiring the woman to endure long-term hospitalization and intravenous feeding of dietary supplements.

In case 4, gestation is likely to exacerbate the patient's CF symptoms, shortening her already-reduced lifespan. Maggie McGee is also less likely than most women to become pregnant regardless of whether she obtains medical assistance because the fertility of women with CF is much lower than that of unaffected women.

Regarding case 2, the health risk of pregnancy for Lily Tighe is probably no greater than it would be for a healthy woman who does not have her impairment. In case 3, the principal health risk for Paula Seitz is the long-term consequences to her of the retroviral treatment that she would be advised to take for the sake of her offspring. These include the possibility that if and when she becomes symptomatic for AIDS, retroviral drugs are less effective for her.

Theoretical considerations

The term "counseling" is prevalently used in conjunction with a deliberative model of the physician-patient relationship—that is, when respect for the patient's autonomy is paramount, but the practitioner offers specific advice about her health risks and health prospects. This advice often includes recommendations about lifestyle practices and prognoses, as well as treatment alternatives. At times, women also seek counsel from health practitioners about nonmedical issues.

Whether they should provide counseling on these matters is an ethical question in its own right. Respect for the patient's autonomy supports a positive response as long as the patient's autonomy still prevails, that is, as long as she is not unduly influenced by the physician or others. Ethically, counseling is intended to facilitate, not impede, autonomy.

In the context of preconception counseling, professional advice is often sought with regard to the condition and health prospects of the potential offspring as well. Practitioners with different positions about the morality of abortion and obligations to children already born may counsel patients prior to conception or fertilization; in both cases, however, standpoint theory argues that the clinician should be aware of, and their patients should be informed of, others' standpoints that may affect their care or counseling. Those who are morally opposed to prenatal terminations, for example, may support preconception sex determination but oppose attempts to become pregnant if there is high risk of transmitting an anomaly. And those who are unopposed to abortion may refuse to perform sex determination prior to conception while supporting the right to become pregnant even if there is high risk of transmitting an anomaly.

In case 1, the doctor's belief that Tara should not attempt another pregnancy may be based on the extreme physical demands of pregnancy for her and the high probability that she will have another severely impaired child. Beneficence toward Tara supports this belief but is overridable by respect for her autonomy (maxim 2). Beneficence toward the potential child may also support the physician's belief, but only if it is better for a child with maternal PKU not to be conceived than for that individual to be conceived, gestated, and eventually born. From an egalitarian perspective, this rationale is morally problematic whether counseling occurs before or after conception. Since Tara already has a child with maternal PKU, her standpoint is informed not only by her own experience of caring for an affected child but also by her ongoing observation of how the disease affects a particular child and her family. Unless the physician has had comparable experience, his belief that pregnancy should be avoided in these circumstances is not similarly informed. While counseling Tara, therefore, the physician should impute privileged status to her standpoint not only as principal caregiver but also as, probably, a better judge of whether the burden of life with maternal PKU outweighs the potential benefit of that life to her potential child.

The remaining cases raise questions about the capacity of a potentially pregnant woman to raise the desired child. Physicians as such are not experts in determination of qualities required for competent parenting. Nonetheless, their expertise regarding physical and mental capacities of potential parents is relevant to such determinations, and their counseling may be based solely on that expertise. Integral to the patient's decision in this regard is the availability and willingness of others to assist in parenting. Successful parenting is rarely if ever accomplished by lone individuals, whether fully able or not.

Although some clinicians believe they should avoid making judgments about parental competence, they inevitably contribute to the parenting decisions of women through preconception counseling. Depending on the extent and quality of the counseling, the practitioner thus assumes some responsibility for the woman's decision. By failing to mention a specific risk, for example, he may encourage a decision the woman or couple might not otherwise make. In cases 1, 3, and 4, therefore, the risks of pregnancy to the women themselves should be clearly indicated; in case 1, the high risk to the fetus, while probably explained in previous pregnancies, needs to be articulated again.

In case 2, the physician apparently has few concerns about health risks to Lily and her possible child. Instead, she is likely to be concerned about how Lily can adequately parent a child despite her blindness. This case illustrates the regrettable fact that economic status may be a crucial variable in assessing parental competence. Because Lily is not only highly intelligent but has a reliable income, she could probably pay for the practical assistance she needs to provide adequate care for a child. That basic child care is often provided by less-affluent women instead of biological mothers who are affluent but not disabled is hardly a new phenomenon in history or in current practice. From an egalitarian perspective, the regrettable part of this scenario is that basic child care is so minimally rewarded and respected that those who provide it for others are poorer than those who do not. Poor women in general do not have options comparable to those of affluent women regarding either child care or medical treatment. If Lily Tighe could not cover the cost of artificial insemination, for example, she could probably not achieve her goal of motherhood even if she were physically, mentally, and emotionally fully capable of raising a child without others' assistance.

To the extent that responsibility for children is shared with others, relationships between the intended biological mother and those who might assist her are relevant to preconception counseling. In case 3, for example, the fact that Paula Seitz's partner and parents oppose her plan suggests that they are unwilling to assist her in fulfilling her goal of parenthood. Preconception counseling should explore the possible reasons for their opposition, to make sure that it is not based on faulty understanding of Paula's HIV status and its implications for her and a possible child.

If her partner remains opposed to her plan, Paula may have to choose between her relationship with her partner and her goal of parenthood. Assuming her partner is male, his opposition calls into question the means by which Paula intends to become pregnant. From an egalitarian perspective, deliberately attempting to conceive a child through this relationship without his agreeing to the plan is unjustified. While giving priority to Paula's standpoint, the physician should facilitate her consideration of the impact of her decision on others and on her relationships to them. Maximizing respect for her autonomy calls for maximizing her understanding of this impact.

The health risks of pregnancy are probably greater for Maggie McGee in case 4 than for patients in the other cases, but she apparently is so desirous of becoming a biological mother that she is willing to undertake them. Preconception counseling in this case would not only include warning about these risks but also discussion of alternative routes to motherhood: adoption and "surrogate" gestation, with or without her own ova. From an egalitarian perspective, whether Sam supports Maggie's desire is morally relevant to her decision because he may be the main caregiver for the possible offspring. As with Paula's partner, his consent is not only practically but morally necessary to achievement of her goal. Unless Maggie needs medical assistance, however, the practitioner may not legally or morally interfere with her decision. As maxim 2 reminds us, respect for the autonomy of the patient has priority over beneficence and nonmaleficence toward her.

Preimplantation genetic diagnosis

Cases

1. On referral from their doctor in Montreal, Sue and Dave Leblanc visit an infertility clinic in the United States, seeking preimplantation genetic diagnosis (PGD) of the embryos that remain from their in vitro fertilization (IVF) treatment in Canada. Their son Luke was born as a result of that treatment, but was diagnosed soon thereafter with Tay Sachs disease. Since Luke's death at age 3, the couple have wanted to have another child through transfer of the remaining embryos, but they are unwilling to attempt this if they cannot ensure that the child would not have Tay Sachs.

2. Sophie Horwitz is a 30-year-old fertile woman whose partner, Hank, had two children before they met. Recently, Sophie underwent genetic testing because of a family history of Alzheimer disease and learned that she is likely to develop the disease before she turns 40. The couple would like to have a child without Sophie's susceptibility to early Alzheimer's, but they are morally opposed to abortion as a means by which to accomplish this.[3] Their physician encourages them to undergo IVF and PGD.

3. Josephine Barat is an affluent 32-year-old woman with no particular risk factor in her pedigree. She requests preimplantation diagnosis for whatever conditions or genetic propensities are currently detectable through the procedure. Her goal is to select for transfer only those embryos that are likely to produce phenotypes that are socially advantageous. If possible, she says, she would like her potential child to be physically attractive, smart, and athletically talented.

Empirical considerations

Preimplantation genetic diagnosis takes place in vitro before early embryos or blastocysts are transferred to a woman's uterus or fallopian tube. Any condition that may be identified after implantation is potentially identifiable prior to transfer, and undesired embryos may be discarded, frozen, donated to others, or used for research. Typically, the procedure is preceded by ovulation stimulation, retrieval of ova, and in vitro fertilization. Single cells are removed from blastocysts for analyses; the remaining cells are capable of continuing development if they are transferred to a woman's body. Analysis of the second polar body of the unfertilized egg has also been attempted as a means of identifying specific conditions prior to implantation; this method avoids the question of disposal of affected embryos but has been less successful in providing definitive results.[4]

A woman who undergoes PGD incurs not only the cost of the test but also the cost and risks of the procedures required to make embryos available in vitro. The procedure is considerably less costly and invasive in case 1 than in the other cases because embryos have already been obtained. In all of the cases, however, prenatal diagnosis could yield the desired information with less cost and invasiveness than PGD. The main advantage of PGD is that it allows women to avoid the distress and invasiveness of prenatal testing and pregnancy termination, assuring them from the onset of gestation that their potential child will not be affected by the conditions identified. If the woman is fertile, successful embryo transfer, implantation, and gestation are more likely than they would be for an infertile patient, but less likely than they would be if fertilization occurred in vivo.

All three cases involve a desire on the part of potential parents to avoid having a child with certain conditions. In cases 1 and 2, the conditions for which testing is done entail physical or mental burdens for those affected; in case 3, the conditions to be avoided are not only diseases but traits of appearance, character, and aptitude that could reduce the potential child's prospects for success in life; the conditions to be promoted are not only good health but also characteristics that are "socially advantageous." Obviously, what characteristics are "socially advantageous" depends on the values a particular society imputes to specific traits.

The diseases mentioned in cases 1 and 2 have different symptoms and variable impact on those affected. Tay Sachs is an incurable autosomal recessive disorder[5] for which Ashkenazi Jews are at greater risk than the general population. Extensive carrier testing of Ashkenazi Jews has significantly reduced the number of Tay Sachs children in this group. Although non-Jewish French Canadians living near the St. Lawrence River (and in the Cajun community of Louisiana) are also at greater risk of Tay Sachs than the general population, Sue and Dave Leblanc were apparently unaware that they were carriers for the disease until Luke was born. Today, most cases of Tay Sachs occur in populations not thought to be at high risk.

At birth, children with Tay Sachs appear normal, but their development slows at about 6 months of age; thereafter, neurological deterioration sets in, and the infant regresses both mentally and physically, eventually becoming paralyzed and nonresponsive. Death usually occurs by age 5, even with optimal management of symptoms. As with other autosomal recessive disorders, if both potential parents are carriers, they carry a 1 in 4 risk in every pregnancy of having an affected child.

Although most cases of late-onset Alzheimer disease are sporadic and occur after age 65, a relatively rare form may have its onset much earlier.[6] Ordinarily, Alzheimer's cannot be definitively diagnosed until after death, but clinical symptoms provide grounds for a probable diagnosis. Laboratory tests such as lumbar puncture and electroencephalogram can support the diagnosis. Although the impairments associated with Alzheimer's escalate at a variable rate, it eventually leads to an earlier death than would otherwise occur.

PGD for specific mutations in cases 1 and 2 may be definitive, but the possibility of Alzheimer's cannot be wholly ruled out by prenatal testing or PGD. Testing for the traits that Josephine Barat (case 3) wants to maximize is at best a matter of increasing the probability of their expression in her offspring. In fact, this probability is low because most traits, such as intelligence, personality characteristics, and physical abilities, are produced not only by multiple genes but also by the interactions between genes and environment. Even if the embryos examined were cloned from adults whose phenotype was already manifest, traits such as these could not be definitively predictable because the environment of the clone would inevitably be different from that of the cloned individual.

Theoretical considerations

If abortion is considered morally wrong, different definitions of abortion are relevant to ethical assessment of how affected embryos are disposed of after preimplantation diagnosis. If abortion means termination of an embryo or fetus at any stage or site of development, destruction of affected blastocysts constitutes abortion. If abortion means termination of a previable pregnancy or gestation, which has not yet occurred when PGD is made, destruction of in vitro embryos is not abortion.

Regardless of how abortion is defined, different starting points regarding the moral status of the fetus lead to different conclusions about "disposition" of embryos after PGD.[7] If they are consistent, those who believe the embryo is a person, even at blastocyst stage, oppose its destruction even if they do not construe this as abortion. From the standpoint of those who believe that the embryo gains moral status through the course of development, destruction of in vitro embryos is obviously more acceptable than late termination during pregnancy. For those who support maximal criteria for personhood, termination at any stage is morally unproblematic unless other relevant variables are introduced.

Even the maximalists may consider PGD more justifiable for Sue Leblanc than for Josephine Barat. The variables that suggest this ordering, based on beneficence or nonmaleficence, are the risks and costs of the procedure, which are greater in case 3 than in case 1. The verity that makes PGD most problematic in case 3 is that of justice: testing and selection for traits suggests the potential for social harm or injustice through positive eugenics. The same verities make case 2 more problematic than case 1. Termination for Tay Sachs avoids symptoms that lead to death very early in life; termination for susceptibility to Alzheimer's seems to disvalue many years of life without symptoms.

From an egalitarian perspective, case 3 is most problematic because the goal of testing is promotion of desired traits rather than prevention of disease. Nonetheless, physicians have long provided treatment to patients for nonmedical reasons. As long as the health risks do not clearly outweigh the expected social benefits desired by the patient, such treatment can be justified on grounds of the risk/benefit ratio, as well as respect for the patient's autonomy. However, respect for autonomy applies to clinicians as well as patients, and no practitioner is morally bound to provide treatment that she considers opposed to the patient's medical interests. If the risk is small (as in cases of cesarean section for nonmedical reasons), the physician *may* acquiesce to the patient's wishes or recommend that her care be transferred to that of another physician. If honoring the patient's request is likely to exacerbate societal discrimination, however, the verity of justice overrides respect for the patient's autonomy.

When PGD is performed, respect for autonomy applies not only to the woman but also to the other potential parent, if there is one. However, if the autonomy interests of the partners are at odds, maxim 1 gives greater weight to her decision, as the one most affected, than to her partner's decision. Balancing obligations of beneficence toward the woman, her partner, clinicians, and the embryo or potential child, as well as respect for the autonomy of all of those affected, is obviously a complicated matter, resolvable only by applying the verity of justice to the variables of each case. When decisions are made about disposal of affected embryos, positions about the moral status of in vitro embryos are an unavoidable variable also. Discard or termination of undesired embryos is morally acceptable to those who impute no moral status to them, but not to those who believe the early embryo has full moral status.

Although the variable of cost is not mentioned in the preceding case descriptions, it is undoubtedly relevant from an egalitarian perspective. In many places, in vitro fertilization and PGD are not available as "standard of care" procedures covered by government or private insurance. If Sophie Horwitz were not affluent enough to pay for her treatment and test, she probably would be denied them for that reason alone. For Sue and Dave Leblanc, the cost of in vitro fertilization has already been covered, and they have a compelling medical rationale for PGD. However, this option would probably be unavailable to them if they could not pay for it themselves.

Another variable not mentioned is the marital status of the woman or couple. Some practitioners do not offer in vitro fertilization, a prerequisite to PGD, to single women. The denial of tests and treatment on grounds of marital status is legally as well as morally challengeable, as is also the denial of infertility treatment on grounds of sexual orientation. Practitioners may not know or even have a right to know whether a woman is married or heterosexual. In cases where these and other variables apply, benefits and risks may be equal, and autonomous preferences may be the same. Justice, as a mediating principle despite its susceptibility to different interpretations, is crucial to adjudication of competing interests.

Prenatal testing

Cases

1. Because of a strong family history of breast cancer, Clare Jones, a 33-year-old pregnant woman, underwent testing for susceptibility to breast cancer three years ago. Although the test result was positive, she has shown no signs of the disease. At 15 weeks gestation, Clare requests amniocentesis and genetic testing to determine whether her fetus is a carrier for any of the known mutations for breast cancer. If the test is positive she plans to terminate her pregnancy.

2. During her first pregnancy at age 25, Beth Brown learns through a simple screening test that she has an elevated risk of Down syndrome (trisomy 21) in her fetus. She requests prenatal testing to determine whether her fetus is affected, intending to terminate the pregnancy if the test is positive. The test and termination would both be covered by her insurance.

3. Same case as above, but Beth indicates she would not terminate the pregnancy if her fetus has Down syndrome; she simply wants to know whether the fetus is affected to help her prepare psychologically for its birth.

4. Same case as above, but chromosomal analysis reveals that the fetus has trisomy 13 rather than trisomy 21.

5. Sheila Smith is a 31-year-old whose prenatal ultrasound at 18 weeks gestation is normal except for the presence of small bilateral choroid plexus cysts in the fetus. The physician is reluctant to reveal this finding to Sheila because the cysts usually disappear during the third trimester of pregnancy; she feels that the disclosure will only create unnecessary anxiety in her patient.

Empirical considerations

The procedures currently available for testing pregnant women vary considerably with regard to the duration of gestation at which they may be safely and effectively performed, the specificity and sensitivity of test results, the invasiveness and discomfort of the procedure, and its cost and health risks to the woman and her potential newborn. Ultrasound may be performed early or late in gestation with virtually no risks; it is routinely performed at low cost in comparison with other tests. For conditions such as hypoplastic left heart syndrome and achondroplasia, ultrasound may be diagnostic. Because of its low sensitivity, however, it is often used as a screen, that is, to determine whether more definitive but invasive tests should be done or to facilitate those procedures through visualization.

Prenatal tests commonly offered to patients such as Beth Brown are chorionic villus sampling (CVS) and amniocentesis. CVS is usually performed between 9 and 13 weeks gestation, amniocentesis between 14 and 20 weeks. Both tests are usually definitive but carry a small risk of fetal loss and vaginal bleeding. CVS has been controversially associated with limb defects when the procedure is performed before 9.5 weeks.[8] Prenatal tests such as fetal biopsies and percutaneous umbilical blood sampling (PUBS) are definitive but more invasive and risky; these can only be done later in pregnancy.

The goals of prenatal testing may differ for patients and practitioners. The latter, for example, may want the information to help determine the mode of delivery or for research purposes. Beth Brown may want to learn whatever information is obtainable through the test to prepare herself psychologically and to facilitate the provision of optimal treatment of her newborn. However, most women who seek prenatal testing for Down syndrome choose to terminate their pregnancies if the test results are positive.[9]

Clinically, the usual criteria for offering prenatal testing are maternal age and family history of genetic or chromosomal disorder. In the United States, pregnant women 35 years of age or older are routinely tested. The risk of Down syndrome at this age is 1 in 385; the risk of another chromosomal anomaly is 1 in 434, making the total risk of chromosomal anomaly in the fetus 1 in 204. As maternal age advances, the risk of anomaly increases but the risks of testing usually remain the same. With early or midtrimester amniocentesis, the fetal loss rate is 1.2 and

0.5 percent, respectively; with transcervical CVS, the loss rate is 0.5 to 1 percent over the general population risk.[10] The risks of prenatal testing are probably lower in centers where the staff is highly trained and experienced with the relevant procedures.

Testing for chromosomal trisomies or single-gene disorders generally yields definitive results. In other situations, however, the test may only indicate susceptibility to a disease, and the disease may not manifest itself until adulthood. Among those who test positive for susceptibility to breast cancer such as Clare Jones, about 15 percent never become symptomatic.[11] In contrast, individuals who test positive for Huntington disease will surely become symptomatic if they live long enough.

Although conditions such as breast cancer may be preventable or curable, the majority of diseases or disabilities identifiable prenatally are not. Some are disabling, some are lethal, and some are both disabling and lethal. Down syndrome involves cognitive impairment but is not life threatening unless other anomalies exist. Medical problems such as cardiac defects and leukemia are present more often in children with Down syndrome than in other children. Depending on where the lesion occurs and when it is treated, spina bifida is physically disabling but not necessarily mentally disabling. Trisomy 13, in contrast, is not only mentally and physically disabling but usually lethal within months after birth.

Incidental findings such as those discovered by Sheila Smith's doctor are a recurrent phenomenon in medical practice, especially in the context of prenatal diagnosis. The main empirical variables associated with this issue are the physician's knowledge and experience regarding the anomaly, the patient's capacity to understand and deal with the relevant information, and the quality of the relationship between the physician and patient.

Theoretical considerations

To maximize respect for patient autonomy, terms commonly used in genetic prenatal diagnosis (e.g., "autosomal recessive" and "carrier status") often need to be explained to patients. In addition, terms such as "lethal" and "high risk" merit discussion because different meanings are attributed to them by those involved. For example, when told that the fetus has a "lethal" anomaly such as trisomy 13 or 18, some potential parents assume that the newborn with this condition will die within a matter of hours or days, no matter what is done. In contrast, clinicians familiar with these trisomies realize that affected infants may survive for several months, and some even survive past 1 year of age. Similarly, when women older than 35 are told that they are at "high risk" of having a child with Down syndrome, many are likely to view the incidence as much higher than it is. Efforts to identify and avoid misinterpretation of the language used in counseling patients about prenatal diagnosis are demanded by respect for their autonomy because people can only exercise autonomy if they adequately understand the context and implications of their decisions.

The obligation of disclosure or truth telling is ordinarily required by respect for the autonomy of the individual to whom the content to be disclosed is relevant. Her standpoint should be privileged not only because of her nondominant status but also because of the impact of the decision on her. In case 5, however, respect for the patient's autonomy may be at odds with nonmaleficence toward her. Apparently, the physician's reluctance to reveal the unexpected finding to Sheila Smith stems from this concern. If the physician has grounds to assume that Sheila herself would not desire disclosure of incidental findings, respect for her autonomy may also support nondisclosure. Generally, acknowledgment to patients of what is unknown is as basic a responsibility as disclosure of what is known because both are pertinent to the patient's decision-making. It is wrong-headed paternalism to refrain from giving bad news, or even neutral news, solely on grounds of producing anxiety in patients. Just as patients have an a priori right to access their own medical records, Sheila has an a priori right to information gathered through tests she undergoes.

Cases 1 through 4 illustrate the fact that women may seek prenatal testing regardless of their age or family history. Women who can pay for their tests out of pocket may be tested for conditions for which they have no known risks. Even for those at risk such as Beth Brown, however, merely "wanting to know" may not justify the expense and risk of the procedure, regardless of the condition to be identified. On utilitarian grounds, the rationale for termination in case 4 is more compelling than the rationale for termination in case 2 because the life prospects of a fetus with Down syndrome are considerably more positive than those of one with trisomy 13. Arguably, termination in the latter case may be regarded as fetal euthanasia, and it may be defended or opposed based on one's positions about the moral status of the fetus and about the practice of euthanasia toward severely impaired individuals.

Respect for autonomy supports women's decisions for prenatal testing and for termination or continuation of pregnancy in all of the cases described. If the fetus is imputed to have moral status, however, that verity may be subordinated to beneficence or nonmaleficence toward the fetus. Testing followed by termination seems most problematic for Clare Jones because an affected offspring could live her entire life without becoming symptomatic; moreover, if the offspring became symptomatic, her condition might be successfully treated. As with Huntington disease, termination for prenatal diagnosis of diseases that manifest themselves in adulthood ignores or negates the value of the life lived earlier. Such disvaluing is obviously at odds with an egalitarian perspective.

Testing and termination to avoid the birth of a child with an impairment such as mental retardation is ethically problematic because it suggests that life with this impairment is not worth living. If a sharp distinction is drawn between moral obligations to born individuals and obligations to those who are not born, this implication is avoidable. If fetuses are assumed to have a right to life, however, the implication is supported. In either case, social variables undoubtedly influence the decisions of women to undergo tests for fetal anomalies and terminate affected fetuses. Only when full social and economic supports are available to any woman who has a child who is impaired will women's decisions in this regard be fully autonomous. The verity of justice clearly calls for such supports.

Misattributed paternity and carrier testing

Cases

1. Marilyn and Bill Dunn, both 27 years of age, visit the obstetrician when Marilyn is 2 months pregnant. Because they tell the doctor that their son Rick had died from cystic fibrosis at 4 years of age, tissue samples are taken from both so that a prenatal diagnosis of CF can be made as accurately as possible. Results of the test indicate that Marilyn is a carrier for the most common mutation associated with CF. Bill is not a carrier for this mutation, and no other CF mutation is detectable in either partner. Marilyn has two unmarried siblings; Bill has one brother who recently married.

2. Keisha Jackson is 26 years old, 10 weeks pregnant, and recently divorced from the man through whom she became pregnant. Although her mother, brother, and nephew all have sickle cell anemia, she and her sister have no symptoms of the condition and have never been tested to determine whether they are carriers. Keisha's former husband is indifferent to whether she continues the pregnancy. She does not know his carrier status, and he is unwilling to be tested for sickle cell trait, which denotes carrier status. Keisha's physician wonders whether she should offer her patient carrier testing or prenatal testing.

Empirical considerations

If an individual or couple are at risk of an autosomal recessive disorder such as cystic fibrosis or sickle cell anemia, testing both partners for their carrier status is a means by which to avoid prenatal testing and its associated risks or to improve the definitiveness of prenatal testing if this is undertaken. The former goal is served if either partner is identified as a non-carrier; the latter goal is facilitated by identifying the mutations to be looked for in prenatal testing. Although carriers of CF and sickle cell trait have no symptoms of these diseases, identification as carriers can expose individuals to discriminatory practices and stigmatization. The history of sickle cell testing in the United States during the last century is replete with examples of such discrimination.[12]

Cystic fibrosis is the most common autosomal recessive disease affecting Caucasians throughout the world; sickle cell anemia is the most common autosomal recessive disease affecting African Americans and also has a high incidence among Hispanic Americans. The incidence of Caucasian carriers for CF is about 1 in 25; the incidence of African American carriers of sickle cell trait is about 1 in 12.[13] As with other autosomal recessive diseases, every pregnancy for carrier couples has a 1 in 4 risk that the fetus is affected, a 1 in 2 risk of being a carrier, and a 1 in 4 risk of being neither affected nor a carrier. Both diseases are currently incurable, and symptoms are variable but relievable.

The symptoms of CF include airway obstruction, chronic infections, pancreatic insufficiency, biliary tract obstructions, and, for men, congenital absence of the vas deferens. The major symptoms of sickle cell disease are recurrent pain crises and occlusion of the blood supply to various organs, making them vulnerable to permanent damage. Life span is usually foreshortened, but not as greatly as with CF. Pregnancy may exacerbate the symptoms of both diseases. Unless both partners have already been tested, they may not learn that they are carriers until they have an affected child. At that point, prenatal testing is ordinarily recommended for future pregnancies. Preimplantation diagnosis may also be recommended, but this entails greater costs as well as the rigors and risks of ovulation stimulation, IVF, and embryo transfer, while reducing the probability of establishing and maintaining gestation.

Misattributed paternity has been estimated to occur in 10 to 15 percent of the population.[14] With some conditions, genetic tests can definitively establish whether someone is genetically related to an affected offspring or fetus, but CF is not one of these conditions. Currently, prenatal tests for CF can detect over 90 percent of known mutations for the disease. Although it is possible, albeit highly improbable, that Bill contributed a nondetectable, rare mutation to Rick, there is no genetic test that could verify this. If Bill is not Rick's genetic father, the risk of CF in the fetus Marilyn is currently carrying is so slim that the risk of the intervention itself, to both Marilyn and her fetus, outweighs it. To provide accurate predictive data regarding the risk of CF in this fetus, the obstetrician faces the question of whether to disclose potentially disturbing information about undisclosed or misattributed paternity to either or both partners.

In their training, genetic counselors are encouraged to anticipate the question of what to do with information about misattributed paternity by ascertaining from clients prior to testing whether such information should be disclosed to either, both, or neither of them. While helpful, this strategy doesn't necessarily eliminate the ethical dilemma of whether or to whom unrequested information should be disclosed. The male partner is often absent from the discussion, and the impact of the information differs for each. Raising the possibility of misattributed paternity may introduce concerns that women in particular would like to avoid.

Although Bill is probably not the biological father of Rick, he is apparently the potential father of the child to whom Marilyn expects to give birth. Since Bill's carrier test is negative, prenatal diagnosis is not medically indicated because the risk of the procedure is not balanced by the potential medical benefit. Nonmedical benefits may nonetheless attach to nondisclosure of the test results or to testing that is not medically warranted. These include the avoidance of possible harm to Marilyn and her family if the information is disclosed to Bill.

Illustrating the fact that genetic knowledge of one person typically entails knowledge about the genome of another, the information about Bill is relevant to Bill's brother and his wife. While assuming that both Bill and Marilyn are CF carriers, he and his wife may seek testing to learn of their carrier status before deciding to have a child together. If Bill is not a carrier, such testing is not medically warranted.

Given Keisha's family history, she has a high probability of being a carrier for sickle cell anemia, and if she and her former husband are both carriers, the fetus Keisha is currently carrying has a 1 in 4 chance of having the disease. If she tests positive, her physician would surely like to know her former husband's carrier status because this would facilitate definitive prenatal testing or provide grounds for avoiding it. Without knowing that result, if her former husband is African American, the risk of sickle cell anemia to her fetus is 1 in 40.[15]

Theoretical considerations

The American College of Obstetricians and Gynecologists advises physicians to offer CF testing to three groups of people: (1) individuals who have a family history of the disease, (2) reproductive partners of affected individuals, and (3) couples in whom one or both partners are Caucasians and who are planning a pregnancy or seeking prenatal care. The college also recommends that screening be available to couples in other racial and ethnic groups who are at lower risk.[16] Because costs of screening or tests for those who are not at high risk are unlikely to be covered by insurance, poor or uninsured women and couples are basically precluded from these procedures. Their preclusion avoids the issues that arise from detection of misattributed paternity but prevents some women from obtaining information relevant to their decision-making. The latter result is obviously at odds with the verity of justice.

If the same criteria are applied to sickle cell carrier testing, Keisha's family history places her in the first category of those to whom genetic testing should be offered. If she and her former husband are both African American, this provides another criterion for offering testing, regardless of whether her partner is tested. On egalitarian grounds, she may be viewed as more deserving of the test than are women in their late thirties, who are routinely offered prenatal testing, because the risk of sickle cell disease in her fetus is far greater than the risk of chromosomal anomalies in their offspring. If chromosomal anomalies have more harmful impact than sickle cell anemia, access to prenatal testing is more compelling for the former than for the latter; in both cases, however, testing is supportable on grounds of respect for the patient's autonomy. If the affected fetus lacks moral status, terminations are also justified after positive diagnoses.

The Institute of Medicine report on genetic testing recommends "that information on misattributed paternity be communicated to the mother, but not be volunteered to the woman's partner."[17] Presumably, this recommendation is based on the priority of respect for the autonomy of, and the interests of, the pregnant woman as one whose standpoint should be privileged. Confidentiality toward her must be upheld because she is the person most affected by the information (maxims 1 and 2). Despite their usual depiction of "couples" and "families" as their clients, geneticists and genetic counselors tend to agree with this recommendation; they thus reject the idea that both partners have equal rights to disclosure of genetic information. Their concern, apparently, is that disclosure of such information to the male partner might precipitate family breakup or physical harm to the woman and her children. Along with their recognition that confidentiality is a necessary component of respect for autonomy, their rationale is based on beneficence and nonmaleficence.

From an egalitarian perspective, the case for or against disclosure of misattributed paternity to male partners cannot be adequately made without attention to variables that the Institute of Medicine does not address in its official position. Nor does that position shed light on the practical issue of how to respond to the direct question of a male partner about whether the test affirms his paternity. Some cases require disclosure while others do not, whether by clinicians or by the women involved. Justice requires that women who already know the information consider the impact of disclosure or nondisclosure on others besides themselves.

Prominent among reasons for disclosure is the relevance of this information to others who are genetically related to the individual who is tested. The information about Bill's carrier status is relevant not only to Bill's brother and his wife but also to Bill if he and Marilyn separate and he subsequently wants to have a child with another woman who may be a carrier. Disclosure of misattributed paternity is probably unavoidable in any honest explanation of why prenatal testing is not medically appropriate. If the explanation is not proffered, the false assumption that Bill is Rick's father could be preserved by testing the fetus anyway, and then giving the couple the "good news" that it is not affected. On egalitarian grounds, this strategy is wrong not only because it introduces unnecessary costs and duplicity but also because it introduces a risk of fetal loss in a (presumably) wanted pregnancy. Moreover, the information will continue to be relevant to future pregnancies in which Bill is Marilyn's partner.

Disclosure is also supportable on grounds that both partners have a right to information obtained by testing them as individuals. The argument here is stronger than when prenatal tests are done without prior testing of the male partner. In practice, disclosure to both partners of prenatal test results is often impossible because women seek and obtain these tests in the absence of their partners. Another reason for disclosure of prenatal findings to male partners stems from the lack of evidence that it leads to family breakup or domestic violence. It may also be argued that if couples split after misattributed paternity is disclosed, they may be better off than they would be if they stayed together solely because the male partner thought (erroneously) that he was genetically related to his child or children. In the case of Bill and Marilyn, we simply have too little information by which to judge whether disclosure would have harmful results to them as individuals, as a couple, or as a family.

Although women and men may be counseled together, it simply isn't true that they are equally patients in the context of prenatal testing of the fetus. Women undergo the testing through their own bodies, while men do not. Moreover, women usually bear the main burden of childcare. These factors support the priority of the women's interests and standpoint if there is conflict between them and their partners (maxim 4). That said, it is also possible that Bill was the main caregiver of Rick before his death and would be the main caregiver of a future child born to Marilyn, regardless of his genetic tie or lack thereof. Unless we subscribe to a merely genetic definition of parenthood, it seems wrong not to recognize Bill as Rick's father if he fulfilled this role.

Sex selection

Cases

1. Ann and Robert Jones have three sons and very much want to have a daughter. Before attempting another pregnancy, they visit Ann's obstetrician to ask for advice on whether and how to ensure that a fourth child is female.

2. Andy White, 41, and Roberta Black, 35, already have a daughter and very much want to have a son. On grounds of maternal age, Roberta's obstetrician recommends prenatal testing, indicating that the test is covered by her insurance. When she is informed of the risk of chromosomal anomaly (1 in 204) and the risk of miscarriage (0.5%), Roberta declines to have the test. However, at 14 weeks gestation, after learning that the test would also reveal the sex of the fetus, she changes her mind and asks to be tested.

3. Mary Murphy, a 27-year old lawyer, is 10 weeks pregnant when she asks for prenatal diagnosis for sex selection. She says she cannot be an adequate (single) parent to a male child. If the fetus is male, therefore, she intends to terminate the pregnancy.

4. In the course of infertility treatment, Hilda Fine and Ray Ramirez are told that nine of their embryos have been successfully fertilized in vitro. To reduce the risk of multiple gestation, the reproductive endocrinologist plans to return only three of the embryos to Hilda's uterus. The couple asks him to ensure that only male embryos are selected for transfer. "As long as we can choose," they say, "we would like our first child to be a boy."

Empirical considerations

Until recently, methods available for sex selection prior to gestation (e.g., timing of intercourse, ovulation induction medication, artificial insemination) were generally unreliable. A better success rate has been reported from in vitro separation of X-bearing sperm and Y-bearing sperm by gradient techniques, but this method has not yet been validated by molecular techniques or controlled clinical trials. A newer method, sperm separation by flow cytometry, is more reliable. Because it is less expensive and less invasive than other methods, some authors believe that flow cytometry for sex selection will be sought, offered, and used more widely in the future.[18]

Sex selection of embryos is possible after in vitro fertilization; this method is expensive as well as invasive unless the embryos are already available in vitro, as in case 4. After implantation, the sex of the embryo is determinable through chorionic villus sampling, amniocentesis, or ultrasound. In some developing countries, prenatal sex selection, while illegal, is increasingly undertaken through ultrasound.[19] In the developed world, clients sometimes pursue sex selection under the guise of a medically accepted reason for prenatal testing, such as maternal age, through which they may learn not only the chromosomal status of the fetus but also its sex. If the fetus is not of the desired sex, they may then ask for termination of the pregnancy, to which they have legal access even when the fetus is free of a detected anomaly. Because most genetic counselors oppose prenatal testing for sex selection, they tend to feel manipulated by this modus operandi. In recent years, however, the number of counselors who support the client's right to sex selection has been increasing.[20]

Sex selection for medical reasons may be undertaken in cases where sex is a marker for an anomaly such as Duchennes muscular dystrophy or hemophilia.

Nonmedical reasons offered by geneticists around the world in support of prenatal sex selection of offspring include respect for the autonomy of the potential parent (in the United States), avoidance of harm to female offspring and their mothers (India), and the potential reduction in the number of abortions that might occur if sex selection were not available (Hungary).[21] In some countries, the practice of sex selection has led to a disproportionate number of males in the population. In China, for example, 118.5 boys are born for every 100 girls, and in Korea nearly 116 boys are born for every 100 girls.[22] Sex selection may be undertaken after birth as well as before conception or during gestation, the latter through neglect or undertreatment of female infants.[23]

Theoretical considerations

Sex selection for nonmedical reasons is often construed as sexist, which puts it at odds with the verity of justice. According to the *American Heritage Dictionary*, sexism involves (1) "discrimination based on gender, especially discrimination against women" and (2) "attitudes, conditions, or behaviors that promote stereotyping of social roles based on gender."[24] Because it assumes that one sex is superior to the other, such discrimination denies the essential equality between men and women. Like racism and classism and other manifestly unjust "isms," sexism thus asserts a dominance that, on grounds of standpoint theory, calls for privileging the standpoint of those over whom the dominance is asserted. Absent any impact on sex inequality, however, sex selection is not necessarily sexist and may be morally neutral; if it reduces inequality, it may even be morally commendable.

According to the Ethics Committee of the American Society for Reproductive Medicine, sex selection for "family balancing" (having children of both sexes) is permissible as long as the individuals who request it know the risks, affirm that they will accept a child of the opposite sex, and are counseled about unrealistic expectations.[25] Some authors refer to this rationale as "sex complementarity."[26] Sex selection in cases 1 and 2 is supportable on this basis more compellingly for Ann and Robert, who already have three sons, than for Andy and Roberta, who have only one daughter. Although selection of females, as in case 3, is sexist if it is based on the assumption that males are inferior to females, it is less problematic than selection of males, as in case 4, because the latter practice is more likely to reaffirm or reinforce the male dominance that already prevails.

Although the intentions of individuals who seek sex selection may not be sexist, it may be impossible to determine whether this is so. Even if the intention is not sexist, the consequences of sex selection may be sexist. In countries where the practice has led to a predominance of males, subjugation of women has not declined; nor is there any evidence that sexism has been reduced in countries where females outnumber males. The verity of justice requires scrutiny with regard to both intention and consequences. In an egalitarian ethic, if the consequences are likely to be sexist, respect for the autonomy of potential parents to choose the sex of their offspring should be subordinated to gender justice.

Sex consistency has also been proposed as a valid basis for sex selection. Presumably, this is why Mary wants sex selection in case 3. Her expectation that she could not be an adequate parent to a male child may be challenged in its own right, but not necessarily on sexist grounds. From an egalitarian perspective, this rationale is less problematic than the rationale of those who legally terminate pregnancies for reasons unrelated to the welfare of the potential child or to the health or welfare of others.

Sex selection prior to conception, as desired in cases 1 and 4, is less problematic than sex selection during gestation or after birth, but it may still be sexist and therefore morally objectionable. The added onus of sex selection during gestation, as in case 3, is that abortion is the means through which having a child of the undesired sex is avoided. Yet more problematic legally as well as morally is sex selection practiced after birth through neglect of the undesired offspring. Regardless of whether sex selection is practiced before conception, during gestation, or after birth, it is morally wrong if it is sexist.

As mentioned above, respect for autonomy is paramount for those who defend the right to sex selection in the United States. For those who defend it in other countries, the paramount verity may be nonmaleficence—that is, the avoidance of harm to potential daughters and their mothers, or reduction in the number of abortions performed. The latter rationale is less compelling than the former if abortion is morally acceptable. The priority of respect for the autonomy of potential parents is also supportable if abortion, whether of male or female fetuses, is morally acceptable. For those to whom the moral status of the fetus increases over the course of development, sex selection is increasingly problematic as gestation proceeds.

An egalitarian approach to all of the issues in this chapter gives priority to the interests of those most affected. Whether fetuses or embryos are to be counted among those whose interests are at stake depends on one's position about the moral status of fetuses or embryos, whether in vivo or in vitro. With complex issues such as sex selection and misattributed paternity, just solutions require careful attention to additional variables. In general, an egalitarian perspective eschews discriminatory practices and attitudes such as sexism, racism, classism, and ableism. Prenatal or preimplantation testing to avoid having a child with certain attributes may be discriminatory but need not be. Whether it is unjust depends on the intention and on the consequences of such testing.

5

Medically Assisted Reproduction

Pregnancy and childbirth are normal and desired experiences for many women in their reproductive years. However, for a substantial number (about 15%),[1] the usual route to pregnancy through sexual intercourse with a married, loved partner is blocked through infertility. For those who are fertile, the usual route may be impeded by social factors or by elevated risks to their health through pregnancy or childbirth. For others, although the usual route is available, options provided only through medical technologies are preferred for nonmedical reasons or to avoid health risks or disabilities in a potential child.

Most infertility patients and their practitioners consider infertility a disease or disability, which, as such, deserves treatment. This view is best supported in circumstances in which fertility is the norm—that is, during the usual reproductive life span of women. For women for whom menopause is a normal, healthy condition, and for a minority of younger women who prefer not to have biologically related children, infertility is neither a disease nor a disability; some may even view it as desirable. When treatment is sought for reasons unrelated to the woman's health, practitioners sometimes attempt to bypass ethical quandaries through the informative model of the physician-patient relationship: by merely informing patients of the risks and potential benefits of treatment and proceeding according to their wishes. As discussed in chapter 2, however, this model is ethically inadequate because both practitioners and patients are responsible for what they do or don't do.

After the birth of Louise Brown, the first child conceived through in vitro fertilization (IVF), methods by which to treat infertility expanded and became increasingly complex. Although men are no less likely than women to be the infertile partner, intracytoplasmic sperm injection (ICSI) has led to greater success in treatment of male infertility. Regardless of whether the man, woman, or couple together are the cause of infertility, however, treatment mainly occurs through women's bodies. In addition to the risks and pain of pregnancy and childbirth, women undergo numerous, invasive procedures that enable them and their partners to have biologically related offspring. Moreover, unlike men, whose contribution to infertility treatment is usually pleasurable, women experience these burdens even when they do not intend to raise the child to whom they are related through gestation or genetics. In light of this discrepant impact, women deserve privileged status in decisions regarding medically assisted reproduction.

In this chapter I identify four "pockets of issues" involving medically assisted reproduction: reasons for seeking or denying infertility treatment, gamete "donation" or "surrogacy," disposition of in vitro embryos, and the increased risk of multiple gestation through infertility treatment. From an egalitarian perspective, variables and standpoints other than, or in addition to, those illustrated by the cases could lead to different ethical decisions.

Criteria for patient selection

Cases

1. Gina Shore, a 35-year-old nurse who has never been pregnant consults her gynecologist about reversal of her sterilization. Eight years earlier she had been diagnosed with HIV infection after a needle stick injury. Due to her apparently limited life expectancy and the risk of transmission to a fetus, tubal sterilization was recommended and performed. Since then Gina has been in good health with no AIDS-defining illnesses; her blood counts have been stable and in normal range. Now married, she and her husband, who is HIV negative, would like to have children. They have considered adoption but feel strongly about having a genetically related child. As long as a couple or woman can pay for their services, the hospital permits physicians such as Gina's gynecologist to determine for themselves whom they shall treat.

2. Kris Gil is a 34-year-old receptionist who visits the infertility clinic because she has not conceived despite three years of unprotected intercourse with her partner. She was diagnosed with lupus at age 11 and has been taking immunosuppressive drugs since she underwent cadaveric kidney transplantation at age 20. Five years ago Kris terminated an unplanned pregnancy because of her health risks at the time. Currently in remission, her remaining health risks include hypertension, mild renal insufficiency, upper respiratory infections, and kidney infections. A maternal-fetal medicine specialist recommended against conception because pregnancy presents significant risks of loss of function in the transplanted kidney, lupus flares, preeclampsia, and other complications. Risks to the fetus include exposure to teratogenic drugs and prematurity. Kris and her partner indicate that they understand these risks and wish to proceed with infertility treatment.

3. Amy Asche is a 30-year-old woman who lost both of her legs through a freak accident at age 5. After graduating from college, Amy was employed by a privately funded organization that advocates for people with disabilities. Two years ago, she married John, a paraplegic war veteran who works for the same organization. John is infertile due to congenital bilateral absence of the vas deferens. They visit the infertility center to ask for assistance in having a child.

4. Same case as above, but Amy is mildly cognitively impaired rather than physically impaired, unmarried but in a loving relationship with John, who is also cognitively impaired. They live in a state-funded assisted-living facility and work on an assembly line in a nearby factory. Amy and John intend to marry and would like to have a child together, but they require medical assistance because of John's infertility.

Empirical considerations

While cases of autoimmune deficiency syndrome (AIDS) and human immunodeficiency virus (HIV) infection have increased across the globe, the increase has disproportionately affected women and minorities. Between 1999 and 2003, the estimated cases of AIDS diagnoses in women increased by fifteen percent and in men by one percent.[2] Many more women are HIV positive, and of these, about 80 percent are of childbearing age, and 80 percent are Hispanic or African American.[3] Over time, the proportion of HIV-positive and AIDS cases attributable to injection-drug use has declined, whereas the proportion of cases from heterosexual contact has increased. Health practitioners face an additional risk (~0.3%) of HIV infection due to needle-stick injury.[4]

Preventive efforts have decreased the overall rate of HIV infection, and new drug combination treatments have improved the rate of survival after onset of AIDS, not only for those affected but also for their offspring. Given these advances, the same physician who recommended tubal ligation for HIV-positive women a decade ago would probably not offer that advice today. If Gina's sterilization is reversed and she becomes pregnant, she has a good chance of maintaining her own health and of having a healthy child. By taking antiretroviral drugs during pregnancy and avoiding breastfeeding after she gives birth, she can cut the risk of HIV transmission to her infant to about 2 percent.[5] Although her own risk of AIDS remains, improvements in drug regimens may prolong her life span if and when she becomes symptomatic.

Kris Gil faces greater health risks through pregnancy, regardless of whether she obtains medical assistance to become pregnant. Because neither lupus nor renal transplantation precludes her ability to conceive, her infertility is probably due to other causes, including, possibly, her partner's infertility. Pregnancy is usually well tolerated in women with good pre-pregnancy graft function, and no specific pattern of malformation has been identified in babies born to women who continue to take immunosuppressive drugs during gestation.[6] Moreover, kidney transplantation can restore ovulatory menstrual cycles and fertility, which is often impaired while on dialysis.[7] Pregnant women with lupus and kidney transplantation must nonetheless be closely monitored because of their increased risks. About 50 percent of lupus pregnancies are completely normal, but 25 percent lead to premature delivery and the remaining cases involve spontaneous or newborn loss.[8]

Congenital bilateral absence of the vas deferens (CBAVD), a major cause of male infertility, is an atypical form of cystic fibrosis. As cases 3 and 4 illustrate, the condition sometimes exists in the absence of other symptoms of CF. Through the availability of ICSI, some men with CBAVD can have genetically related children, despite their extremely low semen count. If Amy is not a carrier for CF, she and John are not at risk of having a child with CF; if she is a carrier, prenatal testing can determine whether the fetus is affected with CF.[9] Because neither Amy's nor John's disability is due to inherited anomalies, their potential offspring have no special risk of these impairments. Unless other factors are present, the only risks that may be of concern to practitioners who offer them infertility treatment are those associated with the physical disabilities of the potential parents.

Case 4 differs from case 3 because the potentially relevant impairments are cognitive rather than physical. If the impairment of either Amy or John has a genetic origin, this would place their potential offspring at risk of similar impairment. Regardless of heritability, however, cognitive impairments cover a broad range of possibilities with regard to the ability of people to care for themselves or others. According to the American Association of Mental Deficiency, mental retardation may be mild, moderate, severe, or profound. Those who are mildly impaired are educable to at least the level of a mentally normal 10- or 11-year-old.[10] With training and supervision, adults with mild cognitive impairment are generally able to lead productive and satisfying lives. Depending on the complexity of the issue addressed, they are also able to make at least some informed and autonomous decisions about matters that affect them.

Theoretical considerations

From the clinician's standpoint, all of these cases are probably more complicated than they would be if the woman were already pregnant or did not require medical assistance to become pregnant. If medical assistance were not required to achieve fertility, the clinician would not share responsibility for the risks that pregnancy involves for the woman or her potential child. From the standpoint of women, however, many ethical decisions must be made prior to pregnancy. If a woman decides to obtain medical assistance to become pregnant, she needs to choose among methods of treatment, how long and at what expense to pursue them, whether to involve third parties, and how to dispose of embryos that may remain after treatment. Potential parents have different standpoints as well as different risks than their practitioners.

Except for John's infertility, Amy could probably become pregnant regardless of physical or cognitive impairment. Except for Gina's sterilization, she could have become pregnant despite her HIV-positive status. And Kris could probably become pregnant without medical assistance with a different partner, as she did in the past. Her lupus and kidney transplant do not account for her failure to conceive after three years of unprotected sex with her current partner. Regardless of which partner is infertile, however, an egalitarian approach to treatment starts with recognition that "couples" are not a single person but two different moral agents whose disparate burdens and potentially different preferences need to be weighed as such.

No clinician is morally obliged to provide treatment for nonmedical reasons, but infertility is sometimes construed as a medically abnormal condition calling for treatment. Even so, on professional as well as moral grounds, clinicians are obliged *not* to provide treatment, even if requested, if its risks clearly overwhelm its expected benefits to the individual. Whether this description fits the situation may be a judgment call, depending largely on how desirable it is to potential patients to have a biologically related child. The risks of pregnancy for Gina and Kris are clearly higher than they would be for healthy women, and especially high for Kris. From both women's standpoints, the benefit of having a biologically related child is apparently worth the risk, and their doctors may concur in that opinion.

The standpoint of clinicians who provide infertility treatment is different from that of those who treat patients who request treatment that is unrelated to a possible pregnancy. This difference arises from the fact that infertility practitioners have some responsibility for potential children who could not otherwise be conceived, gestated, or born without their assistance. In the cases cited, the potential parents of the potential children may be unable to care for them adequately because of their own ill health, limited life span, or disabilities. The question of whether infertility treatment may or should be withheld on grounds of beneficence or nonmaleficence toward the potential child arises even for clinicians who impute no moral status to embryos or fetuses.

Infertility specialists as such have no special expertise for assessing whether a potential mother or couple would make adequate parents, but they play a crucial role in bringing some children into the world. Because infertility treatment is elective, they may legally refuse to provide it even if the potential child would probably be well-parented. Once a care relationship has been established, however, no physician may refuse to continue serving in that capacity unless continuity of care is provided through another practitioner.

Inability to pay for infertility services is one of most common reasons for refusals to provide treatment. In the cases cited, physicians' refusal to provide infertility treatment may be defended on moral as well as legal grounds relevant to the potential child. Whether the defense is adequate depends on the availability of resources that may enable physically or mentally impaired parents to care for their child. In case 3, for example, Amy and John are apparently able to function independently and could probably care adequately for a child despite their physical disabilities. In case 4, John and Amy may lack the ability to adequately parent a child by themselves. But if others, such as their parents, are willing and able to assist them in caring for potential offspring, concerns about the welfare of the potential child would be alleviated. In cases 1 and 2, the main concerns regarding obligations to the potential child are based on the possibly limited life span or health problems of the potential mother. In both cases, the potential success of ongoing treatment, as well as the involvement of a healthy partner, reduces those concerns considerably.

Gamete "donation" and "surrogacy"

Cases

1. Flora Farmer is a college freshman who works part time to cover expenses beyond those that her student loan can afford. Her poor grades are due, she thinks, to the limited time she has to study. Responding to an ad in the college newspaper for egg donors, she comes to the infertility clinic and indicates that she would like to be a donor. Her hope is that the "compensation" obtained from participation in the program will allow her to quit her job and have more time to study. Helping an infertile couple to have a child "of their own" is an added motivation.

2. Elaine Flynn is a 26-year-old single woman who dropped out of high school when she was pregnant with her first child. Two years later she had twins. Having no child support from the father of her children, she supports them by cleaning offices in the evenings and on weekends. Her mother looks after the children when she is working. After hearing about several controversial but well-publicized cases of "surrogate motherhood," Elaine decides that pregnancy for another woman is a means by which she could obtain enough money to quit her job and return to school. Besides leading eventually to more gainful employment, she believes this would allow her to spend more time with her children and set an example for them in their own school work

3. Aida Gambell is a healthy, postmenopausal, 53-year-old who recently married a 48-year-old business associate. Although Aida has a 23-year-old daughter from a previous relationship, her husband has never had a child, and the couple "would like to have a child together." She visits her gynecologist and asks for treatment that would allow her to gestate an embryo formed from a donated egg and her husband's sperm.

4. Elinor Eames is a 30-year-old who was recently diagnosed with premature ovarian failure. Her husband is indifferent to whether the couple has children, but she has long wanted to be a mother. Although Elinor is unable to have a child with her own ova, she would like to experience pregnancy and give birth. Her sister, she says, is willing to donate her eggs to be fertilized in vitro with sperm from Elinor's husband.

5. Ferosha Patel, a 35-year-old neonatologist at a leading university hospital, was unmarried and had not dated for several years. Attempts to adopt a child had been unsuccessful. While aware that health problems of her own would be exacerbated by pregnancy, she asks her gynecologist, a colleague at her medical center, for artificial insemination from an anonymous donor. "More than anything else, I want to be a mother," she says, "and time is running out on my biological clock."

Empirical considerations

For over 100 years, artificial insemination (AI) has made it possible to produce children without going through the usual route of sexual intercourse.[11] AI has also made it possible for a couple to have a child whose biological father is unknown to her or to either of her legal parents. However, not only sperm "donation" but all of the currently available methods for treatment of infertility involve at least two biological parents as progenitors. A third biological parent is possible if the woman who gestates is different from the one who provides the ova, and a fourth is possible in rare cases, such as if one woman provides the nuclear DNA and another provides the mitochondrial DNA. (This technique has been pursued as a means of avoiding mitochondrial disorders.) Social or rearing parents need not be biologically related to the child they raise; neither do they have to be married or of the same sex. In many cases, children have only one social parent, usually the mother, who may or may not be biologically related to them.

In general, medically assisted reproduction carries more health risks than unassisted reproduction. The risks mainly apply to the women who are directly involved through gestation, ova provision, or both, regardless of whether they themselves are infertile and regardless of whether they intend to be social mothers of the offspring produced through their participation. The health risks to women who undergo ova stimulation and retrieval to provide gametes for another are the same as those experienced by women who undergo these procedures to have children they intend to raise. To assist other women to become mothers, they subject themselves to hormone injections, ovarian enlargement, and curtailment of ordinary activities for several weeks following the injections, as well as increased risks of severe ovarian stimulation syndrome, which sometimes requires hospitalization.[12] The health risks to women who gestate for other women are not only those experienced routinely in any pregnancy but also the risks and rigors of hormonal treatment and embryo transfer. The latter procedures usually involve cramping and increased risks of tubal pregnancy, bleeding, infection, multiple gestation, hypertension, and diabetes.[13] Depending on whether women who provide eggs or gestation for another are "compensated" for their bodily assistance, they may derive emotional or moral satisfaction from this exercise of their reproductive capacity. However, ovarian stimulation limits the availability of ova for future pregnancies, whereas the availability of sperm is virtually unlimited.

Some countries, such as Israel, cover the costs of medically assisted reproduction for its citizens. In the United States, the costs of technically sophisticated methods of assisted reproduction are not covered, or only partially covered, by insurance and are generally too high (e.g., averaging $12,400 per IVF cycle in 2006)[14] for many infertile couples to afford. AI and ovulation stimulation without IVF are the least expensive and most widely available forms of treatment. Compensation for women who gestate for others (averaging $20,000 in 2006) does not include additional expenses paid by the "commissioning couple" for each IVF or insemination attempt, prenatal and maternity care, legal fees, and so on.[15] The success rate of IVF, as measured by the probability of giving birth after one egg retrieval, is about 30 percent[16] if ICSI is included in the calculation. Because ovulation diminishes as women approach menopause, the probability of pregnancy is considerably reduced as they get older—unless the ova are obtained from younger women.

"Compensation" to women who gestate or provide ova for another varies considerably.[17] Those with traits specifically desired by affluent potential parents have been paid $50,000 to undergo ova stimulation and retrieval of their gametes for potential parents. A more typical "compensation" is about $3,000, and some women are uncompensated beyond coverage of the expense of treatment or lost income. Like sperm "donation," egg "donation" is legal in most countries, and in some it is encouraged because fertility is a national or cultural priority.

The legality of "surrogacy," whether gestational only or genetic as well, also varies. In the United States, some states outlaw so-called commercial surrogacy—contracts in which the "commissioning couple" or potential parents agree to pay the "surrogate" a specific fee for her "services." Most states have no laws prohibiting either remunerated or unremunerated surrogacy arrangements. Physicians are thus legally free, in most cases, to decide for themselves whether they wish to assist individuals or couples to have biologically related children.

Several studies indicate that many women attach greater importance to the gestational tie to children than to the genetic tie.[18] Most men, in contrast, attach greater importance to the genetic tie to children, not only for themselves but also for their partners. The separability between genetic and gestational ties through ova retrieval and IVF makes it possible for couples who are both carriers for autosomal recessive diseases to be biological parents without the 1 in 4 risk that any of their potential children will be affected by the disease. Fertilizing a non-carrier donor egg with the potential father's sperm and transferring the resultant embryo to the potential mother allows her to be biologically related through gestation while her partner is related to their offspring through genetics.

Premature ovarian failure (POF), which affects 1 to 3 percent of the reproductive population, involves the onset of menopausal symptoms in women younger than 40 years of age.[19] Although genetic and infectious causes of the condition are probable, its exact etiology is not yet clear. Affected individuals occasionally resume normal or irregular ovulation, which may lead to pregnancy. However, along with other symptoms and risks associated with menopause, the major harm for the relatively young women who suffer from POF is that they no longer produce ova and are therefore infertile. If they wish to have biologically related offspring, this makes them prime candidates for ova donation.

Theoretical considerations

Terminology commonly employed in discussions of assisted reproduction is sometimes misleading or inaccurate. The term "surrogate," for example, literally refers to someone who stands in the place of another, suggesting that a "surrogate mother" is not a real mother. Yet throughout history, a woman who gestates and gives birth has been regarded as the "real" mother of her offspring. While it is generally assumed that she is also genetically related to her child, this is no longer necessarily true because of the separability of genetic and gestational ties through ova retrieval, IVF, and embryo transfer. Just as men who "donate" sperm to infertile couples become biological fathers to children they never know, women may be biological mothers, through gestation *or* genetics, to children they do not raise. Unlike the gamete provider, however, the gestator always knows that she is the biological parent of the child to whom she gives birth. An irony here is that postmenopausal women, who are unable to have genetically related children, may nonetheless become pregnant and give birth after egg donation and are generally referred to as "mothers," not "surrogate mothers." In contrast, women who agree to give their offspring to others to raise, but are themselves both gestational and genetic mothers, are typically referred to as "surrogates." The end points or goals of these different participants in the reproductive process obviously affect the standpoints from which they make ethical decisions about the process.

The term "donation" is also used misleadingly in cases of gamete or embryo provision to others. Embryos no longer desired by their progenitors, for example, may be "donated" to defray costs of the "donor's" infertility treatment. With regard to egg "donation," remuneration may be a compelling motivator for women who agree to undergo its rigors and risks, as in case 1.[20] Similarly, the "compensation" attached to "surrogate" arrangements is seen by some women as a means by which to obtain needed income, as in case 2. The class difference between those who do the work of gestation or egg provision and those who "buy" their labor, inconvenience, risk, and pain is evident in the contrast between these cases and case 3.

"Preembryo" is another problematic term. If it is understood as a shortened form of "preimplantation embryo," the interpretation is accurate. If instead "preembryo" is understood to mean that the organism is not yet an embryo, it is misleading because, in fact, the preimplantation embryo or blastocyst contains the entirety of the embryo—that is, all of the genetic material necessary for development into a mature organism, along with the extraembryonic material which becomes placenta after transfer to a woman's uterus.

In addition to economic differences between "donors" and recipients of reproductive assistance, the cases described in this section also illustrate the variables of age and health status of potential recipients. Because reduced ovarian function is naturally associated with aging, egg "donation" from younger women is sometimes recommended for treatment of older women. In case 3, the patient herself requests it as the only means through which she and her husband can "have a child together." At 53 years of age, Aida Gambell is apparently healthy but incapable of having a child conceived with her own ova; she is nonetheless capable of gestating and giving birth because she still has a uterus. Aida is not only age-appropriately postmenopausal but has already had a child, presumably through the usual means. She has a different standpoint than Elinor Eames, who has not had a child and whose infertility at age 30 stems from a disease rather than a normal healthy condition. From an egalitarian perspective, Elinor is more deserving of infertility treatment than Aida, even if Aida is able to cover the costs of treatment and Elinor is not. Other variables may shift the moral calculus—for example, if additional health problems augment the medical risks for Elinor; in general, however, the health risks of induced pregnancy are considerably greater for a woman who is 53 years old than for one who is 30.

The health risks of induced pregnancy even by the relatively unsophisticated method of AI are also a significant variable in case 5. Despite the usual priority of respect for the patient's autonomy, it may be morally wrong for the physician to provide treatment that could exacerbate health problems already faced by this patient. Some risks are small enough to permit invasive, harmful interventions solely on grounds of well-informed and fully autonomous consent because they offer nonmedical benefits to the patient. Other risks are simply not small enough to warrant such risks even if those conditions are met. In the case described, there is insufficient information to assess whether the threshold of safety is met. Even if it is met, the standpoint of the practitioner is also relevant, and she is not morally obliged to provide treatment that opposes her moral convictions or poses unnecessary medical risks to the patient. In such circumstances, respect for the clinician's autonomy should prevail.

Case 5 also illustrates the fact that fertile individuals at times seek infertility treatment. Some fertile patients are single or lesbian, and some are married fertile couples who want treatment by which they can reduce genetic risks or choose specific characteristics for their potential child. Justice is again the verity that ought to govern ethical responses to these situations, and justice demands consideration of the interests of the potential child as well as the potential parents. Ethically, the right to have a biologically related child, which is supportable by respect for the autonomy of the potential parents, is less compelling than obligations incurred on grounds of justice toward children already born, regardless of whether they have biologically related parents. It follows that the adoption option should at least be presented to infertile individuals or couples as an ethically desirable route to parenthood. Ferosha Patel, the neonatologist in case 5, apparently considered adoption a preferable route, albeit a route that was not successful for her.

Finally, justice demands examination of the different goals of women who gestate or provide ova for others. To look only at "compensation" aspects is to miss the ethically significant variable of intentionality. Cases 1 and 2, for example, depict individuals whose goals or end points are consistent with those that women in their age groups are expected to pursue and may even be obliged to pursue. Neither woman is seeking enrichment for herself beyond a level that should be available to everyone in a just society. Elaine Flynn, moreover, is apparently choosing "surrogacy" as a means by which she can provide better parenting for her children. Lest it be thought that a desire for economic remuneration renders ova "donation" or "surrogacy" morally suspect, the potential link between these activities and morally praiseworthy intentions needs to be acknowledged.

Disposition of in vitro embryos

Cases

1. Jackie and Mark Sylvester, 35 and 37 years old, respectively, are the biological parents of 5-year-old twins, conceived through IVF. Ovulation stimulation and IVF had produced eleven embryos; three of these were transferred in their first (unsuccessful) pregnancy attempt, and four were transferred in their second (successful) attempt. The remaining four embryos were frozen for possible future use. Having decided not to have more children, the couple are considering their options regarding disposal of the remaining embryos.

2. Same case as above, but Jackie and Mark divorced two years after the birth of their twins. Mark is now remarried and his wife is pregnant. Jackie and Mark disagree about disposition of the embryos: Mark would like them destroyed; Jackie wants them to remain frozen.

3. Over the past decade, an infertility center has acquired about 100 frozen embryos for which it has no instructions from the gamete providers regarding disposal if the center loses contact with them. Renewed efforts by phone and mail to contact the gamete providers to ascertain their wishes have been unsuccessful. Most of the gamete providers had initially agreed to pay for cryopreservation, but when contact with them was lost, the cost of maintaining the remaining embryos was covered by the center. The freezing facility must now be dismantled to prepare for a move to a new building. To facilitate the move, the director of the center would like to destroy the "abandoned" embryos.

Empirical considerations

Ovarian stimulation through administration of hormones is routinely performed in conjunction with infertility treatment, regardless of whether the woman herself is fertile. The goal of the procedure is to produce multiple ova to be fertilized in vitro so that several embryos can be transferred and future transfers may be performed without resorting to further stimulation and retrieval procedures. Typically, a superfluity of embryos is produced—that is, more than the infertile woman or couple wish to use for their own treatment. The options for "disposition" or "disposal" of the surplus embryos include freezing, donation to another woman or couple, donation for use in research, and "destruction" of the embryos. Women whose religious or ethical convictions are opposed to any of these options have asked to have their unused embryos returned to their bodies through the vagina, to be reabsorbed in a manner that precludes the possibility of pregnancy.

In 2003, a study by the Society for Assisted Reproductive Technology reported that nearly 400,000 embryos are stored in cryopreservation facilities across the United States. The great majority of these are maintained to help those who provided the gametes to have children at a later date. Only 4 percent are available for research or donated for use by other infertility patients, and about 2 percent may be thawed without transfer.[21] The study does not indicate how the thawed embryos are disposed of if they are not transferred.

Couples who provide gametes for treatment of infertility are usually asked to indicate their wishes regarding the number of embryos to be transferred after fertilization and the disposition of embryos that may remain after treatment. Most programs require couples who choose embryo storage to give written instructions regarding disposition of the embryos in case of the death of either partner, divorce, separation, failure to pay storage charges, inability to agree on disposition in the future, or lack of contact with the program. If no contact with the program has occurred for a specified period and the couple has not kept the program informed of how to reach them, the embryos are regarded as "abandoned" and the program is permitted to thaw and "dispose" of the embryos. Without consent of the gamete providers, use of the embryos for research or transfer to another woman is not permitted.[22]

Although for the woman undergoing treatment use of frozen embryos is less expensive and less invasive than use of fresh embryos, freezing reduces the success rate of the embryo transfer from about 30 to 20 percent.[23] When ovulation stimulation and IVF produce surplus embryos, however, freezing them is a means by which to reduce the risk of multiple gestations without destroying them. As discussed in the next section, high-order multiple gestations entail grave risks not only for women but also for their potential children.

Theoretical considerations

The terms "disposal" and "disposition" are both rooted in the verb "displace," which means "to put in place."[24] "Disposal" often has a negative connotation, suggesting a means by which material is thrown away or discarded because it is no longer useful to, or desired by, someone. If the material is useful to or desired by others, "disposal" may also have a positive connotation. For example, embryos that are no longer useful to or desired by their progenitors may be disposed of through donation to recipients who do desire them or find them useful. In neither case does "disposal" imply that the potential for development of the embryo is terminated. A term that would imply this is "destruction."[25] To destroy an embryo is to cause it to die: to end its life or its potential for further development.

Given these alternative meanings, the morally available options for disposal of embryos created in vitro are very different from the standpoint of those who impute moral status to the embryo than for those who do not. If the embryo has no moral status, the means of disposal is morally neutral or amoral; if it has full moral status, it may not be directly killed or destroyed. If the embryo has intermediate moral status, it may be permissible to terminate its existence in some circumstances but not others, and whatever means is used should be accompanied by some degree of respect. In other words, for those who impute any or full moral status to the embryo, it should not simply be discarded as trash or as diseased or cancerous tissue. Even if a woman or couple indicated a desire that their in vitro embryos be directly killed or treated in the same way as malignant tissue, a practitioner who views the embryo as having moral status would violate his own moral integrity by responding affirmatively to their request. He would, of course, be respecting the potential parents' autonomy, but, to be consistent, his obligation to practice beneficence or nonmaleficence toward the in vitro embryo would take precedence. From the standpoint of a practitioner for whom the embryo has no moral status, the request of the potential parents has priority.

Cases 1 and 2 illustrate a prevalent dilemma for couples who undergo ovulation stimulation and IVF. Because freezing reduces the chance that a given embryo can develop further, the process is legitimately interpretable as harmful to the embryos. For many, however, freezing is simply a way of extending reproductive options and postponing decisions about embryo disposal. In case 1, since Jackie and Mark have decided against having more children, they must decide whether to continue paying for maintenance of the embryos, to donate them for research or treatment of another infertile couple, or to ask that they be "discarded." The last alternative includes the possibility of allowing the embryos to die rather than directly ending their capacity for further development; in either case, it is possible to treat them with respect rather than as waste material. It is possible, for example, to dispose of in vitro embryos by pouring the test tubes in which they are contained into a garden rather than trash, and even to do so with an accompanying ritual.

Case 2 also illustrates the fact that couples occasionally disagree about how to dispose of frozen embryos. Although this is more likely when the couple divorce, partners may also disagree while remaining together. From an egalitarian perspective, Jackie has a more compelling position than Mark because she contributed more to generation of the embryos. Nonetheless, because the embryos are not within her body, her position in this regard is weaker than it would be if she were gestating them. Destruction of the embryos, as Mark would like, is the least justifiable option for either party if the frozen embryos have full moral status; if partial moral status is attributed to them, justification depends on whether the autonomy of either or both progenitors trumps the degree of moral status imputed to the embryos. Any means of disposal is acceptable if the frozen embryos have no moral status, but if the progenitors disagree, an egalitarian perspective supports whichever position is most likely to contribute to the welfare of others, such as through donation to an infertile couple or to research.[26]

Case 3 shows uncertainty on the part of practitioners or researchers concerning the wishes of gamete providers. The fact that the center is unable to ascertain the wishes of gamete providers suggests that the consent procedures that preceded embryo freezing were inadequate. Had they been adequate, couples might have been required, as a condition of their treatment, to allow the center to determine the disposition of their cryopreserved embryos after a specified period of time, if they could no longer be reached to ascertain their wishes. The embryos that remain in this case may be considered "abandoned" by their progenitors. If the embryos are regarded as persons, their disposition should be determined on similar grounds as those met in behalf of abandoned children: placement in the care of others. A foster care equivalent would be temporary placement through transfer to another cryostorage facility; the adoption equivalent would be permanent placement through transfer to a woman for gestation. As in case 2, other means of disposal are acceptable if the frozen embryos have no moral status and may be acceptable if they have partial moral status. Regardless of who decides about their disposition, the standpoints not only of the progenitors but also of the center director and potential beneficiaries of the remaining embryos, such as other infertile individuals or researchers, are ethically relevant to decisions about them.

Multiple gestations

Cases

1. Alexa Abrams had been an infertility patient for two years before becoming pregnant after taking gonadotropin (an injectable fertility drug). Although she had been advised of the risks of multiple gestation, the possibility of reducing the number of embryos after implantation was not mentioned. When a second heartbeat was detected at 6 weeks gestation, the physician gave Alexa what he considered the "good news" that she was carrying twins. One week later Alexa returned to the clinic and asked for "fetal reduction," a possibility she had heard about from friends. Having often cared for women who had twins, the physician was not only surprised but also somewhat irritated by her request. He had occasionally performed elective abortions, but had never performed "fetal reduction." The doctor told Alexa that an attempt to terminate one of the twins might lead to spontaneous abortion of the other. "If that happens," she said, "I'll try again. But if I can't have just one, I want to end this pregnancy and start over."

2. Vickie Schildress became pregnant after taking perganol, as prescribed by her family physician, and gave birth at term to a healthy daughter. Three years later she visited the same doctor and asked for help to conceive again. While prescribing perganol for her, he reminded her that the drug carries an increased risk of multiple gestation and told her she could undergo "fetal reduction" if this occurred. Vickie took the prescribed dose of perganol and subsequently became pregnant. At 7 weeks gestation, an ultrasound showed seven embryos implanted in her uterus, and her physician explained the risks of continuing to gestate all seven. In response to his recommendation of "fetal reduction," Vicki said "I don't want to kill any of my babies." Her subsequent pregnancy involved placement of a cerclage,[27] two months of bed rest, and medication to forestall prematurity. At 24 weeks gestation Vickie gave birth to seven infants, who each spent at least six weeks in the hospital before going home. Three of the children were later diagnosed with cerebral palsy and one with retinopathy of prematurity.[28]

3. Anita Speck, 42 years old and independently wealthy, had not achieved pregnancy despite three attempts of in vitro fertilization and embryo transfer. In her fourth attempt, five embryos were transferred and, as visualized by ultrasound at 6 weeks, were apparently developing in utero. Informed of the risks of continuing her quintuplet pregnancy, Anita asked that the number of embryos be reduced to two.

Empirical considerations

Until the advent of infertility drugs and IVF, Hellin's Law governed the predictability of multiple births: the natural occurrence of twins in the general population is 1/100, and the frequency of each higher multiple is determinable by multiplying the denominator by 100, so that the frequency of triplets is 1/10,000, the frequency of quadruplets is 1/1,000,000, and so on. The incidence of multiple gestations increased markedly after it became possible to induce greater production of ova than women normally produce. Between 1980 and 1997 the number of twin births in the United States rose 52 percent, and births of triplets or more climbed 404 percent.[29] Older women are more likely to have multiple gestations than younger women, mainly because they are more likely to undergo infertility treatment. But most cases of high-order multiple gestations occur in women who have undergone ovulation stimulation without IVF. The number of embryos transferred after IVF is generally based on the desire of practitioners as well as the potential parents to minimize mortality and morbidity risks while maximizing the chance of having a healthy newborn.

Not surprisingly, risks to the fetus and pregnant woman escalate with each higher order of multiple gestation. For women, the risks include anemia, preterm labor, hypertension, thrombophlebitis, preterm delivery, and hemorrhage. Tocolytic therapy to avoid preterm delivery introduces further risks. For potential children, the risks include intrauterine growth retardation, malpresentation, cord accidents, and the usual sequelae of preterm delivery, such as respiratory distress, intracranial hemorrhage, and cerebral palsy.[30] If a high-order multiple (greater than twin) gestation is established, the risks may be reduced by terminating some of the embryos while maintaining the pregnancy. The most common method of reducing the number of gestating fetuses is transabdominal injection of potassium chloride into the fetal thorax at 9 to 12 weeks gestation. The goal of the injection is to "achieve cardiac standstill."[31] Inevitably, the procedure entails some risk of loss or injury to the remaining embryos. A similar procedure has been used at a later stage of gestation when one of several fetuses is diagnosed with an anomaly such as trisomy 21.

The high costs of IVF and embryo transfer are seldom covered by insurance, whereas ovulation stimulation alone is usually covered or available to infertile individuals who have no insurance. The risk of high-order multiple gestations is reducible in IVF cases by transferring only a limited number of in vitro embryos for gestation. For women who undergo ovulation stimulation alone, care for the infants born to them is routinely covered by government or private insurance programs. For poor or economically disadvantaged infertile individuals, the only route to having a biologically related child may be the one that poses the highest health risk to them and to their offspring. Societal costs for this care are obviously higher than they would be for care of healthy or fewer infants.

If ovulation stimulation occurs without IVF, high-order multiples may still be avoided by ultrasound monitoring of the maturation of follicle cells and refraining from administration of a second drug that would trigger the release of eggs. Alternatively or additionally, the woman may agree to refrain from intercourse until her next cycle, when modification of her drug dose would reduce the risk of multiple gestation. These are measures by which women may reduce risks to themselves and their potential children, and those who are opposed to abortion may preserve their moral integrity. Although the costs and risks of ongoing infertility treatment are thus increased, these are still less than the societal costs of care for high-order multiples.

Theoretical considerations

The terminology used for procedures to reduce the number of developing embryos or fetuses during gestation is controversial. Among the terms used are "selective birth," "selective abortion," "selective reduction," "fetal reduction," and "multifetal pregnancy reduction."[32] "Reduction" suggests either that fetuses are reducible or that pregnancy is reducible. In fact, however, it is the number of fetuses or embryos that is reduced rather than any fetuses themselves, and pregnancy is not reducible because a woman is either pregnant or not, regardless of how many embryos she gestates. A non-misleading definition would indicate that the procedure involves terminating some embryos or fetuses while preserving others. "Selective birth" is accurate if it is assumed that fetuses do not develop to birth unless a woman chooses to carry them to term. If abortion is defined as termination of a fetus instead of termination of pregnancy, "selective abortion" is accurate, but this term fails to indicate that the pregnancy is not terminated. "Selective abortion with pregnancy preservation" is more precise.

Ironically, an ethical rationale for the physician's positive response to Alexa Abrams's request is the desire to save at least one embryo.[33] This would not only uphold respect for her autonomy but also nonmaleficence toward her and the fetuses that might be harmed by continuing the multiple gestation. Since Alexa has indicated she will terminate both embryos if she cannot obtain the procedure, her physician might reason that the value of life in this case can only be affirmed by permitting the death of one to preserve the life of the other. This line of reasoning implies that the end justifies the means, which is problematic even if one does not impute moral status to embryos.

Another relevant variable in case 1 is the physician's lack of experience with the procedure. Respect for Alexa's autonomy doesn't necessarily override nonmaleficence if his lack of experience in performing the requested intervention would compromise her welfare or that of her potential offspring. Although her standpoint should be accorded privileged status, the physician's standpoint is also ethically relevant. An egalitarian perspective requires that the verities should be maximally upheld with regard to all of those affected. In this case, respect for the autonomy of both physician and patient can be maintained by referral to a practitioner whose experience in performing the procedure is more likely to lead to the desired outcome. Nonmaleficence toward Alexa as well as the surviving fetuses would thus be maximized also. For those who support minimal criteria for personhood, however, "fetal reduction" is never morally justified.

Case 1 also illustrates the possible moral relevance of a physician's emotional stance regarding patient requests. Having considered her treatment successful because the patient is now pregnant with twins, Alexa's doctor is irritated that she apparently does not share this view. Practitioners may try, and are sometimes indoctrinated, not to let emotional factors influence their treatment of patients, but it may be impossible, and sometimes undesirable, for them to do so.[34] In this case, the physician's negative feelings about the patient's request strengthens the argument for referral to another.

Although twin gestations are more risky than singleton gestations, they are highly likely to lead to healthy outcomes for both the woman and her potential children. Except for the woman's plan to abort both embryos if she cannot obtain the procedure, this makes the intervention more difficult to justify for Alexa than for Anita Speck, for whom the morbidity and mortality risks are considerably higher.

The septuplet pregnancy of Vickie Schildress might have been avoided by the methods mentioned above. On grounds of risks to the woman and her potential children, the practitioner and couple should have followed these procedures. The choice of ovulation stimulation without IVF may have been triggered by economic concerns, but it could also have been based on the fact that perganol alone had proved successful in the patient's previous treatment. Even if IVF had been performed, a patient who regards her in vivo embryos as babies might also have requested that all of her in vitro embryos be returned to her, and maxim 1 would require that her request be honored. Based on maxim 2, the risks to potential offspring of high-order multiple gestation are offset by the benefit of life, which, even if accompanied by impairment, is generally a greater value than never to have been born.

The topics and cases discussed in this chapter provide only a small sampling of the ethical complexity raised by ongoing advances in treatment of infertility. In addition to topics untreated (e.g., posthumous reproduction, ovarian tissue transplants), more variables could be mentioned for each of the cases described, and these could lead to different ethical conclusions, based not only on different starting points about moral status but also on the assignment of different weights to the relevant ethical verities with regard to those affected. In light of this variability and complexity, clinicians need broad guidelines to help them apply the verities to the nuances of cases. Guidelines such as those already available through the American Society for Reproductive Medicine and other professional organizations facilitate respect for the autonomy of patients, as well as avoidance of harms and promotion of benefits to them and their potential offspring. Professional guidelines do this in part not only through consideration of the welfare and autonomy of patients and potential patients but also by respecting the autonomy of competent infertility practitioners. On grounds of justice, however, guidelines are not enough. Regulation of infertility practice is also needed to ensure that inequalities in treatment are minimized.

6

Noncompliance during Pregnancy

On legal and moral grounds, it is generally recognized that a competent adult is (or should be) free to refuse any recommended medical treatment if she is adequately informed of its risks, possible benefits, and the expected consequences of refusal. The same rationale applies to deliberate noncompliance with behavior recommended for the sake of her health. An exception to the duty to respect such refusals may occur if others' lives or health are jeopardized by the refusal. Although most ethicists support the priority of respect for the autonomy of patients who refuse treatment, this position is sometimes at odds with the commitment of health caregivers to sustain lives and promote the health of their patients.

A classic example of cases in which refusal of treatment must legally be honored despite significant health risks to the patient is that of Jehovah's Witnesses who, on religious grounds, are unwilling to accept blood transfusions necessary for their health or survival. This legal requirement does not apply to Jehovah's Witnesses who refuse transfusions judged medically necessary for their minor children. As maxims 2 and 3 affirm, respect for autonomy outweighs beneficence or nonmaleficence when these verities apply to the same individual, but when the interests of incompetent others are at stake, their interests may outweigh respect for the autonomy of those who care for them.

This chapter focuses on the unique complexity of cases in which a pregnant woman refuses treatment intended to benefit her potential child. If fetuses do not count among those whose welfare might override the autonomy of competent, informed adults, these cases are analogous to other cases of refusal of treatment for oneself. If fetuses have partial moral status, justification for refusal of treatment on their behalf is less compelling. Even if fetuses are considered persons, however, it may be legally and morally wrong to treat pregnant women coercively. Women may be legally and morally obliged to accept treatment or comply with behavioral recommendations on behalf of their potential children, but this does not imply moral justification for forcing them to do so. The moral argument for overriding refusal of treatment to benefit another is surely more compelling when the potential beneficiary is uncontroversially a person.

Refusal of hospitalization

Cases

1. Joan Blackstone is a 31-year-old pregnant woman with a history of rheumatic heart disease. At 25 weeks gestation she is admitted to the hospital in atrial fibrillation (AF). After extensive testing, she is diagnosed with heart failure, probably due to cocaine use. Her fetus is slightly small for gestational age but apparently in good health. Over a two-week period, Joan is stabilized and seen by a social worker, who learns that her partner and family members use drugs routinely. At discharge, she is cautioned about the importance of taking her cardiac medications and avoiding cocaine use, for her own sake as well as that of her potential child. Three days later Joan comes to the walk-in clinic, again in AF, acknowledging that she has used cocaine and failed to take her medications. When hospitalization is recommended, she refuses. In light of the risks her refusal poses to her and her potential child, the physician asks to have her involuntarily hospitalized until fetal lung maturity can be demonstrated and the fetus delivered.

2. Betty Barry, a 28-year-old with type 1 (juvenile) diabetes and a long history of noncompliance with her diet and insulin regimen, supports herself through part time work as a housekeeper. She became pregnant through a short-lived relationship with a neighbor. Despite being counseled extensively about the need for compliance with medical recommendations for her own sake and that of her potential child, Betty was hospitalized twice for poor glycemic control and once for diabetic ketoacidosis (DKA) at 27 weeks gestation. One week later, after being stabilized through fluid management, the attending physician recommended prolonging her hospital stay to ensure dietary and insulin control. Betty refused and requested discharge. Her competence for decision-making was not in doubt. Clinicians who had treated Betty considered the health risks to her and her potential child extremely high if she did not remain hospitalized.

Empirical considerations

Circumstances in which hospitalization of pregnant women is recommended include the need for persistent monitoring, diabetic noncompliance, premature labor, preeclampsia, and cardiomyopathy. Optimal treatment for these conditions depends in part on the duration of gestation. At 25 weeks, the fetus may be viable but is likely to be harmed by premature delivery. Several weeks later, the probability of a good outcome for the fetus is considerably improved, but prolonging gestation is still desirable for the sake of the potential child.[1] An added risk for the fetus in case 1 is that it is small for gestational age. In case 2, the fetus is more likely to be macrosomic, larger than normal at birth, which increases the obstetric risks.

Atrial fibrillation is a common cardiac arrhythmia, found more prevalently in men but more likely to be fatal in women. Although its mortality and morbidity are often associated with stroke, AF is usually treatable successfully, and some patients never develop symptoms. Risk factors include advancing age, preexisting hypertension, heart disease, and recreational drug use. When AF occurs in pregnant women, which is rare, it threatens the potential child as well as the woman,[2] but optimal treatment of the woman is ordinarily optimal for her potential child also. The risks of drugs associated with teratogenicity (birth defects) when taken during the first trimester or of fetal hemorrhage in later stages of gestation are avoidable through use of other drugs that are equally effective.

Diabetes is the sixth-deadliest disease in the United States, affecting approximately 9 million women. It is caused by lack of, or inability to use, the insulin necessary for glucose to enter the bloodstream and produce energy. The prevalence of diabetes is twice as high among African American, Hispanic/Latino, American Indian, and Asian/Pacific Islander women as it is among Caucasian women.[3] Once diagnosed, the mortality and morbidity associated with diabetes is reducible through compliance with medical recommendations regarding diet, exercise, and insulin replacement. There are three types: juvenile onset (type 1), adult onset (type 2), and gestational diabetes.

Diabetics who do not comply with medical recommendations face health risks such as ketoacidosis.[4] The risks escalate during pregnancy, when risks of preeclampsia, spontaneous abortion, obstructed labor, and polyhydramnios also increase.[5] Risks to the potential child include congenital malformations, hypoglycemia, respiratory distress syndrome, and jaundice. Fetal and neonatal loss as well as major congenital malformations are two to three times greater in diabetic pregnancies than in normal pregnancies.[6]

The preceding cases differ with regard to the probability that the patient is fully autonomous in her decision-making. In case 2, the patient's competence for decision-making is evident, whereas in case 1, the patient's ongoing use of cocaine may impede the voluntariness of her refusal of hospitalization. Addiction to drugs is recognized as a disorder in the diagnostic manual of the American Psychiatric Association,[7] but the extent (if any) to which it reduces the capacity for autonomous decision-making is unclear and controversial. It is possible that Joan Blackstone's autonomy is compromised further by the fact that those on whom she depends for support also use drugs. To the extent that this is so, she may lack the ability to render a fully informed and voluntary refusal of the recommended care. Legally, the clinician risks charges of liability regardless of whether the patient is hospitalized, especially if the outcome involves morbidity for her or her newborn.

Although hospitalization generally involves undesired restrictions on behavior, it is not always viewed as harm by patients such as pregnant women to whom the hospital provides a respite from demands of home and workplace. The patients mentioned in cases 1 and 2 are obviously not in this group. Resistance to hospitalization is sometimes triggered by patients' mistrust or fears of doctors and treatment, and sometimes by dependence on harmful drugs that would be denied them if they were hospitalized. Pregnant women who are socioeconomically disadvantaged are more likely than other pregnant women to be treated coercively.[8] For some, the refusal to follow medical recommendations is based on different priorities than those of health care practitioners. Women may be particularly prone to assume health risks for themselves in order to address the needs of other family members.

Theoretical considerations

Two variables are crucial to determination of whether Joan Blackstone should be involuntarily committed and Betty Barry should be discharged: the decision-making capacity of each, and the risk of harm to them or others. If the risk of harm is grave, a paternalistic rationale may be invoked to justify involuntary commitment or opposition to discharge. This rationale is at odds with maxim 2, which gives priority to the decisions of adequately informed and autonomous patients, even if their decisions entail serious harm to themselves, as long as their decisions do not disproportionately harm others. If the latter situation prevails, their decisions are overridable on utilitarian grounds. From an egalitarian perspective, a paternalistic rationale is neither needed nor desirable in either case.

As already mentioned, whether the fetus counts among the others whose risk of harm may justify opposition to a patient's autonomous decision is a question that people with different starting positions on its moral status answer differently. From the standpoint of those for whom fetuses are persons, the answer is clearly "yes." For some who attribute partial moral status to fetuses, the answer is "yes" if the fetus is probably viable, but this does not imply that coercive hospitalization is either morally or legally justified. Even if a woman has a moral obligation to accept medically recommended treatment, this variable alone does not justify coercing her to do so.

Viability is an important variable even for clinicians who deny moral status to fetuses because it implies that they can fulfill their responsibility to safeguard the pregnant woman's health and support her decision to terminate her pregnancy while also promoting the interests of the potential newborn. Some, however, give priority to the pregnant woman's choice not only with regard to pregnancy termination but also with regard to the fate of a fetus that could survive the termination; for them, the most important clinical variable is neither viability nor the risks of refusal but simply the determination of whether the woman's refusal is fully autonomous, that is, a decision freely made, based on adequate understanding of the implications of her decision for herself and her potential offspring.

Even if fetuses are not persons, a health threat to women and their potential children provides a rationale for hospitalizing women against their wishes. Accordingly, Frank Chervenak and Laurence McCullough claim that coercive treatment of pregnant women is justified if it is intended to promote the health of both the fetus and the pregnant woman. To them, the verities at stake are the autonomy interests of one patient and the beneficence interests of two patients. The doubling of the beneficence interest, they argue, trumps the single autonomy interest of the woman.[9] As discussed in chapter 2, these authors also believe coercive interventions are justified solely on grounds of fetal viability. Both arguments may be convincing to those who share their view that the fetus and woman are separate patients. Chapter 2 discusses reasons for disagreeing with this position.

Because of her drug use and her social situation, the autonomy of Joan Blackstone's refusal is probably compromised but not eliminated, and her health risks are based on the expectation of caregivers that she will neither avoid drug use nor take her medication unless she is hospitalized. Betty Barry's health risks are based on a comparable expectation: that she will continue the behavior that endangers her and her potential offspring unless she is hospitalized. Joan's refusal may not reflect what she would decide if her judgment were not impaired through drug use. Arguably, therefore, her refusal may be overridden on grounds that it probably does not express what some have called her "authentic" self.[10] On this rationale, her consent to treatment to benefit her and her potential offspring may be reasonably presumed. Although the merit of this position depends crucially on the probability of the premises, the argument itself is valid.

A similar argument cannot be offered for coercive hospitalization of Betty. Legally and morally, opposition to her requested discharge can only be defended on paternalistic grounds relevant to the patient (reducing risk to her by overriding her autonomy) or on grounds of beneficence or nonmaleficence toward the fetus or potential child. The former rationale is inconsistent with the long-standing practice of allowing competent patients to leave hospitals against medical advice (AMA) even when their departures will probably lead to their demise; the latter rationale rests on the assumption that some people may be coercively treated for the sake of others, a practice that is inconsistent with the legal impermissibility of coercing someone to be tested or treated for the sake of another through virtually non-risk procedures such as buccal smears or blood donation. An egalitarian perspective requires consistency with regard to the permissibility of coercive practices toward pregnant and nonpregnant individuals whose autonomous refusals may impugn the welfare of others.

In most jurisdictions, if an incompetent adult lacks decisional capacity, physicians are legally and morally bound to make treatment decisions based on the patient's best interest. If her capacity for decision-making is questionable, however, an adult may be involuntarily committed on an urgent basis to avoid risks to her health or life. Joan Blackstone may be temporarily hospitalized on this basis, but if she is subsequently judged competent, her hospitalization cannot legally be continued without her consent, nor may she be coercively medicated.

Refusal of treatment likely to avoid a bad outcome in the newborn is distressing to most practitioners. Nonetheless, the American College of Obstetricians and Gynecologists agrees with U.S. courts that no competent, adequately informed patient should be treated without consent, even if her refusal of treatment is likely to harm her potential offspring. While recommending that "every reasonable effort should be made to protect the fetus," the college insists that "the pregnant woman's autonomy should be respected."[11] Medical organizations and the U.S. legal system thus affirm that competent, adequately informed, autonomous pregnant women have at least as compelling a right as do other adults to refuse hospitalization or treatment for their own or others' sakes. The claim that no one should be coercively treated or hospitalized is in essence a pro-choice standpoint. From a strictly pro-life standpoint, this position is unacceptable. If life is a more important value than choice, nonpregnant as well as pregnant patients should be treated coercively if this is the only way by which to save another's life.

Dietary noncompliance

Cases

1. Tara Gwinn is the woman with PKU discussed in chapter 4 in connection with preconception counseling. In light of her previous history and her high risk of having another child with maternal PKU, her physician advised her to avoid another pregnancy. Encouraged by her husband, however, she has now become pregnant and visits her obstetrician for prenatal care. Although she hopes for a son, she says she would be happy to have another daughter. She indicates that she wants very much to have "a healthy baby" and will "try hard" to avoid the "wrong" foods. Having had so difficult a hospitalization in her previous pregnancy, however, Tara is unwilling to be hospitalized again for percutaneous feeding with phenylalanine-restricted protein supplements. Her obstetrician wonders whether she may be legally or morally coerced to comply with the recommended diet so that she will not have another child with maternal PKU.

2. Nina Torres is a 34-year-old single woman who developed gestational diabetes during her first pregnancy at age 15. Five years ago, she was diagnosed with type 2 diabetes and advised of the importance of following medical recommendations regarding diet, exercise, and insulin, especially if she became pregnant. Early in her current pregnancy, she sought an abortion but subsequently changed her mind. As gestation continued, she failed to comply with her recommended diet, and her insulin level became critical. At 16 weeks gestation, she lapsed into diabetic coma and was transported to the hospital where she underwent two weeks of intensive care but remained comatose. A neurologist consulted on the case concluded that it was "highly likely that Ms. Torres will either die within the next few weeks or survive in her comatose state for years." Told of her prognosis, her parents and fiancé said they wanted "everything done to help Nina" and did not want her treatment to be compromised for the sake of the fetus. In light of her prognosis, the obstetrics team questioned whether to attempt to prolong her pregnancy.

Empirical considerations

PKU and diabetes are conditions for which preconception counseling is routinely recommended to facilitate the reduction of risks for the woman and her potential child. Most adults with PKU have been successfully weaned from the restrictive diet of childhood, but women with PKU are more likely to have unaffected offspring if they return to the restrictive diet before becoming pregnant.[12] Similarly, risks to women with type 1 or type 2 diabetes are lower if their blood sugar levels are in good control before as well as during pregnancy.

PKU is a genetic condition for which newborns are routinely tested so that severe cognitive impairment can be avoided in those who test positive through strict adherence to a phenylalanine-reduced diet from infancy through adolescence. Although Tara Gwinn apparently benefited by early testing and dietary restriction, her successful treatment did not preclude the risk of maternal PKU in her offspring. Despite her attempts to comply with the restrictive diet in previous pregnancies, she did not reach the desired phenylalanine level either time. Her first child fell within the small percentage of offspring who are not affected; her second daughter was not as fortunate.

Lest it be thought that dietary compliance is a simple thing to expect of pregnant women, the case of Tara makes plain that this is not necessarily so. Because phenylalanine concentrates in the fetus, the diet recommended for pregnant or potentially pregnant women is even more restrictive than the diet required for children who test positive for PKU. Women find it particularly difficult to adhere to the diet because, as adults, they have usually become accustomed to a normal diet and the social expectations surrounding it. Moreover, the recommended diet often fails to provide enough protein to support fetal development. As in Tara's case, feeding through a nasogastric tube with phenylalanine-reduced protein supplements may be required to avoid growth restriction in the fetus.

Gestational diabetes occurs in about 1 in 20 pregnant women but generally disappears following childbirth. Up to 50 percent of women with gestational diabetes develop type 2 diabetes within ten or fifteen years.[13] Long-term diabetics are usually accustomed to the burdens of dietary compliance and checks on their own glucose control and knowledgeable about the consequences of "out-of-control" blood sugars. Pregnancy often increases the motivation of pregnant women to conform to these practices, but socioeconomic circumstances sometimes exacerbate the difficulty of doing so. The risks of continuing noncompliance, as indicated in the previous section, are significant. DKA is a medical emergency for which effective treatment is needed immediately to avoid death or long-term morbidity; it occurs twice as often in women than in men.[14] With treatment through modern methods of fluid management, the mortality rate is about 2 percent for pregnant women and 9 percent for their fetuses.[15]

Theoretical considerations

Treatment decisions in the above cases are clinically and ethically more complicated than they would be in the context of preconception counseling. Once pregnancy is established, practitioners with different starting points about moral status have different standpoints on ethical issues regarding treatment or nontreatment. In case 1, for example, physicians who regard embryos or fetuses as persons cannot in good conscience advise a patient to end her pregnancy even if her potential child were certain to have maternal PKU and she would otherwise be required to undergo severe dietary restrictions and months of hospitalization. In case 2, physicians who hold this view would probably advocate interventions to prolong the woman's pregnancy even if this were no longer medically optimal for her. Those who attribute no moral status to embryos could conscientiously encourage the patient to undergo abortion in both cases, and those who impute intermediate moral status could do so if the termination were early enough and the rigors of treatment or compliance were severe. Most of the latter group would probably agree with Nina Torres's family and fiancé that her interests should not be compromised for the sake of the fetus.

From the standpoint of those who attribute personhood to fetuses, coercive treatment in case 1 is ethically defensible. The case is thus analogous to that of a parent who deliberately places a child in harm's way, or allows the child to remain in harm's way, when this can be avoided. Regardless of the physician's starting point, however, other variables are also ethically relevant: whether the requirements of avoidance are reasonable, how reliable they are in securing avoidance, the severity of the harm to be avoided, and the beneficiaries of its avoidance.

Dietary compliance through exclusion or addition of certain foods is obviously not as strenuous or invasive a requirement as nasogastric infusions, prolonged hospitalization, or placement of a gastrostomy tube through which nourishment is supplied directly to the stomach. Even so, family relationships and economic constraints may make a change in diet much more difficult for some than for others. The ethical and professional challenge of clinicians who treat patients in such circumstances is to facilitate rather than enforce compliance.

In Tara Gwinn's case, despite the extreme demands of dietary compliance and related procedures, it may be argued that the outcome is worth the rigors in terms of benefits to the potential child as well as the parent who cares for the child. Ultimately, this rationale implies that respect for the woman's autonomy may be overridden by beneficence when the latter is applicable to both parent and potential child. Maxim 2 opposes this rationale unless the fetus counts as a person; otherwise maxim 3 prevails because two individuals stand to benefit, overriding the autonomy of one. As for the potential father's benefit, this is subordinated to the impact on the pregnant woman because he is not directly affected by what is done or not done to her.

Two ethically relevant features are applicable to case 2, but not to case 1: Nina Torres is (a) clearly incompetent and (b) highly unlikely to survive or be able to care for a child to whom she might give birth if treatment is prolonged. Because of her comatose state, respect for her autonomy is impossible unless this is interpreted as respect for her previously indicated wishes. Privileging her standpoint requires efforts to ascertain these wishes. The fact that her last known decision was to continue her pregnancy suggests that she wanted her fetus to survive, but this decision was probably made with the expectation that she herself would be able to raise the child. Had she anticipated the current circumstances, her decision might have been different. Although there is now no way by which to ascertain her wishes, her parents and fiancé should be asked what they think *she* would want regarding prolongation of treatment for the sake of the fetus. Their answer could in fact be different from what they themselves would want.

If a patient's wishes or standpoint are unknowable, beneficence and nonmaleficence toward her have priority. "Doing everything to help Nina," as her parents and fiancé have requested, is obviously consistent with this priority, but what constitutes "help" for an apparently dying, comatose patient is not clear. An egalitarian perspective argues that she should be treated in the same respectful manner as any other patient who is probably dying and comatose: She may be removed from life support and allowed to die in a dignified manner. The removal may be postponed briefly for the benefit of her loved ones or to facilitate organ transplantation, but at some point, continuation of mechanical support can no longer be defended as respectful of the dying patient. In Nina's case, it is too soon to determine whether that point has been reached. With proper management, patients in diabetic coma can recover, and comatose pregnant women have given birth, albeit rarely, to healthy children.[16]

"Helping Nina" in this case is interpretable as prolonging treatment that postpones her probable death for the sake of the fetus if that outcome is in fact realistic and consistent with her wishes insofar as they are known. The duration of gestation is critical to determination of whether fetal survival to viability is a realistic possibility. If it is, supporters of an intermediate position about moral status, as well as those who consider fetuses persons, should support efforts to prolong treatment that the patient herself may validly, although not infallibly, be presumed to desire. The standpoint of family members should only be given priority if it is based on the patient's own interests, including her presumed wishes (maxims 1 and 2).

From an egalitarian perspective, concerns about the impact on others may override respect for an individual's autonomy, as well as obligations of beneficence and nonmaleficence toward individuals (maxim 3). Accordingly, some may argue that the societal costs of caring for a severely impaired child with maternal PKU or of a child whose mother has died or is irreversibly comatose are an unfair imposition on the rest of society. If the only costs considered are economic, this may be true. But "costs" have a broader meaning, encompassing the psychological and moral impact on society of policies or decisions that would prevent the birth or curtail treatment of groups of people based on costs of caring for them. An egalitarian society imputes the same value to those who are physically, mentally, socially, or economically able as to those who are disabled in any or all of these respects.

Refusal of cesarean section

Cases

1. Zoe Mazur, a 30-year-old nurse in her thirty-eighth week of an uncomplicated pregnancy, came to the obstetric service with spontaneous rupture of membranes. She had had uterine contractions during most of the day. The fetal monitor showed "nonreassuring fetal heart rate tracing," indicative of persistent fetal distress. An epidural line was placed for administration of anesthesia. When Zoe was told that delivery was imminent and a C-section might be necessary to avoid significant neurological impairment in her newborn, she said she wanted to deliver vaginally despite the risk.

Oxytocin, a drug intended to promote labor, was administered, but fetal tracings continued to show prolonged fetal bradycardia (slowing of heart rate). Over the next three hours, the patient's vaginal examination remained unchanged, and oxytocin was therefore discontinued. When C-section delivery was recommended to prevent fetal demise or severe impairment in the newborn, Zoe again refused consent. Her physician restarted the oxytocin and attempted to facilitate delivery through manual dilatation, but severe fetal distress continued. While checking on the patient in the presence of her husband, the physician acknowledged his anxiety and worry about the outcome. He told Zoe he had made preparations for an emergency C-section but would not operate without his patient's consent and then left the room. After the couple discussed the matter further, Zoe changed her mind, and an emergency C-section was performed. The newborn showed signs of neurological compromise; whether this was the result of delaying surgical delivery could not be determined.

2. Angela Carder was a 28-year-old woman whose aggressive recurrence of cancer was discovered during her twenty-fifth week of a wanted pregnancy.[17] After learning that she probably had only weeks to live, Angela discussed the prognosis for her potential newborn with a neonatologist and agreed to treatment likely to improve the chance of healthy survival for her newborn. She also indicated, however, that she wanted her physicians to continue to treat her optimally. One week later, Angela's death was judged imminent, and C-section was recommended for the sake of the potential child. At that point, the probability of viability was 50 to 60 percent, with less than 20 percent risk of serious impairment in the newborn. After being informed of the risks, Angela declined consent for the C-section; her family members and clinicians agreed with her decision.

The hospital's legal counsel asked the court to clarify the hospital's responsibilities. Following a hearing at which lawyers represented Angela, the fetus, and the hospital, a judge ruled that the C-section should be performed for the sake of the fetus. In accordance with this ruling, Angela underwent surgical delivery. Her newborn expired after two hours despite aggressive treatment; Angela succumbed two days later.[18]

Empirical considerations

Surgical interventions are commonly perceived as more drastic than other modes of treatment. George Annas's description of coercive cesarean section as "the most unkindest cut of all"[19] is consistent with this perception. From the standpoint of most pregnant women, however, even very invasive, prolonged, and painful treatments or behavioral modifications are acceptable if they are the only means by which to promote the health of their offspring. Occasionally, some women have religious objections or other reasons for refusing recommended treatment. A first step in addressing the above cases and all of the cases in this chapter, therefore, would be to explore the woman's reasons for noncompliance to ensure that they are not based on inadequate understanding of the risks and benefits of the recommended treatment or behavior.

Refusals to follow medical recommendations for oneself or others are not adequately autonomous unless the relevant implications are understood.

When physicians offer medical advice, they are usually already convinced that the benefits of following it outweigh the harms or risks of not following it. Women, however, may assign quite different values to different kinds or degrees of harm to themselves or their potential children, and they usually weigh risks and benefits in more than medical terms. Moreover, while medical factors may justify medical advice, following the advice does not guarantee the desired result, and practitioners' predictions of dire consequences sometimes prove wrong. For example, a court in Georgia authorized a C-section on grounds that it was necessary for the health of a woman as well as her potential child; during the time that the order was appealed, the woman vaginally delivered a healthy infant and left the hospital sooner than she could have had the order been implemented.[20] Most practitioners have experienced multiple cases in which, for better or worse, outcomes that they predicted with virtual certainty did not materialize.

When the fetus is considered viable, C-sections may be recommended on grounds that surgical delivery is medically better than vaginal delivery for the woman, her potential child, or both. As indicated in chapter 3, viability connotes a point in development beyond which others can ensure that the newborn, if delivered, survives and is adequately cared for. By dates and examination, the fetus in case 1 was viable and the fetus in case 2 was potentially viable. In the United States, most laws affirm an "interest" in the viable fetus even though it is not legally a person, and this "interest" precludes nontherapeutic abortion.

Cesarean section is major abdominal surgery involving different and sometimes disproportionate risks and benefits for the woman and her potential child. Although the maternal mortality associated with the surgery is low, it is usually greater than the mortality associated with vaginal birth; other risks for the woman include infection, hemorrhage, transfusion, injury to other organs, anesthesia complications, and psychological sequellae. Risks to the fetus include prematurity, respiratory distress syndrome, intensive care, and delayed mother-infant bonding. On average, a cesarean delivery is more costly than vaginal birth, but the latter is not without risks, and these, in some cases, outweigh those posed by surgical delivery. When a C-section is medically indicated, it can be life saving as well as health promoting for both the woman and her potential child. This is not the situation, however, in either of the above cases, and in case 2, the surgery carries the additional risk of hastening the death of an already dying woman.

Although the World Health Organization recommends a C-section rate no greater than 15 percent, the rate in the United States is more than twice that.[21] To reduce the rate of surgical deliveries, vaginal birth after a C-section (VBAC) is sometimes performed, but this is not always medically preferable or appropriate. Cesarean rates are also influenced by nonmedical factors. Rates are higher, for example, for women who have private medical insurance; obtain their care at private rather than public clinics; and are older, married, well educated, and in a high socioeconomic bracket. Because these women are usually agreeable to, sometimes even desirous of, surgical delivery, they rarely object to it. The women for whom court orders have been sought to perform C-sections are patients at clinics of teaching hospitals or on public assistance.[22]

The main medical reasons for C-sections in North America are routine repeat sections; nonprogressive labor, breech presentation, and fetal distress. As discussed in chapter 7, C-sections are also performed for reasons unrelated to maternal or fetal well-being.

Theoretical considerations

Legal rulings in the United States and elsewhere support the position of the American College of Obstetrics and Gynecology which, while encouraging physicians to counsel patients thoroughly about the risks of refusal, opposes coercive C-section. If the risk of harm to the fetus is the same as or less than the risk to the woman, maxim 1 supports this position even if the fetus is viewed as a person. In case 1, however, the risk to the potential child is probably greater than the risk to the woman, and her refusal may only be supportable on grounds that she is unquestionably a person and the fetus is not. In case 2, the fetus probably has a greater chance of survival than does the already-dying pregnant woman.

From the standpoint of those who support maximal criteria for personhood, coercive treatment of the woman, a moral agent, for the sake of the potential newborn is nonetheless unjustifiable. For those who hold a minimalist position, coercive treatment of a pregnant woman for the sake of her potential newborn is justifiable on the same grounds as it may be supported after birth. For those who impute some but not full moral status to late-term fetuses, justification for coercive treatment of pregnant women requires weighing the extent of the harm to be avoided against the degree of infringement on autonomy that the treatment entails.

If the verity of justice is invoked to resolve apparent conflicts between the interests of the potential child and those of the pregnant woman, another factor to consider is whether treatment may be imposed coercively for the sake of another in other circumstances. Recognizing the need for consistency, a judge in the state of Washington observed: "A fetus cannot have rights in this respect superior to those of a person who has already been born."[23] In other words, if no born person may be forced to undergo a medical procedure for another, then neither may a woman be coerced to do so for her fetus. Cesarean section is decidedly more invasive and risky than bone marrow retrieval, for example, but the latter has never been legally mandated, even for one's (born) child or spouse. This difference argues that the opposite situation should prevail: that is, that refusal of C-section should be managed less coercively than refusal of bone marrow donation. On egalitarian grounds, obligations to respect the refusal of a medical procedure are more stringent when consent to it involves greater risk.

Any of three alternatives would remedy the inconsistency between opposition to coercive tissue donation in circumstances in which the potential donor is the only match for the potential recipient and support for coercive treatment of pregnant women for the sake of the potential newborn. First, from the standpoint of those who cite maximal criteria for personhood, both positions should be upheld. Second, from the standpoint of those who give priority to respect for autonomy, both positions should be opposed; while consistent, this view is at odds with maxim 3 and an egalitarian perspective. Third, from the standpoint of those who impute a right to life to potential bone marrow recipients but not to fetuses, coercive bone marrow donation, but not coercive C-section, is permissible.

Legally and morally, the right to refuse treatment for oneself is not equivalent to the right to obtain treatment and, a fortiori, to obtain treatment that is not medically indicated. While physicians are generally obliged to respect refusal of treatment, they are not obliged to provide treatment that is medically unwarranted. Requests for C-section for nonmedical reasons fall into the latter category. As long as the risks of C-section are small, physicians *may* perform the surgery for nonmedical reasons; if the risks are high in a particular situation, surgery should not be performed. Importantly, respect for autonomy applies to both the physician and the patient, and in the latter cases, respect for the physician's autonomy and nonmaleficence toward the patient override the obligation to perform the surgery solely on grounds of the woman's request.

In both cases, clinicians are less likely than family members or partners to know what the patient would want done or not done. As indicated earlier with regard to Nina Torres, the input of relatives or others close to the patient should be sought if she is unable to articulate her own standpoint. In asking for such input, however, clinicians err if the question they pose is "What do *you* want us to do?" Ethically, the appropriate question is "What would *she* want us to do?" An answer to the former question does not fulfill either the legal requirement of informed consent or the moral requirement of respect for the patient's autonomy. Among possible surrogate decision makers, the one whose answer to the latter question should prevail is the one most likely to know the patient's wishes or standpoint. In the cases described, the potential father apparently fulfills this criterion.

Case 2 is legally and ethically complicated not only because the patient is pregnant but also because she is dying. A simplistic interpretation of utilitarianism may be invoked to justify intervention for the sake of the fetus, even though it might shorten the life of the pregnant woman: the fetus has the potential for a long and healthy life, whereas Angela Carder is likely to die soon, no matter what is done or not done. But if "utility" is defined more broadly—for example, as encompassing the network of relationships that have already been established for the pregnant woman, and taking account of the number of people likely to suffer through her death—the opposite position is supportable. Either position could be dubbed "act utilitarian" because it is based on the consequences of a particular act.[24]

Rule utilitarianism and deontological reasoning also argue against a simplistic interpretation of utility as grounds for compromising care of Angela for the sake of her potential child.[25] The rule underlying such a decision is objectionable to utilitarians because it negates the basic claim that every individual counts as one and not more than one. Moreover, it implies that some persons are not equal to others or some actual persons deserve less care than potential persons. This rationale could hardly satisfy the Kantian imperative of universalizability. From an egalitarian perspective, even if the fetus counts as a person, care for a dying patient is as morally incumbent on caregivers as is care for those expected to survive for many years.

In all of the cases in this chapter, the apparent conflicts in provision of care to pregnant women involve their refusal to comply with recommended lifestyle changes or treatment modalities. Although these situations are typically labeled "maternal-fetal conflicts," they are seldom if ever conflicts between women and their fetuses but, rather, between pregnant women and their physicians.[26] As already mentioned, such conflicts are more likely to occur between women who are socioeconomically disadvantaged and their physicians than they are between physicians and patients whose socioeconomic status is closer to theirs. This difference is suggestive that a power differential may impede physicians' trust of patients as well as patients' trust of physicians. From both sides, trust needs to be earned and cultivated.

From an egalitarian perspective, overtreatment may be as unjust as undertreatment, regardless of the patient's socioeconomic status. Overtreatment may be requested and even demanded by patients, and financial concerns may serve as additional incentives to practitioners to offer or provide unnecessary treatment or suboptimal treatment for particular patients. To avoid overtreatment, physicians and patients alike need to recognize tendencies to display "overtrust"—confidence that exceeds the inevitable limits of clinical judgment and expertise. Overtrust is ethically problematic on both sides of the relationship.

7

Decisions at Parturition and Birth

Decisions during and immediately after childbirth are generally less controversial than decisions about prenatal testing because, at that point, the fetus or the newborn is much more likely to be considered a person by those involved. Even if birth threatens prematurely, the probable viability of the fetus is morally significant not only to those who subscribe to a minimalist view of personhood but also to those who support a woman's decision to terminate her pregnancy. Childbirth, whether or not it involves medical assistance, is the inevitable termination of a pregnancy that has not been spontaneously or deliberately interrupted before viability. Despite the prevalent perception (or misperception) that doctors deliver babies, pregnant women always have and always will deliver them.

Practitioners who care for pregnant women have a legal and moral responsibility to promote the welfare of the potential child of a woman who intends to carry her pregnancy to term. However, whether this responsibility outweighs their obligation to promote the interests of the pregnant woman if and when these appear to be at odds with those of the potential child is disputed. Whether parents may refuse or insist on treatment of their neonates is also disputed.

The cases in this chapter illustrate variables relevant to ethical decisions about modes of delivery, elective cesarean sections, decisions for impaired neonates, and sex assignment at birth. As most women know from their own diverse experiences, many other issues arise during the momentous event of childbirth and its sequellae.

Mode of delivery

Cases

1. Nan Ost was near term during her third pregnancy. Ultrasonographs taken early and late in gestation indicated the absence of skull formation or calcification around the fetal brain. To optimize the chance of neonatal survival, Nan wanted to undergo operative delivery. After exploring postdelivery options, a medical team concluded that survival of the newborn was virtually impossible, no matter how aggressive the treatment during delivery and after birth. In light of this conclusion, the obstetrician considered it "medically irresponsible" to perform a cesarean section. "Operating on this patient," he said, "violates my professional duty to do no harm." But Nan persisted in her request for operative delivery; she thought the team's medical opinion might be incorrect, and vaginal delivery would be more painful for the fetus.

2. Lee March was a 26-year-old with Eisenmenger syndrome. She was diagnosed with this condition soon after birth, and her mother was told she required surgery as an infant to correct the disorder. Unfortunately, the child did not return for treatment until she was 12 years old, when the correction was no longer possible. At that point, the cardiologist warned her that she should never become pregnant because pregnancy "could be fatal" to her. When Lee became pregnant at age 24, she contacted the same cardiologist she had seen as a child and asked for his advice. Her condition had already deteriorated to a point where her remaining life span was estimated at about two years. The physician urged her to have an abortion, but Lee decided otherwise. As she approached term, a decision was needed regarding the method of delivery. On learning that the optimal method for her potential child might not be optimal for her, Lee stated that she wanted what was best for the baby regardless of the risks to her. Her family disagreed with this decision, indicating that they would much prefer to have her with them for whatever time she had left.

Empirical considerations

Both of the preceding cases[1] illustrate the tendency of the majority of pregnant women to maximize the welfare of their potential children even when this entails avoidable health risks to themselves. At parturition, the risks are often greater than they are earlier in pregnancy, and the mode of delivery may reduce or exacerbate these risks. Depending on their underlying condition, risks are greater for some women and sometimes also for the potential newborn. Occasionally, optimal timing of delivery is different for the pregnant woman than it is for her potential newborn; this happens in cases of toxemia or preeclampsia.

Another variable relevant to decisions about mode of delivery is the experience and expertise of the practitioner. Some physicians, for example, are more skilled than others with rotation procedures (to move the fetus into a position more conducive to delivery) or with use of forceps. Patients seldom question this aspect of their care. In case 1, Nan might have requested operative delivery solely on grounds that it would be less painful for the fetus, whose survival is apparently impossible no matter what mode of delivery is chosen. In case 2, Lee might have asked for whatever assistance was most likely to ensure survival of her infant, even if that method posed risks to her, possibly even hastening her death.

The fetal condition described in case 1 is a congenital malformation called acrania or exencephaly. It involves the absence of skull rather than absence of brain development, and the brain itself may be normal. If nerve centers are sufficiently developed, the fetus at term may experience pain. Even with very aggressive treatment after surgical delivery, however, it is virtually impossible for a newborn with acrania to survive. The risk of cesarean section to Nan is small but greater than that of vaginal delivery. Although surgical delivery is probably less painful than vaginal delivery to a mature fetus, the latter is usually warranted on grounds of its minimal risk to the newborn as well as the pregnant woman (nonmaleficence). In this case, neither is expected to benefit medically by surgical delivery, and the pain or discomfort of vaginal delivery may be adequately addressed through provision of pain relief for both.

Eisenmenger syndrome is a progressive condition that develops from a congenital heart defect, the most common of which is patent ductus arteriosis (PDA), an opening between the aorta and pulmonary artery that normally closes shortly after birth. If the newborn has this life-threatening problem, its expression may be thwarted through surgical correction during infancy. Clinically, the essential features of Eisenmenger syndrome are pulmonary hypertension (elevated blood pressure in the lungs) and abnormal blood flow (from right to left instead of left to right). Medication is the primary treatment option if the condition is not corrected early in life; in rare cases, heart-lung transplantation is possible. Because of the very high mortality for pregnant women with uncorrected Eisenmenger's (30%–70%),[2] avoidance or early termination of pregnancy is commonly recommended.[3] If a pregnancy continues, parturition is particularly dangerous for the woman; risk for the fetus is increased but not as acute and largely depends on the woman's condition and treatment. To reduce the woman's mortality risk as much as possible, the least physiologically stressful mode of delivery is normally chosen.

Theoretical considerations

Legally, even at term, respect for the pregnant woman's autonomy and beneficence toward her trumps other verities with regard to the fetus.[4] Nonetheless, no practitioner is morally or legally obliged to provide treatment that is more harmful than beneficial to the woman's health, even if she requests it. In both of the cases here, the woman's choice is at odds with beneficence toward her. To put it bluntly, the main conflict the physician faces is between nonmaleficence toward the woman and respect for her autonomy. In both cases, fetal welfare is paramount from the woman's own standpoint. Accordingly, the physician should assure Nan of adequate pain relief for her probably sentient fetus during the course of vaginal delivery, which is medically recommended for her. If she still wishes cesarean delivery, the physician may, but is not obliged, to operate, on the same grounds that cesareans are permissible in cases such as those discussed in the next section. The overall benefit to Nan would then be calculated on nonmedical as well as medical grounds.

Beneficence or nonmaleficence toward the potential child supports the woman's request more compellingly in case 2 because the fetus has a reasonable chance of survival without severe, incurable morbidity. Just what mode of delivery is most respectful of the woman's request is unclear. Ordinarily, an uncomplicated vaginal delivery is preferable to surgical delivery on medical grounds relevant to both the woman and the fetus; it should therefore be pursued unless respect for the woman's autonomy countermands it. If fetal complications arise, C-section may be recommended for the sake of the potential child.

Unlike cases in which the risk to the woman is acceptable because it is slight, surgical delivery in case 2 could entail a high mortality risk to Lee. If the risk of C-section to her is greater than the risk of vaginal delivery to the potential newborn, beneficence and nonmaleficence should prevail on behalf of Lee even from the standpoint of those who consider her fetus a person. In this case, however, respect for her autonomy adds moral weight in support of surgical delivery. If Lee had declined surgical delivery, knowing as fully as possible its risks and benefits to her and her potential child, respect for her autonomy would tip the scale in the opposite direction. Either decision could be made from altruistic motives on her part. From her privileged standpoint, a decision to promote her own survival could be made out of a sense of obligation to those already born, even as one made on behalf of the fetus would be made to promote the welfare of her future child.[5]

Another possibility in case 2 is that labor is so protracted and stressful to Lee that cesarean delivery is recommended for her sake. Respect for her autonomy as well as beneficence toward her would then support the surgery, which could also optimize the outcome for her potential child. Practitioners who impute full moral status to the fetus, or at least to the viable fetus, may disagree with the legal requirement that a woman's refusal of a mode of delivery intended to benefit the fetus should be respected. Those who consider birth the crucial demarcation point should have no moral problem with this requirement, but they are likely to feel uneasy about any apparent risk to the potential child.

Respect for autonomy is relevant toward all of those affected by health care decisions, including family members and practitioners. It may be argued that the autonomy of the potential father in case 2 deserves priority because, in such dire circumstances, he is most likely to be the only parent who can care for the newborn. Still, he is not directly affected because he is not the patient, as is Lee. To fail to respect her wishes on grounds that she may not survive implies that a person who is or may be dying is no longer as worthy of respect as other persons. Obviously, an egalitarian standpoint is at odds with this position.

Cesarean sections for nonmedical reasons

Cases

1. Carolyn Jacobs is a 29-year-old woman who at 40 weeks gestation requests a C-section to avoid possible problems with bladder or bowel function after vaginal delivery. As a professional triathlete, she is concerned about the effect incontinence would have on her career. She has had an uncomplicated pregnancy, the fetus is in the cephalic position, the estimated fetal weight is appropriate, and her pelvis is judged adequate for vaginal delivery.

2. Brittany Smith, mother of two, has recently been treated for genital herpes simplex virus (HSV) infection. She requests a C-section delivery at 39 weeks gestation. Brittany has no active herpetic lesions and understands that the risk of vertical transmission (mother to infant) is low in the absence of these lesions. Still, she says she "doesn't want to take any chances" because HSV infection can be devastating to an affected newborn. Brittany's previous vaginal delivery was uncomplicated.

3. Evelyn White is a pregnant woman who asks for a C-section because she had previously experienced a difficult labor and painful vaginal delivery requiring use of forceps. Complications of that delivery included a significant perineal tear,[6] urine retention in the month after delivery, and pain during intercourse. Her newborn had low Apgar scores and required observation in the nursery for 24 hours before discharge; he is now developing normally.[7] Through operative delivery, Evelyn hopes to prevent further perineal damage and to avoid the anxiety and pain she experienced with her previous delivery.

4. Jennifer Young is a 25-year-old woman who has had an uncomplicated first pregnancy. At 38 weeks gestation, she is told that her cervix is still closed and firm. Realizing that she will reach 39 weeks gestation on December 31st, she requests a C-section on that date if her cervix is still "unfavorable" and she has not yet gone into labor.

Empirical considerations

Because of its risks, costs, and invasiveness, C-section has traditionally been viewed as a last resort for situations in which vaginal delivery is unlikely or unsafe for the woman or for her potential child.[8] These situations arise, for example, when a woman with a small pelvis is delivering a large infant. Other obstetrical indications for C-sections include active HSV infection, breech presentation, and fetal anomalies that make vaginal delivery hazardous. In the absence of such conditions, women have routinely been counseled and expected to undergo a "trial of labor" leading to vaginal delivery. Approximately 25 percent of these women do not delivery vaginally but undergo C-sections after their trial of labor.

Recently, an increasing number of women have asked for C-sections for reasons other than obstetrical indications.[9] The grounds for such requests, prevalently described by practitioners as "patient choice cesareans," are sometimes health related. The health-related rationale of Carolyn Jacobs, for example, was her desire to avoid the possible risk of damage to the muscles of the pelvic floor, which may cause urinary or fecal incontinence.[10] There are as yet no studies that prove this correlation. Fear of complications from vaginal deliveries is another health-related reason that women request C-section deliveries. But complications experienced in a previous vaginal delivery do not increase the likelihood of delivery complications in a subsequent pregnancy.

Some women, such as Brittany Smith, request C-sections out of concern for their potential child rather than themselves. In her case, however, there are no data to show that vaginal delivery poses greater risk of HSV infection to newborns than C-section poses. The case of Jennifer Young is intended to illustrate the increasing number of instances in which women seek C-section delivery for reasons unrelated to either their own health or a future child's health. While the rationale for her request is not explicitly indicated, the desire to ensure a newborn's arrival prior to the beginning of a new year may be based on the desire to obtain a tax deduction for a child born in the antecedent year.

Support for C-sections in elective cases may come from recent debate about the risks of vaginal birth after a woman has already had a C-section delivery (VBACs). Because the risk of uterine rupture associated with maternal or perinatal death is low, policy makers and insurers have encouraged practitioners to perform VBACs to reduce the overall rate of cesarean delivery. However, data suggesting a small increased maternal and neonatal mortality risk through uterine rupture[11] have led obstetricians and other policy makers to agree, almost unanimously, that women with a prior C-section should be given a choice about whether or not to undergo a trial of labor during a subsequent pregnancy. They recommend that women be presented with this option only after extended discussions of the risks and benefits of alternative modes of delivery. From the obstetrician's and the policy makers' standpoint, therefore, repeat cesarean and VBAC are both appropriate in many cases.

Theoretical considerations

As with other choices women make regarding childbirth (such as whether to undergo anesthesia), elective C-sections may be ethically justifiable even though the immediate medical risks are greater than those of vaginal delivery. However, an important variable in determining whether C-sections should be performed in the above cases is the probability that it will have the desired outcome. If the woman is highly likely to have an uncomplicated vaginal delivery after a trial of labor, the burden of justification for C-section is obviously greater than it would otherwise be. In case 1, for example, estimates of the size of the fetus and the dimensions of the woman's pelvis indicate (albeit imperfectly) that she is able to deliver vaginally with fewer medical risks than she would undergo through C-section. Similarly, in case 2, the probability of a successful vaginal delivery is high. Obstetricians may be reluctant to perform C-sections on such patients because surgical intervention seems medically unwarranted. These cases stand in contrast to those in which the surgery is clearly warranted—for example, when a very large fetus or a very small pelvis is suspected, making eventual C-section probable.

The reluctance of some practitioners to perform an elective cesarean on patients likely to have a safe vaginal delivery is supported by the Hippocratic dictum: to do no harm, that is, the verity of nonmaleficence. These practitioners prefer not to expose the patient to the risks of surgery unless these are outweighed by the expected medical benefits. Moreover, if a patient were to suffer a complication such as hemorrhage requiring transfusion as a result of elective C-section, a physician could be held liable for an avoidable harm resulting from unnecessary surgery.

The key questions that arise when considering the ethics of elective C-section are to what degree a woman's request for cesarean is autonomous and, if it is, under what circumstances a request for this mode of delivery should be honored. The woman's degree of autonomy is dependent on another variable: her understanding of the relevant data and the voluntariness of her decision. Whether her request should be honored solely on grounds that it is autonomous depends on the invasiveness and risks associated with alternative modes of delivery. In the hands of experienced, competent physicians, surgery may be less invasive and risky than the alternatives. If the risk is greater but not high, respect for patient autonomy may nonetheless justify C-section for nonmedical reasons.

In none of the above cases is cesarean delivery as justified on medical grounds as it is in procedures that may reduce mortality as well as morbidity. While exploring delivery options, frank disclosure and discussion of the available data, disparate risks of surgical versus vaginal delivery, and efforts to reduce possible lack of understanding or anxiety are ethically warranted. However, as long as there is lack of clear evidence about the risks of C-section versus vaginal delivery, determining the method of delivery from the standpoint of the affected woman is paramount. Arguably, the standpoint of the potential child is relevant also, but the alternatives considered in these cases entail substantially equal risks and benefits for both the woman and her potential child.

Case 1 illustrates the link between a health-related rationale and a rationale related to other aspects of women's lives. Women themselves are prevalently aware of this linkage; inevitably and appropriately, it informs their standpoints. Avoidance of urinary or fecal incontinence is not typically considered a sufficient reason for major surgery instead of vaginal delivery, but if there were data demonstrating a greater risk of this problem through vaginal delivery, surgical delivery would be defensible on grounds that incontinence impedes one's quality of life. It would be even more justifiable for Carolyn Jacobs, whose career might be jeopardized by incontinence. However, the fact that incontinence is an impediment to any woman's quality of life argues for the importance of obtaining data that will either prove or disprove that vaginal delivery carries a greater risk of incontinence than C-section delivery.

The fact that Evelyn White in case 3 has already undergone vaginal delivery suggests that she is more informed about what this involves than she would otherwise be; this strengthens the argument for respecting her autonomy and privileging her standpoint. However, most obstetricians and many multiparous women are well aware that childbirth experiences can vary greatly in the same individual.[12] Adequate respect for autonomy requires the practitioner to inform the woman that, despite her previous experience, vaginal delivery in her current pregnancy could involve a much more positive experience and outcome than cesarean delivery. If the woman remains anxious about vaginal delivery, this in itself is medically relevant. At its extreme, a "bad birth" experience may result in a condition known as "tokophobia," and refusal of C-section for women with this condition has apparently triggered severe psychiatric problems.[13]

In the absence of the potential for psychiatric sequelae or other medical harms, is a physician justified in offering or performing a C-section solely on nonmedical grounds? By considering this question from the standpoint of the woman, a C-section performed to improve the birth experience is justifiable as long as its risks to her are minimal. Even if the woman's rationale is completely unrelated to her health, as in case 4, the benefit to her may be worth the medical risk, and her standpoint should be privileged in determining how one weighs against the other. Only if the medical risk is clearly high is the physician obliged, on professional as well as moral grounds, to refuse to perform the C-section.

Decisions for impaired or very premature newborns

Cases

1. A full-term infant born in Bloomington, Indiana, had esophageal atresia and Down syndrome (trisomy 21). The obstetrician told the parents they might either consent to surgery to correct the blockage or decline their consent and request that the infant not be fed so as not to prolong his dying. The parents chose the second course. On report of their plan to hospital lawyers, a legal opinion was sought at county and state levels. Both jurisdictions affirmed the obligation of practitioners to abide by the decision of the parents. Although an attempt was made to reverse the ruling by appeal to the U.S. Supreme Court, the baby died before a hearing could be held, at 6 days of age.[14]

2. At 22 weeks gestation, Clarisa Barnes is sent from the emergency department to the labor and delivery floor because doctors believe she is "threatening" to give birth. On arrival, the fetal torso and lower extremities are visible in her vagina. The obstetrics resident tells Clarisa she is having a miscarriage and should begin pushing to deliver the fetus. She does so and delivers a living but extremely premature infant. No efforts are made to extend the life of the newborn, who dies within 10 minutes of birth.[15]

3. At an estimated gestational age of 23 weeks and 3 days, a baby is delivered vaginally at a rural hospital and immediately intubated (breathing tube inserted into the trachea). Informed of the slim chance of survival, and probable morbidity if their daughter does survive, the parents, Max and Millie Mancini, ask the doctor to extubate (remove the breathing tube) to allow the baby to die.

4. Tamika LeMoyne, 32 years old, was referred to the medical center at 34 weeks gestation for evaluation of bilateral fetal hydronephrosis (swelling or dilated kidneys) and myelomeningocele (a severe form of spina bifida). Ultrasound examination confirmed these findings and showed, in addition, a triangular shaped head and cupping of the left ear, symptoms associated with the presence of an extra chromosome. Fetal weight was estimated at less than the tenth percentile for gestational age.[16] Amniocentesis was performed, revealing a male fetus with trisomy 13. Tamika was told that her fetus had a "lethal anomaly" for which treatment after birth was "inappropriate." Three weeks later, she delivered an infant with multiple anomalies and requested that "everything be done" to save her son.

Empirical considerations

Three variables are crucial to the newborn's prognosis in the above cases: duration of gestation, underlying health status, and availability of effective therapeutic options. Prematurity often brings health complications, but some premature infants have a better prognosis than infants who are delivered at term, and those born in or near tertiary care centers[17] usually have a better chance of survival than those born in rural settings, as in case 3. Even if the newborn in case 4 is treated aggressively with the best expertise and equipment available, he is unlikely to survive for long because his underlying life-threatening condition is incurable. Trisomy 13 is a genetic disorder that involves severe mental retardation, low birthweight, abnormal features, sensory deficits, and other health problems. Various cardiac abnormalities occur in about 80 percent of cases; myelomeningocele and hydronephrosis are also associated with the condition.[18] Infants who have any of the associated conditions, but not trisomy 13, are routinely treated after birth. In those with this anomaly, however, treatment for the associated problems is usually foregone unless it is deemed necessary for the child's comfort. The median survival for trisomy 13 is fewer than three days,[19] but some survive for months and, rarely, even years.

In contrast, the infant with Down syndrome in case 1 might have lived for many years if his esophageal atresia had been surgically corrected.[20] If this newborn did not have trisomy 21 and were otherwise healthy, the physician would probably have sought and obtained a court order authorizing the surgery over the parents' objection. Survival of a full-term infant with trisomy 21 and an operable life-threatening lesion is relatively easy to ensure unless there are other medical problems. In contrast, survival of the infant delivered at 22 weeks in case 2 would be extremely unlikely, no matter how aggressively treated, even if the child were chromosomally normal. Apparently, the physician in this case anticipated the newborn's demise and considered delivery unpreventable. Technically, Clarisa Barnes experienced premature labor and birth rather than a miscarriage. Clinical texts define miscarriage as spontaneous abortion or termination of pregnancy before 20 weeks of gestation.[21]

According to one neonatologist, infants born at 23 weeks gestation have a 10 to 15 percent survival rate, but rates of survival increase fairly rapidly after that. At 24 to 25 weeks, the chance of survival is about 40 to 60 percent, depending on the neonate's prior health status and available medical care.[22] Survival is not the only concern of practitioners and parents in decisions about very premature infants. About a third of these infants have serious medical problems such as cerebral palsy, hydrocephalus, seizures, neurological problems, or developmental delay; another third have chronic problems such as visual impairment or mild cerebral palsy. During their prolonged hospitalization, very premature infants are also at risk of intracranial hemorrhage and intestinal damage.[23] By 28 to 30 weeks gestation, the risk of these complications is much lower, and for infants born between 32 and 35 weeks, most medical problems are short term and may be resolved by the time they go home.

Regardless of gestational age, health status, and prognosis, every newborn is legally a person, who as such has as much right to medical treatment as any other person. In other words, infants are independently patients. In the United States, pregnant women enjoy relatively full legal rights to determine whether they are treated for the sake of their potential newborns, even after viability, but this right is limited once the fetus is externalized, when it is no longer a fetus but a newborn even if its remaining life span is severely limited. Regardless of parental consent, the law may mandate treatment of infants who are developmentally younger and sicker or more impaired than some fetuses. Birth is thus a crucial legal threshold; whether it should be so is morally debatable.

Theoretical considerations

The verities of nonmaleficence and beneficence toward newborn patients have priority in decisions made by parents or practitioners on their behalf. Respect for parental autonomy is ethically relevant, but not with the priority that respect for patient autonomy has in decisions made by pregnant women, who are directly affected by decisions about fetuses. After birth, an egalitarian perspective argues for respect for the father's autonomy as well as the mother's, but both are subordinated to the welfare of the newborn. In decisions that affect them directly, the interests of infant patients are paramount.

Admittedly, the interests of an infant are sometimes difficult to determine, even for parents who generally want what is best for their child. In case 1, however, the child's interests are fairly clear through data showing that most people with Down syndrome find life worth living.[24] Although the infant as such is unable to articulate his interests, the standpoint of the nondominant group to which he belongs, older children or adults with Down syndrome, should be given privileged status in determining his interests.

If their biological parents are unable or unwilling to raise them, infants with trisomy 21 may be adopted by others. During the six days of life of the infant described in case 1, a number of couples, including two who already had a child with Down syndrome, attempted to adopt him. Two years after the infant's death, federal (U.S.) legislation was passed to prevent other infants with impairments from being denied treatment routinely provided to other infants. This law, which remains in effect, views treatment refusal in such cases as discrimination against people with disabilities. Exceptions to the legal requirement to provide "medically indicated treatment" to all newborns are situations in which "the infant is irreversibly comatose or the treatment would be futile and inhumane or would only prolong dying."[25]

The other three cases are scenarios in which treatment may justifiably be denied on grounds of the infant's interests. In case 4, however, Tamika requests aggressive treatment for her son despite the high probability that treatment will be futile. Parental *insistence* on treatment that is not medically recommended is not unusual; it may occur more often than parental *refusal* of medical treatment for their children. Regardless of whether parents or practitioners insist on treatment, however, the primary verities to be implemented are beneficence and nonmaleficence toward the patient. Respect for the autonomy or welfare of others becomes ethically more compelling when the interests of the infant cannot be clearly determined, for example, when prolonging the newborn's life through treatment *may* be a greater burden to the infant than allowing him or her to die.

If it is impossible to determine whether treatment or nontreatment is best for the infant, parental decisions on behalf of the newborn should be given priority. Two reasons support this: parents are more likely than others to have the best interests of their child as their own priority, and they are more affected by the consequences of the decision than anyone except the infant. As long as the treatment that Tamika requests for her newborn does not entail a preponderance of harms over benefits to the child, it should therefore be provided. At whatever point (if any) it is clear that continued or new treatment is more detrimental than supportive of the infant's interests, her request should not be honored. Consistent with maxims 1 and 4, palliative treatment assumes a priority in cases in which an infant is suffering from an incurable, lethal anomaly such as trisomy 13.

The terms "lethal" and "futility," both used above, are open to different interpretations on the part of parents and practitioners. Although trisomy 13 is commonly described as "lethal," family members sometimes think this means that death will occur inevitably within hours or days. However, if in response to the parent's request "everything is done" in case 4, the infant will probably survive for a considerably longer period of time, and even this inevitably shortened duration of life may be a greater benefit for both parents and child than an earlier death. Considering such treatment "futile" seems to miss this possibility. The meaning of futility depends on the goals against which it is measured, and these may include quality as well as quantity of life factors. To forestall miscommunication with parents of impaired infants, physicians need to be explicit about what they mean when they use these terms. In case 4, for example, Tamika should be informed that about 10 percent of affected newborns survive past the first year of life.

In light of the extreme prematurity of the infants in cases 2 and 3, treatment was futile as measured against the single goal of survival beyond a few hours, with or without treatment. The likelihood of demise during parturition or immediately upon delivery in case 2 was so high that the physician apparently tried to shorten the duration of trauma to Clarisa as well as her infant by asking her to push. Although this was consistent with maxim 4, it neglected a key element of respect for Clarisa's autonomy—that is, that she be accurately informed of the medical situation. Had he explained his morally defensible request on grounds of reducing suffering to her newborn, instead of misleadingly characterizing what was happening as a miscarriage, respect for her autonomy would have been upheld.

Case 3 illustrates the priority that should be given to parental decisions as long as the interests of the infant are not clearly determinable. The principal ethical question here is whether being allowed to die is a kinder or more loving option for a severely impaired infant than is ongoing invasive, painful treatment that would prolong life without contributing anything to its quality. If this question cannot honestly be answered despite efforts to learn as much as possible about the anticipated outcome, either alternative is morally legitimate, and parents should be allowed to choose the one they think best for their child. On considering their options, Tamika and her husband may conclude that the preponderant experience of their newborn would probably consist of more harm than benefit to him if he is not extubated and allowed to die. In other words, treatment is more harmful than helpful in these circumstances. It may also be argued that the parents' own interests support extubation, since they may thereby avoid prolonged caregiving responsibilities. This argument is never adequate in its own right, but it may buttress the former argument, especially if the parents' capacity to care for other dependents would be severely taxed by new caregiving responsibilities.

Intubation is always appropriate if more time is needed to assess the situation. Extubation decisions are often more difficult emotionally, although the paramount ethical criterion is the same in both situations: the interests or standpoint of the patient. Too little information is provided in case 3 to tell whether extubation is justifiable on grounds of the infant's interests (maxim 1). Occasionally, but probably not in this case because of the extreme prematurity of the neonate, extubation is not followed by demise; parents need to be aware of this possibility, and practitioners should consider how they might respond to it. However, no physician should offer the option of extubation on grounds other than the infant's own interests. If prolonged intubation is associated with unrelievable pain and no realistic expectation of improvement, the physician should not only offer but recommend extubation. Continuing treatment in such circumstances does more harm than good to the infant patient.

Sex assignment at birth

Cases

1. Jill Brown, 30 years old, had two uncomplicated pregnancies before being referred to perinatal specialists during her third pregnancy. Ultrasound showed possible dysplastic (nonfunctional) kidneys and fetal anhydramnios (lack of amniotic fluid). The sex of the fetus was indeterminable. The infant to whom Jill subsequently gave birth had severe pulmonary hypoplasia (lung immaturity), no external genitalia, and no observable anus. After inspecting the infant, the obstetrician told Jill he could not definitively tell her the baby's sex. A neonatologist, also present at delivery, informed her that an emergency interdisciplinary evaluation would be initiated as soon as possible to help clarify the issue for the parents. While the evaluative work-up was being arranged, the baby was aggressively but unsuccessfully treated for pulmonary hypoplasia, from which the child succumbed during the first day of life.

2. George and Gladys Simpson, 36 and 30 years old, had been offered amniocentesis early in the third trimester of Gladys's pregnancy, after prenatal ultrasound failed to establish whether the fetus was male or female. The couple were informed of this uncertainty and that its possible explanations included abnormal enlargement of the clitoris or a small phallus and bifid (split) scrotum. Although Gladys declined amniocentesis at the time, she later changed her mind and requested the procedure prior to delivery. This prompted the obstetrics team to arrange for a genetics consultation at which the differential diagnoses were discussed with the couple. Amniocentesis was recommended and performed to avoid the delivery room/nursery confusion about assignment of gender and to facilitate efficient coordination of the relevant clinical work-up.

Empirical considerations

Unless the sex of their offspring has already been learned through prenatal diagnosis, the first statement that a physician often utters to parents after the birth of an infant is "It's a boy" or "It's a girl." "A healthy baby" may instead be the practitioner's first utterance, but if this is not linked to disclosure of the infant's sex, the question that immediately follows is "What is it, Doctor?" Given the importance to most people of learning the sex of a newborn, and the linguistic difficulty of talking about an infant (or any human being) without knowing this, the preceding cases illustrate the difficulty faced by clinicians when an infant is born with ambiguous or absent genitalia.

Ambiguous or atypical genitalia occurs about once in every 4,500 births.[26] Although sex is normally determined at fertilization, its physical expression is communicated through development of the gonads, which manufacture hormones crucial to the expression of genital tissues and structures specific to males or females. Any deviations along the route of development can cause ambiguous genitalia. One deviation is androgen insensitivity syndrome, in which fetal tissue does not respond to the stimulus of male hormones; another is congenital adrenal hyperplasia, in which excessive male hormones are produced. The former condition may lead to a newborn with both testicles and female reproductive organs, whereas the latter may produce an infant whose female genitals are masculinized. In some cases, an androgen-secreting tumor in the pregnant woman or lack of a particular enzyme in the placenta may trigger an excess of male hormones, resulting in the masculinization of a genetically female offspring. Chromosomal causes of atypical genitalia include combinations of male and female chromosomes, inactive genes on the Y chromosome, and attachment of a small Y segment to the X chromosome.[27] Presumably, these possibilities and their implications would be discussed with Jill Brown and Gladys and George in the cases sketched above.

Although the sex chromosomes of the majority of people are either XX or XY, other chromosomal arrangements occur in individuals who are unambiguously male or female. As mentioned in chapter 1, for example, Turner syndrome occurs in females who have only one X chromosome, and Klinefelter syndrome occurs in males who have an extra X along with their Y chromosome. Sex *assignment* appears necessary only in cases in which the phenotypic features that establish one's sex are not clearly discernible at birth.[28] The sex chromosomes in such cases may be XX or XY, but this may not be known at delivery, as in case 1. Even if it were known through amniocentesis, as in case 2, that information alone would not preclude a different sex assignment in an infant born with ambiguous genitalia.

Amniocentesis offers definitive diagnosis of chromosomal sex, but this could not be done in case 1 because of the anhydramnios. Even if it could be done, amniocentesis does not show whether a particular fetus has its full complement of male or female organs or genitalia. Ultrasound, especially late in gestation, is helpful but not definitive in this regard. In both of the above cases, physical exam in the birthroom might lead to a preliminary diagnosis, but further tests would be needed to confirm it. Hormone analysis, genetic tests, and X-ray analyses take several days or longer. Because surgical reconstruction is usually more successful in fashioning female genitalia, the usual recommendation for genetic males with ambiguous genitalia is that they be raised as females. Increasingly, however, the issue of whether sex assignment or reassignment is morally appropriate has been questioned on grounds that it is more harmful than helpful in the long run to the unconsenting patient. Contrary to the expectation of practitioners and the hope of parents they counseled, some individuals who underwent surgical reconstruction as infants and were raised according to an assigned gender different from their genetic or chromosomal sex claim they have been more hindered than helped by those early decisions.[29]

To those who distinguish between "sex" as biologically determined and "gender" as psychosocially determined, "gender assignment" describes decisions in these cases more accurately than "sex assignment." The "assignment" is intended to settle ambiguity about whether the infant should be raised as a boy or girl. At times it is a "reassignment" because the decision reverses an earlier designation of the child's sex, usually on grounds that the child will adapt more readily to the reassigned sex. From the standpoint of parents, "reassignment" exacerbates the confusion and anxiety they experience in these situations.

Whether clinicians learn about the possibility of ambiguous genitalia prior to or after birth is an important variable because learning sooner rather than later allows them to prepare, and help parents prepare, for the birthroom situation. Either prenatally or postnatally, a major responsibility from the standpoint of the attending physician is to facilitate decision-making by enlisting the assistance of a multidisciplinary team that includes pediatric endocrinology, genetics, neonatology, pediatric urology, and psychology. Karyotyping (chromosome analysis) should be done not only to determine the genetic sex but also to determine whether other anomalies may be present. Some experts recommend that the genetic sex not be disclosed to potential parents because they tend to "psychologically 'bond' to the chromosomal gender," making it more difficult for them to deal with a potentially different sex assignment after birth.[30] They also recommend that the infant be admitted to the newborn intensive care unit as "baby," not "baby boy" or "baby girl." The latter strategy is hardly likely to succeed in reducing anxiety in people who are unable to overcome the need to use gender-specific language or symbols (e.g., pink or blue hats or IDs).

Theoretical considerations

The very fact that sex or gender designation seems essential in the newborn setting attests to the practical need to develop ethically appropriate clinical strategies for dealing with these situations. Case 2 offers the possibility of preparing clinicians and parents ahead of time, but even with such preparation, these cases are emotionally as well as clinically and ethically difficult. Although truthful disclosure of what is known and not known is demanded by respect for autonomy, answering the question "What is it, Doctor?" truthfully may be at odds with nonmaleficence or beneficence toward parents. A truthful answer similar to the statement of Jill Brown's physician is "We don't know yet." Some experts recommend telling parents that their fetus or infant "has a sex that is incompletely developed and has yet to be determined."[31] Words alone, however, rarely communicate as fully or clearly as does the demeanor of the speaker. What is often forgotten in discussions of honest disclosure is that the manner of disclosure may determine whether an individual is harmed or helped through what is revealed. The same words used sensitively by one practitioner may be used insensitively by another: in one case diminishing the burden, in the other increasing it.

As maxim 1 suggests, the focus in the above cases ought to be the child whose sex or gender assignment will affect his or her entire life. "He" or "she" is surely the one whose standpoint is paramount, and parents' or clinicians' or anyone else's need to know the sex or gender of an offspring takes second place to this. A newborn with ambiguous genitalia is obviously unable to provide "informed consent" to tests, treatment, or sex assignment, and to the extent that this decision must be made as early as possible to maximize its therapeutic potential, parents have an a priori right and responsibility to decide what they think best for their child. Unless there is evidence that their decision opposes the infant's interests, their decision should be supported, not only because they are likely to have the child's best interests as their own objective but also because they themselves are more impacted by the decision than anyone other than the child.[32]

Although ambiguous genitalia is considered an impairment, it is a different type of impairment than those discussed in the previous section. Most important, the condition does not in itself constitute a threat to an individual's health or life, as does pulmonary hypoplasia in case 1. It is often but not always associated with infertility, but infertility is not a disability for some people, and it is treatable for others through various modes of reproductive assistance. A higher incidence of other medical problems is associated with atypical genitalia, some treatable and some not, but these problems also occur in individuals whose sex and gender are definitively established. Case 1 illustrates the importance of acknowledging that sex assignment is not as crucial as other medical needs of patients. The verity of beneficence often demands prioritizing health needs requiring intervention so that those most crucial to survival are treated first or most aggressively.

The development of secondary sex characteristics and the ability to have sexual intercourse may also be impaired by ambiguous genitalia, but here, too, medical interventions may overcome these deficits in individuals who are treated later in life. In recognition of the possibility that some individuals may not want the treatment when they are competent to make their own decisions, a key question from the clinician's standpoint is whether effective treatment may be deferred until then. If not, the presumption that a parental decision on their behalf should be supported is well-founded. In other words, respect for parental autonomy is probably consistent with respect for the autonomy of the future adult or mature adolescent, whose standpoint should be imputed privileged status.

From an egalitarian perspective, the linguistic and psychological need to know definitively the sex of a particular offspring is problematic in its own right because it thwarts recognition that people who have characteristics of both sexes, or phenotypes that don't match their chromosomal sex, are just as valuable as those who are clearly "he's" or "she's." Clinicians who care for infants with ambiguous genitalia and their parents thus face the dilemma of how to practice beneficence and respect for the autonomy of those who are personally affected while avoiding complicity in the discriminatory practices and attitudes associated with nonconformity to gender stereotypes. This dilemma is not adequately resolvable through arguments for one position or the other because clinicians are morally and professionally obliged to do what is best for a particular infant in a way that takes account of societal and parental limitations, including social prejudice. Fulfillment of this responsibility inevitably risks complicity in prejudice. But clinicians are also moral agents and citizens whose clinical commitments do not excuse them from responsibility to promote justice or at least reduce the injustice of discrimination in their community.

Partial resolution of this dilemma may require a kind of schizophrenic ethic, that is, one in which the clinician does one thing in the clinic and another in political or social life. Accordingly, in the clinical setting a practitioner may recommend sex assignment that theoretically condones sex or gender stereotypes that the same practitioner opposes and attempts to reduce in public venues—for example, by supporting equal rights for gay and lesbian individuals. From an egalitarian perspective, treatment should not be withheld from an individual for whom such treatment appears to be the only way by which to avoid the disadvantages associated with heterosexism. Dominant individuals who support gender justice in public policies are not thereby entitled to hold nondominant individuals hostage to their political critique.

Many of the cases considered in this chapter deal with newborns rather than fetuses, but there can be a great deal of ethical complexity in decisions made immediately after birth as well as prior to it. Choices about modes of delivery are complicated by the fact that both the potential child and the pregnant woman are affected by what is done or not done, and burdens and benefits to both are therefore, unavoidably, ethically relevant. The variables illustrated in the cases discussed are merely suggestive of the complexity that real people face in the highly charged settings in which women deliver babies.

Depending on one's position about the moral status of the fetus, resolution of cases involving fetuses, even term fetuses, may be decided quite differently than cases involving newborns, no matter how impaired or premature they are. For those who impute full moral status to the fetus, at least at term, respect for the pregnant woman's autonomy is clearly less compelling than the obligation to avoid serious harm to the potential child. This does not imply that respect for the woman's autonomy is ignored; it simply means that this verity doesn't outweigh the others in this instance. As suggested earlier, *respect* for autonomy doesn't dictate blind conformity to the woman's wishes; rather, it demands careful consideration of her wishes in an effort to balance their moral weight against the interests of the potential child, and sometimes against her health interests also. For those who attribute full moral status to the newborn but deny it to fetuses, the woman's autonomy will typically be given priority until the fetus is externalized. At that point, for practitioners as well as parents, decisions about newborns, regardless of their gestational age, health status, gender, or expected life span, should center on the child's own standpoint or interests.

8

Treatment of Minors

The "age of majority" generally refers to the age at which, from a legal perspective, a person has all of the rights and responsibilities of an adult. When this occurs varies in different jurisdictions, times, and cultures and may be different for some decisions than for others (e.g., marriage eligibility, voting age). Across the globe, the onset generally ranges from 14 to 18 years of age. A "minor" is one who has not yet reached the age of majority and who, as such, is more deserving of protection before the law than an adult.

A person who is legally an adult is assumed to have decisional capacity—that is, the ability to understand alternatives and their implications, choose one, and assume responsibility for the consequences of her choice. If the decisional capacity of an adult is in doubt, the matter must be adjudicated, and if she is found lacking its essential elements, a guardian may be appointed by the court to make decisions in her best interests. Parents are usually the legally appointed guardians of adult children who are decisionally incapacitated.

Age is an indicator of the probability of competence, and in some cases (infants and very young children) it is a definitive indicator of the lack of decisional capacity. With older children and adolescents, age is not definitive of their capacity for moral decision-making.[1] Other variables, such as reasoning ability, knowledge, emotional stability, experiences the child has had, and the complexity of the content to be decided on, may hinder or enhance this capacity, just as they do in adults. Some adolescents are as psychologically mature as some adults, and some adults are less mature than some adolescents. From a practitioner's standpoint, the moral challenge entailed by respect for autonomy is to recognize whatever capacity for moral decisions is present in any patient of any age. To the extent that this is lacking in minors, beneficence and nonmaleficence toward them have priority, and respect for their parents' autonomy is a means by which to determine this. Parents are surrogate decision makers for their children; as such, they are assumed to act in their child's best interests, but if they do not, their decisions may be legally and morally overridden. As with other patients, the standpoint of minors who are patients also deserves privileged status.

The terms "assent," "dissent," and "consent" are applicable to different levels of competence for decision-making. "Consent" requires that the decision maker be adequately informed of the available alternatives and their implications, free of constraints in making her decision, and able to communicate it to others. "Dissent" refers to the ability of minors not yet capable of consent to refuse treatment that is not necessary for their own health, such as genetic testing for late-onset or untreatable disorders or organ donation to a sibling. "Assent" refers to the capacity of a minor to agree, while lacking full autonomy or full understanding, to medically recommended treatment for herself or others. For those who are clearly immature, assent is desirable as a means by which to respect their developing autonomy; in most cases, it is neither legally nor morally obligatory for treating them.

Exceptions to the legal requirement of parental consent for treatment of minors are situations in which their consent is impossible or obtaining it could be prejudicial to their interests. Examples of these exceptions are requests by teenagers for contraception or abortion, treatment of sexually transmitted diseases (STDs), and drug treatment. Parental notification is sometimes required for abortion, but in most jurisdictions a judge may override this requirement if the adolescent's welfare is threatened by notification. As stipulated by maxim 1, the patient's interests have priority over respect for the autonomy of surrogate decision makers.

In the United States, two legal designations are relevant to clinical decisions regarding treatment of teenagers: emancipated minor status and the mature minor principle. Interpretations of these designations differ among the states. In general, however, emancipated minors are entitled to be treated as adults because they have assumed adult responsibilities such as economic independence, marriage, or motherhood. Mature minors are those to whom decisional capacity may be legally imputed when parental consent to medical care for them is unobtainable or undesirable.[2]

Most of the cases in this chapter deal with minors whose capacity for moral decision-making is uncertain or problematic. Although the topics considered are often applicable to adults as well, I include them here because they occur more often or are more complicated when the patient is a minor.

Teenage pregnancy and motherhood

Cases

1. Eva Castro is a 15-year-old high school sophomore who is popular, bright, and pregnant after her first sexual encounter with her 16-year-old boyfriend, Carl. After missing her period she performed an over-the-counter pregnancy test on herself. When she told Carl and her parents about the positive result, they encouraged her to have an abortion. Neither teenager was interested in marriage, but Eva was unsure about abortion. Her mother scheduled a visit with her own physician and called ahead to ask him to tell her daughter how risky it is to have a child at such a young age, and how unfair it would be to the child to have only one parent. After confirming the pregnancy, the doctor did not tell Eva what her mother wanted him to say. Instead, he told her she had three options to think about, any of which he would help her pursue: "abortion, adoption, or keep and raise the child with your parents' assistance."

2. Loretta Adams is a 16-year-old Caucasian who supported herself through prostitution after her single mother died from a drug overdose. Four months ago, Loretta gave birth to an infant with a large ventricular septal defect (VSD). Chromosome studies were ordered, yielding a diagnosis of trisomy 18. Because the newborn was relatively stable, Loretta was told that "aggressive" treatment would be inappropriate because of the infant's "lethal" anomaly. She took her daughter home where she apparently cared for her adequately. Four months later, she brought her to the clinic because her condition seemed to have deteriorated. The infant was diagnosed with congestive heart failure. Loretta wanted her treated, but the doctors opposed the surgery because of the infant's underlying anomaly.

3. Pat Quinn was a 14-year-old African American who, along with her 16-year-old brother, had been raised by her 70-year-old grandmother since she was 2 years old. Pat's mother was a drug addict who had not seen her children in ten years. The grandmother had legal custody of both children. Based on testing at the special school she attended, Pat had a mental age of 7 years. During a routine visit to the clinic, she underwent a physical exam that showed, unexpectedly, that she was about 2 months pregnant. Options of termination, adoption, or raising the infant were discussed with the grandmother, who, when asked if she knew "how this happened," acknowledged that her grandson might have been sexually active with his sister. The grandmother stated that she wanted Pat to continue the pregnancy and give the baby up for adoption. At this point in her life, she said, she did not feel able to raise another child herself.

Empirical considerations

Although the incidence of teenage pregnancies has declined in recent years in the United States,[3] it remains a matter of concern because of its social and health risks to adolescents and their children. Births to girls younger than 15 constitute a small fraction of all live births. Births to older teenagers, most of whom are 18 or 19 years old, constitute about 11 percent of live births.[4] The health hazards of pregnancy for teenagers are mainly applicable to the younger age group; these include toxemia, ruptured placenta, and complications associated with immaturity of the pelvis. For older adolescents, the health risks of pregnancy are comparable to those of pregnant women in their twenties but less than those of pregnant women over 30 years of age.

For most pregnant teenagers, the social risks of childbearing are greater than the physiological risk because they are likely to have more children and less education than their nonpregnant peers, with concomitant economic hardships such as welfare dependency. These social risks have negative impact on the teenager's overall health, even as they do on the health of pregnant and nonpregnant adults. Adolescents who undergo abortions generally fare better educationally, economically, and emotionally than those who continue their pregnancies to term. According to one study, they also fare better than teenagers who believe they are pregnant but later find out that they are not.[5]

Children of adolescents face increased risks of preterm birth and low birth weight, decreased growth rate, low IQ, suboptimal school achievement, disordered behavior, and interactional difficulties between them and their mothers.[6] Like trisomies 13 and 21, trisomy 18 is associated with older mothers, but its incidence (1 in 6,000–8,000 live births)[7] is higher in newborns of younger women because more children are born to them and they are less likely than older women to undergo prenatal testing and termination of affected fetuses. Prominent among the effects of trisomy 18 are severe cognitive impairment, anomalies of appearance, generalized muscle spasticity, renal anomalies, and cardiac defects. Feeding is often difficult because of some of these anomalies. The median survival time for affected newborns is four days, and only about 10 percent survive beyond the first year of life, usually because of cardiac problems.[8] Invasive treatment for life-threatening problems is routinely withheld, and "comfort measures only" are recommended when these occur. Although trisomy 18 is considered "lethal," survival for years has been reported in rare cases.

VSD, the most common of all congenital heart defects, involves an opening between the lower chambers of the heart. Although the opening prevents the heart from pumping blood correctly, it often closes on its own during the first few weeks of life. Practitioners usually refrain from treatment to allow this to occur. As in case 2, however, if closure does not occur naturally, symptoms of congestive heart failure develop, making corrective surgery necessary for survival.

With regard to case 3, the pain and discomfort of childbirth would probably be greater for Pat Quinn than for someone who is mentally able to appreciate the transiency and purpose of the experience. Late in gestation, the pain and risks of an abortion are comparable to those of childbirth, but at 3 months gestation it involves fewer risks than continuing the pregnancy and giving birth. If Pat's pregnancy continues, the child to whom she gives birth has greater risk of genetic anomalies than one conceived by someone who is not cognitively impaired or incestuously related to the potential father. It is not at all certain, however, that her child will have any serious impairment. Mentally and physically healthy people who are genetically unrelated sometimes face considerably higher risks of having children with a severe genetic disorder. Probably the greatest risk to the potential child in this case is the socioeconomically disadvantaged situation in which he or she is likely to be raised—a set of liabilities similar to those to which Pat and her brother have been exposed.

In the United States, there is an unmet demand for Caucasian infants to be adopted, but considerably less demand when the infant is African American. Further factors that reduce the likelihood of adoption in case 3 include Pat's cognitive impairment and the possibility of incest, which may be confirmed or disconfirmed through DNA testing. If her impairment is due to a genetic abnormality, the possibility of bearing a similarly impaired child is greater regardless of whether her pregnancy is due to incest. Most incestuous pregnancies are electively terminated, but those that are brought to term may result in healthy babies. The majority of infants conceived through "close consanguineous matings" are relinquished for adoption despite the high empiric risk of severe abnormalities.[9] Presumably, many of the adopted infants do not exhibit these abnormalities at birth.

Theoretical considerations

These three cases illustrate the obvious but important fact that teenagers are not all the same. Just as adults differ in intelligence, maturity, socioeconomic circumstances, and life goals, so do they. All of these factors contribute to different standpoints from which decisions are made about health care. Although the interests of the patient has priority (maxim 1), an adolescent's interests are sometimes inseparable from those of other family members, as in case 3; at other times members of the same family have conflicting interests, but each is a patient of the same physician, as in case 1. Confidentiality, addressed in the next section, is at stake as well. Maxim 1 is operable in these cases, but different positions on moral status may point to different conclusions regarding whose interests count most.

Eva Castro's doctor privileged her standpoint when he told her about her three legal options. Even if the physician is unwilling to perform an abortion and may know little about how to arrange an adoption, he should facilitate his patient's access to relevant information about her options. Maxim 1 gives priority to the interests of the pregnant teenager vis-à-vis her partner and her parents, but whether this overrides the interests of the potential child depends on whether the fetus is accorded moral status in its own right.

Although she is only 16 years of age, Loretta Adams may well be more mature than some of her older counterparts. Nonetheless, she is obviously in a nondominant position not only because of her age but also because of her psychosocial circumstances. Deprived of family supports, Loretta has demonstrated an ability to survive on her own, albeit through prostitution, and to care for a newborn with significant needs and an exceedingly grim prognosis. Legally, her status is that of an "emancipated minor" who is entitled thereby to make decisions on behalf of her child. Morally, Loretta's standpoint regarding surgery to close the opening in her daughter's heart should be as privileged as it would be for an adult parent. Only if the surgery is clearly opposed to the infant's own interests should the surgery be withheld (maxim 1). From an egalitarian perspective, the infant patient has as compelling a right to aggressive treatment as does an adult patient with a comparably limited expectation of survival.

Respect for autonomy is inapplicable to Pat Quinn because she is decisionally incapacitated. In such cases, beneficence and nonmaleficence toward the patient have priority, potentially overriding the autonomy of parents or guardians (maxim 1). For those who support a minimalist account of personhood, however, this priority does not settle the matter. As in case 1, clinicians who hold this view should disclose it to those to whom it is pertinent, so that they may seek treatment elsewhere if they choose.

From the standpoint of clinicians who support a woman's right to abortion, the crucial question in case 3 is whether termination or continuation of pregnancy is in the best interests of the impaired patient. Answering this question requires consideration of the health risks of gestation and childbirth to Pat, as well as the impact of the decision on her welfare. Because she depends on her grandmother for her care, the grandmother's wishes are inseparable from Pat's welfare. The risk of sexual abuse by her brother (or anyone else) must be adequately addressed to ensure her safety; he also has needs for caregivers to identify and address. While considering removal of Pat from her home, however, it should be recognized that Pat's interests may be better served through her grandmother's ongoing care of her than through institutional or foster placement. Even a dysfunctional family may be preferable to a situation in which there is no indefinite commitment to care.

Having raised her granddaughter for over a decade, Pat's grandmother is probably more able than others to communicate with her granddaughter and to assist her in dealing with pregnancy and childbirth, but she is apparently unwilling to support her having an abortion. In light of her desire that her potential grandchild be adopted, the grandmother should be informed that racial factors and genetic risks decrease the likelihood that this will occur. Alternatives to adoption and abortion (e.g., assistance in raising the child, placement with another relative, institutional or foster placement) should also be explained.

Confidentiality issues

Cases

1. Tricia Johnson is a 17-year-old who was admitted to the hospital with fever, pelvic pain, and an examination consistent with pelvic inflammatory disease (PID). After 36 hours of intravenous antibiotics, she began to improve. Cultures taken of her cervix were positive for gonorrhea and chlamydia, confirming that her pelvic infection was sexually transmitted. In the absence of her parents, the practitioner had a frank discussion with Tricia about the implications of PID and other STDs for her future health and fertility. Tricia asked that the etiology of her diagnosis not be disclosed to her parents. Because her hospitalization would be covered on her parents' insurance plan, she worried that this might result in their learning why she was treated. When the gynecologist left the room, Tricia's mother asked him: "What is going on with my daughter?"

2. Jamie Jones, 15 years old, was admitted to the pediatric intensive care unit after being found unconscious on the floor of her bedroom with an empty bottle of aspirin next to her. While treating her condition as a suicide attempt, the staff discovers through routine tests that Jamie is pregnant. The attending physician wonders whether to reveal this to Jamie's parents and whether, if he does, he needs Jamie's consent to do so. He also wonders whether Jamie's sexual partner has a right to be informed of the pregnancy.

3. Kim Sawicki is a precocious 14-year-old who visits the pediatrician's office after school to arrange for an appointment. One of the doctors recognizes her and asks how she is. She says she would like to get a prescription for birth control and adds: "Please don't tell my parents." The physician agrees but tells Kim she needs to be examined first. In the interim between this encounter and the appointment, Kim's mother takes her toddler, Kim's sibling, for a check-up, and asks the doctor whether Kim has stopped in to see her recently.

4. Caroline Gandy, 15 years old, is examined by a gynecologist to explore whether there is any medical reason to worry about why she has not yet had a period. Her exam and testing reveal that she does not have a uterus and has an XY genotype, consistent with androgen insensitivity syndrome (AIS). The physician wonders whether he should disclose this information and its implications to Caroline or to her parents.

5. Sue Ryan, nearly 18, has never dated or been sexually attracted to boys, despite encouragement by her parents in that regard. She has felt particularly attracted to Melissa, one of her classmates, who is equally uninterested in boys. At her annual check-up, Sue confides to her physician that she thinks she may be gay. "If I am," she says, this would greatly disturb her parents and make her life "more difficult than it is already." She wonders if anything can be done to help her shift what appears to be her same sex orientation to an orientation towards the opposite sex.

Empirical considerations

Although all of these cases involve the sexuality of adolescents, the health risks posed by them vary considerably. Tricia Johnson has two STDs and has become severely symptomatic. Kim Sawicki appears healthy but is probably at risk of STDs through current or anticipated heterosexual activity. The risks faced by Caroline Gandy and Sue Ryan are mainly psychosocial; as such, they may be impossible to address adequately through medical expertise. Jamie Jones is probably at greatest risk because of her apparent suicide attempt.

Chlamydia and gonorrhea are the most commonly reported bacterial sexually transmitted infections. Both are especially prevalent in younger age groups (e.g., 15–24 years), but treatable through antibiotics. The actual incidence of chlamydia is probably much higher than its reported incidence because three-quarters of infected women and one-half of infected men have no symptoms and therefore do not seek testing until complications develop.[10] In contrast, gonorrhea generally becomes symptomatic within two to ten days after sexual contact with an affected partner. If left untreated, both conditions lead to reproductive and other health problems. Women with untreated STDs have a high risk of pelvic inflammatory disease, which may permanently damage the fallopian tubes, uterus, and tissues surrounding the ovaries. Additional risks include chronic pelvic pain, premature birth, and transmission of these infections to newborns.

In the United States, suicide is the third leading cause of death in adolescents from ages 15 to 24, surpassed only by car accidents and homicide.[11] In the past three decades, while the general incidence of suicide has decreased, the rate for this age group has tripled, in part because of increased availability of drugs and guns. Attempts to commit suicide may be triggered by traumatic or stressful events, such as Jamie Jones's unexpected pregnancy, or by long-standing depression and substance abuse. Girls tend to attempt suicide by cutting themselves or overdosing on drugs and are about twice as likely as boys to attempt suicide. Boys tend to choose more sudden and decisive methods such as firearms or hanging and therefore "succeed" in their attempts three or four times more often than girls. No matter what the method, any suicide attempt indicates a need for professional help.[12]

Androgen insensitivity syndrome (AIS) occurs in about 1 in 20,400 XY births but may not be detected until the affected individual reaches puberty.[13] As discussed in chapter 7, the condition is caused by the inability of a chromosomally male (XY) fetus to respond to the hormones necessary to produce the external male genitalia. The testes develop internally (and female organs do not develop internally), but the external genitalia develop along female lines. As a result, the reproductive organs and genitalia do not match the genetic sex. Because it is a recessive, X-linked condition, women who are carriers have a 1 in 2 chance that any XY child will have AIS and a 1 in 2 chance that any XX child will be a carrier. Treatment generally involves hormone replacement therapy and psychosocial support.

Teenagers who are lesbian, gay, bisexual, or unsure about their sexual orientation, as in case 5, are at greater risk than their peers of substance abuse, depression, and suicide. Most studies regarding the prevalence of homosexuality (5%–10%) involve adults, but these figures are considered applicable to adolescents also.[14] Realization of a homosexual orientation often starts with the absence of attraction toward the opposite sex, and efforts to develop that attraction or suppress the attraction to one's own sex are not uncommon. Fear of ridicule, rejection, and hostility leads many adolescents to hide their homosexual tendencies from others, including clinicians. The fact that Sue has revealed her worry to her doctor provides him with a crucial opportunity to advise her about health risks and facilitate contact with professionals who may help her. Regardless of her sexual orientation, Sue's willingness to seek care is probably dependent on her expectation that confidentiality about these concerns will be strictly observed.

Theoretical considerations

According to the American Academy of Pediatrics, "the issue of confidentiality has been identified, by both providers and young people themselves, as a significant access barrier to health care."[15] Typically, this issue arises in the context of the adolescent's desire that her parents remain unaware of the problem that brought her to the health care system. She is anxious about how her parents would react to this information. Tricia Johnson and Kim Sawicki, for example, may worry that disclosure to their parents would incur their anger, punitive measures, and interference with their intended sexual activity. The efforts of adolescents to avoid disclosure of medical information to parents may also be based on concern for the parents themselves; Sue Ryan, in case 5, explicitly expresses this rationale.

Ethically significant variables in case 2 are not applicable to the other cases: Jamie Jones was apparently suicidal and is currently unconscious as well as pregnant. From a clinical standpoint, the knowledge that a patient is pregnant is pertinent to determination of how to optimally treat her in a way that also minimizes the possibility of harm to her potential child. The option of continuing the pregnancy should be preserved at least until Jamie herself can make a decision in this regard. Parental consent to treatment does not require that the parents be informed of the pregnancy, and Jamie herself should be the determiner of who if anyone is told about this after she recovers consciousness. As with other patients, her standpoint should be privileged regarding disclosure of medical information about her.

The practice of confidentiality imputes privileged status to the standpoint of those who have a need or right to privacy in decisions that affect them alone or only minimally affect others. Although confidentiality toward minors is not legally required for some health care issues, it is morally obligatory if the adolescent is capable of responsible decision-making. From an egalitarian perspective, confidentiality may and should be overridden if its risks or harms to others outweigh its potential benefit to a patient of any age (maxim 4). For teenagers, the expectation of confidentiality is particularly important to encourage honest and adequate communication with their clinicians, facilitating correct diagnosis and effective treatment. In other words, confidentiality serves both therapeutic and ethical purposes.

From the standpoint of caregivers, the question of whether to respect confidentiality often arises from conflicting priorities of different family members. While treating several patients from the same family, the practitioner has an a priori obligation of confidentiality toward each one as an individual. If questions raised by a parent are answered with that priority in mind, the physician may simply indicate that he is unable to answer because he is professionally bound to observe confidentiality, even toward patients who are minors. A common ethical strategy in such situations is to suggest that the parent talk with her daughter about the matter. However, it is sometimes practically impossible to avoid parents' interpretation of a clinician's efforts to preserve confidentiality as tantamount to disclosure. In case 3, for example, if the physician declines to answer the mother's question, she may conclude that her daughter has seen the doctor. But if the physician tells the mother she is not legally permitted to answer questions about patients, even to family members, she fulfills her obligation of confidentiality to Kim without lying. Lying to preserve confidentiality is neither legally nor morally required; whether it is ever permissible has long been debated by moral philosophers.[16]

In case 1, the practical exigency of insurance coverage may make it impossible to avoid parental access to information regarding Tricia's condition. However, the physician would fulfill her obligation of confidentiality by advising the teenager of this probability, and, if it is realistic, the possibility of cash payment in installments by the teenager.

As already mentioned, the law often allows teenagers to seek some forms of treatment without parental consent. In situations such as cases 4 and 5, however, the law offers little counsel. Concerns about confidentiality in these cases mainly stem from the potential harms of social stereotypes regarding gender identity and sexual orientation. Caroline's physician apparently recognizes this harmful potential when he questions whether to disclose information about her genotype to her parents, as well as whether to disclose it to the patient herself. Regarding Caroline, however, respect for a competent patient's autonomy requires disclosure of information that may harm as well as help her, and confidentiality toward his patient clearly has priority over disclosure to her parents.

When and how potentially harmful or hurtful information should be disclosed also needs to be considered by the clinician. If Caroline has a good relationship with her parents, disclosure to them first, or disclosure to them and Caroline together, may reduce the harms or hurts to her through their support. Either approach could be justified on grounds of her probable consent. However, if her parents are unlikely to be supportive or if Caroline would probably object to this mode of disclosure, her consent should not be presumed. Her standpoint is privileged not only on grounds that she is the patient but also on grounds that she is a minor.

Sue Ryan is legally a minor but appears to be as able as many adults to understand and deal with the probability that she is "gay." Counseling should be recommended to assist Sue in clarifying the situation for herself. Her physician has an important educative role to fulfill by informing her that homosexuality does not call for medical interventions because it is not a disease but a condition that occurs naturally in some people. If after counseling Sue concludes that she is "gay," additional supports should be recommended to help her deal with the stigmatization and psychosocial burdens that are associated with a same-sex orientation. If she persists in wanting to avail herself of means by which to "shift" her orientation, this should be explored only as a totally elective, experimental option. Family support should be encouraged, but Sue alone should be the determiner of who, if anyone, learns about her sexual orientation.

In all of these cases, maxim 1 is operable because the interests of teenage patients include promotion of their welfare and of their developing autonomy. In general, however, decisions about whether to uphold or breach confidentiality should be based on whether they maximize all of the verities toward all of those affected, with justice the criterion for prioritization in situations of conflict.

Ritual female genital surgery

Cases

1. Fauziya Kasinga, a 19-year-old woman from Togo, sought asylum in the United States on grounds that she would be forced to undergo removal of her external genitalia if she returned to her country of origin. In Togo, the procedure was usually performed with crude, unsterile objects and no anesthesia. The U.S. authorities were concerned that an affirmative response would incite other women to seek asylum to avoid genital surgery. They also wondered whether permission in this case implied that potential victims of other culturally sanctioned treatments such as government-forced abortions in China or spousal violence in some Latin American and Muslim countries should be granted asylum, if requested.[17]

2. Zara Ali Muku brought her two daughters, ages 5 and 7, to the clinic and asked that they be "circumcised" before returning to Somalia, where this would otherwise be done in her home village. If the procedure was performed here, she said, her daughters would experience much less pain and risk of complications than she had experienced when she underwent the surgery. Although the practitioner told Zara he could not legally perform the procedure, he questioned its illegality on moral grounds. He believed he would prevent greater harm to the children if he performed the surgery in his clinic under safe and sanitary conditions that the children would not have access to in Somalia.

3. Nisha Al-Najar, a 17-year-old, fully veiled young woman from Yemen, came to the clinic and, with her aunt serving as interpreter, told the nurse practitioner that she had severe pain in her abdomen, especially during menstruation. She said her menstrual blood seemed to get stuck, and she had recently noted a white discharge. Thinking that her problems might be related to previous genital surgery, the practitioner said, "I know that some women in your culture have been closed, and sometimes this causes problems like you're experiencing. Were you closed?" In the conversation that followed, the clinician learned that Nisha had undergone infibulation (a type of genital surgery) as an 8-year-old and now had a slow urinary stream. On physical exam, the practitioner observed that Nisha's introitus (entrance to the vagina) was only 5 mm wide, and she had a budding yeast infection with fungal growth. Through treatment with antifungal and anti-inflammatory medications Nisha's pain and discomfort were soon resolved. At a subsequent appointment, ultrasound indicated that she had no retention or accumulation of blood in the vagina. Although she was advised that she could have either defibulation or stretching of her introitus to avoid the recurrence of her problems, Nisha refused both procedures.[18]

4. Eglal Ellighani, an 18-year-old Sudanese woman came to a refugee clinic to have health forms filled out for acceptance in a course on English as a second language. Although she had not been sexually active, she indicated that she had been "circumcised" as a young child. The physician told Eglal that if she were "opened" prior to her first intercourse, the experience would be less traumatic than it might otherwise be. Two weeks later, she returned to the clinic with a man she introduced as her future husband. Eglal said she wanted to be "opened" because her friends had told her that their first intercourse with their husbands had caused considerable pain, bleeding, and other problems.

Empirical considerations

Traditional or ritual genital surgery is practiced widely in parts of Africa; 80 percent of women who emigrate to the United States and Canada from these areas have already undergone the surgery.[19] As in case 2, they occasionally seek genital surgery for their daughters. If immigrant women have not undergone the surgery, as in case 1, they may request asylum in order to avoid it if they return to their home village. Within cultures that endorse the practice, the procedure is often enforced and performed by women on young girls.[20]

The practice of female genital surgery is sometimes referred to as "female circumcision," but the procedure is quite different from male circumcision. Although often considered an Islamic tradition, the practice predates Islam and is not prescribed by the Koran.[21] The principal forms of female genital surgery are excision, which entails cutting or removing part or all of the clitoris, with or without the labia minora and majora; and infibulation (sometimes called radical circumcision), in which, after the excision, the introitus is sutured closed, leaving a small opening for passage of urine and menstrual blood. Local customs dictate the timing and type of procedure performed. Defibulation, cutting or tearing open the scarred vaginal tissue, occurs partially when an infibulated woman has intercourse and more extensively when she gives birth. In many cultures, a husband difibulates his bride after seeing that she is a virgin.

In the home countries of women who undergo ritual genital surgery, the procedure is usually performed by a medically untrained person without anesthesia and with poor or nonsterile equipment. Beyond the trauma of the surgery itself, more than half of those circumcised experience medical complications, especially from infibulation. Harmful consequences often include painful urination or intercourse, blockage of urine and menstrual blood, urinary and vaginal infections, diminished sexual sensation, and obstetric complications. As illustrated in cases 3 and 4, defibulation prior to intercourse and vaginal infections are reasons that circumcised women may seek health care. Despite its risks, the practice of female genital surgery persists not only because it is sometimes (mistakenly) considered a religious obligation but also because it is thought necessary for cleanliness and beautification. Further reasons are its requirement for acceptance by one's social group, as evidence of virginity before marriage, and to increase male sexual satisfaction.[22] Some sexually active, unmarried women are reinfubulated to create a false appearance of virginity.

Theoretical considerations

All of these cases raise the difficult question of how to respect the autonomy of individuals whose identity and values are apparently inseparable from the cultures that have nurtured them. From an egalitarian perspective, the standpoints of women from different cultures should be as privileged, and sometimes more privileged, than those of women who belong to the dominant culture. The practitioners in cases 3 and 4 show respect for the cultural values of their patients through nonjudgmental responses to their refusal of treatment based on western standards. In doing so, they acknowledge that the patient's standpoint is privileged with regard to that of her culture if the two are at odds. Legal and ethical limits to their support for cultural differences are nonetheless necessary if the practice endorsed by the culture is at odds with the patient's own welfare or wishes, or if it disproportionately impedes the autonomy or welfare of others.

Although Fauziya Kasinga is still in her teens, she is legally an adult in most parts of the world. Had she requested genital surgery so that she could return to her native Togo without fear of having to undergo the procedure in a nonsterile environment with no anesthesia, her physician in the United States could have legally and morally responded affirmatively to her request. Maxims 1 and 2 would support this response, making the procedure permissible but not obligatory. However, the chief question raised by this case is not whether to treat or not treat Fauziya electively, but whether she should be granted asylum as a means of avoiding the procedure. This question is mainly one for governmental authorities, whose responsibility extends to all whom their policy decisions affect. The verity that must guide these decisions is that of justice. Clinicians fulfill their responsibility with regard to social justice by providing policy makers with adequate and accurate medical information relevant to potential policies. In this case, for example, the physician could inform them of the risks of genital surgery performed in an African village setting as opposed to the risks of performing the same procedure in his clinic.

At times, social justice requires that the interests of the individual be subordinated to those of the majority. In light of that priority and unless countervailing variables are introduced, asylum should be granted not only to Fauziya but also to other women who face the risk of coercive genital surgery and those who, without asylum, face credible risks of forced abortion or spousal violence. From an egalitarian perspective, the minimal economic cost to the public of providing asylum in such circumstances is outweighed by the benefits of its provision to those who seek it.

Regarding case 2, "circumcision" of children aged 5 and 7 is illegal in most countries. Respect for parental autonomy in treatment decisions regarding their minor offspring should be overridden if the treatment they request is more likely to harm than help the child (maxim 3). As the physician in this case recognizes, performing the procedure prior to the return to Somalia would probably prevent greater medical harms and risks to the children than they would face if the circumcisions were performed in their home village. The case thus illustrates the problematic relationship that sometimes occurs between law and ethics.

Whether an individual practitioner may or should violate a law in order to promote the interests of an individual patient is a larger question than I can adequately consider here. Moral heroes such as Mohandas Gandhi and Martin Luther King Jr. have argued that unjust laws may (morally) be broken and at times should be broken on grounds of fidelity to a higher, just law. On that account, genital surgery *may* be morally justified in case 2 despite its illegality, but more variables need to be examined to determine whether the verity of justice also supports the intervention. Relevant variables include the implications of this decision for other potential patients, the degree of certainty that the family will in fact return to Somalia, and the possibility of postponing the decision until the children are old enough to decide for themselves. Because the children in this case are least dominant and most at risk, their standpoint should be recognized as privileged, and their interests should be given priority (maxim 1).

Although Nisha, the patient described in case 3, is two years younger than Fauziya (case 1), the younger teenager may in fact be more mature and capable of autonomy than her older counterpart. In their native countries, both would probably be considered adults, and in any country, the moral obligation to respect autonomy applies to both. In the United States, the provider could probably offer legal justification for treatment of the 17-year-old on grounds of the aunt's consent "in loco parentis," as well as on grounds of Nisha's apparent competence for consent to necessary treatment. If parental consent is unavailable and treatment is not postponable, maxim 2 calls for its provision even for younger minors.

As already suggested, cases 3 and 4 illustrate circumstances in which circumcised women may obtain medical care consistent with their cultural values. Unmentioned with regard to case 3, however, is the possibility that the aunt who serves as an interpreter may not accurately represent her niece's own values. Use of hospital translators who are adequately prepared and available can reduce the risk of erroneous interpretations of the patient's values. These cases also illustrate the fact that individuals of any age may not subscribe to the values of their cultural milieu or to official teachings of their religion. Knowledge of cultural or religious differences is a means of ascertaining the values or priorities of an individual, but they are not determinative of those values. In cases of conflict, the patient's own standpoint should be privileged vis-à-vis the prescriptions of her culture or religion. Eglal's request to be "opened" illustrates a standpoint that should be privileged in this regard.

Eating disorders

Cases

1. Barb Wright is a shy, bright, athletic and attractive 17-year-old, whose parents have been worried about her anorexic tendencies for the last three years. Her family physician has seen her intermittently, warned her of the dangers of anorexia nervosa, and advised her parents how to interact with their daughter to promote healthy behavior. Barb's weight has now declined to about 20 percent less than normal for her age, and she has had no menstrual periods for three months. She says she doesn't want to eat more because she feels ill when she does so. She is totally resistant to her physician's recommendation of hospitalization for treatment. Although the parents support her recommendation, the physician questions whether, in light of Barb's understanding of her condition and her apparent competence for consent, it is morally justified to hospitalize and treat her coercively.

2. Julie Day is a 17-year-old with cystic fibrosis (CF) and anorexia nervosa. Over the years, she has made friends with other teenagers with CF, some of whom have died from the disease. She became anorexic about two years ago and was recently hospitalized because her weight loss was so severe that it became life threatening. Although Julie has persisted in her refusal of treatment, her mother has authorized the medical team to feed her through a nasogastric tube. Julie has told her mother, her pulmonary specialist, and the consultant psychiatrist that she would prefer to die from anorexia than from CF.

3. Dr. Greg Carson specializes in adolescent medicine. He was recently invited to a statewide conference on "Body Image and Teenagers" to address the question of whether there should be a law requiring advertisers to present more realistic pictures of men and women in their ads. Although he would have been happy to speak about symptoms and treatment of body image disorders, Dr. Carson questions whether it is ethically appropriate for him to address the question posed by the conference organizers.

Empirical considerations

Eating disorders occur in men and women of all ages; approximately 90 percent of those affected are women, and 86 percent of those affected report its onset before the age of 20.[23] Anorexia nervosa, bulimia nervosa, and binge eating all involve a preoccupation with food and body image. Each is a complex, chronic disease with an identifiable progression and predictable symptoms, arising from a combination of genetic, social, and psychological factors. Up to 10 percent of those affected die as a result of starvation, cardiac arrest, or suicide. Anorexia has a mortality rate higher than that of nearly all other mental disorders, 0.56 percent per year.[24] Treatment of eating disorders generally entails psychotherapy and pharmacotherapy, either alone or in combination.

The main characteristics of anorexia nervosa are starvation of oneself and a distorted body image. Although affected individuals are dangerously underweight (< 85% of healthy weight) they see themselves as fat.[25] For some patients, such as Barb Wright, severe weight loss prevents menses, leading to bone loss and reduced muscle mass. All of the major organ systems are threatened by the lack of adequate nutrition. Although bulimics practice binge eating, they face comparable risks because their weight gain is deliberately restricted through methods such as self-induced vomiting, water pills, laxatives, fasting, and extreme exercising. Binge eaters who are not bulimic experience uncontrolled consumption but do not attempt to eliminate the food after consuming it.

Various mental illnesses are associated with eating disorders. Among these, depression is the most common and the most deadly. Independently of their risk of eating disorders, adolescent girls are twice as likely as boys to develop depression. The TV commercials and magazine articles that provide the bulk of their information about women's health typically advertise weight loss mechanisms as a means of becoming more attractive to the opposite sex. As their sense of adult sexual identity is just emerging, these images exacerbate the low self-esteem that often makes them susceptible to eating disorders. Food restriction or purging in pursuit of the false idol of extreme thinness is perceived as a means by which to exert control in the midst of life circumstances that are otherwise uncontrollable.

Patients with CF such as Julie Day find it difficult to maintain normal body weight because of pancreatic insufficiency and malabsorption.[26] A stereotype of muscularity in men may motivate males with CF to achieve adequate body weight despite this difficulty, whereas the stereotype of thinness as beautiful is a disincentive for their female counterparts. Most adolescents with CF are aware of their foreshortened lifespan and have known others who died as a result of their illness. This provides them with a standpoint based on data and experience rather than a false self-image. At 17 years of age, Julie has probably known a number of patients who died from the disease, some younger than she. While she thus has an informed basis on which to judge what it would be like to die from her CF, she is unlikely to be similarly knowledgeable about death through self-starvation.

Refusal of food and water by competent adults is generally legal; this method by which to hasten death has apparently been chosen by a small but increasing number of hospice patients. Clinicians who provide palliative treatment for these patients claim that they usually expire peacefully and painlessly within a few weeks.[27] Regardless of whether an individual dies from starvation or from a disease such as CF, it is usually possible to provide adequate pain relief during the dying process.

Physicians such as Greg Carson are often invited to speak in public fora about policy issues for which their expertise and experience are relevant. Some draw substantial remuneration from these situations, and a few depend on expert testimonies as their principal source of income. As Greg recognizes, however, the type of expertise and experience a physician offers in such situations does not in itself constitute adequate information on which to base policies or legislation. The public good, as potentially different from the good of individual patients, is the primary responsibility of lawmakers.

Theoretical considerations

Barb Wright and Julie Day are legally minors. As such, because neither of their situations is covered by the various legal exceptions to the requirement of parental consent, the law in the United States and elsewhere permits treatment despite their refusal. From a moral point of view, however, the legality of coercive treatment is questionable because respect for autonomy is applicable to them to the extent that they are autonomous and understand the implications of their decisions. With anorexic patients of any age, autonomy with regard to treatment of their condition may be deficient because they are unable to recognize or acknowledge its risks to them. Their capacity for decision-making is selective because it applies to other areas of life but not to their own need for treatment. This selective capacity is particularly pertinent to the clinician's assessment of Barb's competence for consent: she is probably competent enough to make informed and autonomous decisions in other matters but not with regard to treatment of her anorexia. Since her standpoint is distorted by the false image she has of her body, it is appropriate to hospitalize and treat her solely on grounds of her parents' consent. To the extent that she is incapable of an autonomous decision on this issue, maxim 1 is not thereby violated.

Julie Day is probably just as competent for decision-making as Barb Wright, which means that she is just as unable to make informed and autonomous decisions regarding treatment of her anorexia. However, the variable of Julie's prognosis, based on her CF, is morally relevant to her physician's decision about whether to override her objection to treatment. A "reasonable person" standard may be invoked to justify termination of nonpalliative treatment of an incompetent person who is in the terminal phase of a terminal illness.[28] If Julie is in fact in the terminal phase of CF, it would be reasonable to stop treatment and allow her to die with adequate palliative care. In this context, Julie's asking to be allowed to die from anorexia rather than from CF is not in itself unreasonable or inconsistent with a valid standpoint on her part. Respect for her autonomy (maxim 1) may not be applicable to treatment of her anorexia, but allowing nontreatment of anorexia instead of nontreatment of her CF is consistent with maxim 2.

Most physicians who treat patients with eating disorders know that media images of beauty and attractiveness contribute to but are not determinative of these diseases. And most adults are well aware that teenagers are particularly vulnerable to media influences because, insecure about their sexuality and gender identity, they look for models in the media. While images of female beauty tend to be unrealistically and unhealthfully thin,[29] the ideal of masculinity is often a healthy one, promoting physical fitness and strength. Recognizing the important impact of media images on teenage health, the question raised for Greg Carson in case 3 is one that arises in other health-related circumstances also: Should I, as a doctor, publicly address the question of whether and how advertisers should be regulated?

From an egalitarian perspective, it is not only appropriate but, arguably, morally obligatory for Greg to use his experience and expertise as a physician in support of public policies or laws conducive to the health of adolescents. By positively responding to this invitation, he can provide those who develop policies or laws with a basic understanding of the health risks of eating disorders, their complex causality, and the empirical differences between images in ads and healthy individuals in the general population. For clinicians, addressing these topics involves more than description of "symptoms" and "treatment" modalities; it also involves "preventive medicine"—that is, efforts to preempt the causes of specific diseases. Just as doctors have spoken out against the health hazards of smoking, not only for teenagers but for the population in general, they may and should speak out against false, health-endangering, and seductive images of feminine beauty. With regard to the masculine or athletic ideal, clinical experts as well as public figures have spoken out against the hazards of substances that may buy short-term gains with disproportionate risk (e.g., use of steroids). Given the high risks of eating disorders, warnings against practices whose harmful impact can be reduced are just as professionally obligatory. Regulations that encourage the media to present more diverse and realistic images with positive messages about health and self-esteem should thus be supported by professionals who recognize their potential for decreasing the incidence of eating disorders.

If paternalism is understood as undermining or impeding the genuine autonomy of competent individuals, albeit with the intention of helping them, it is hardly justifiable from a moral point of view toward all of those who are younger than 18 years of age, some of whom are more decisionally competent than some adults. The risk of disproportionate harm to others always justifies limitation of the autonomy of those who would inflict the harm; this is justified on grounds of beneficence or nonmaleficence rather than paternalism. Intervention on behalf of people of any age who are not autonomous is not paternalism; it simply constitutes beneficence and nonmaleficence toward them.

A model that may be invoked as a guide in all of these complex cases is that of "parentalism."[30] Obviously, this term derives its meaning from the term "parent," which is applicable to both mothers and fathers. In contrast, paternalism derives its meaning from the Latin *pater* for father, and "maternalism," which some have proposed as a substitute for paternalism, comes from the Latin *mater* for mother. "Parentalism" may be construed as embodying traditional understandings of the roles of both parents: father as protector and mother as nurturer. Although many mothers are more protective of their offspring than their fathers are, the pivotal event that makes a woman a mother is her push of her offspring from womb to world. Cutting the umbilical cord separates the newborn from her, so that the child may grow increasingly less dependent on her. Her essential role is to nurture that development by fostering the child's autonomy.

Regardless of age, all of us need the kind of parenting I've just described: we require (paternal) protection from harm and (maternal) nurturance of our capacity for autonomy. The protective role is fulfilled through the practice of beneficence and nonmaleficence by others; the nurturant role encourages and facilitates each one's autonomy. Most of us are also responsible for parenting others by practicing the same verities toward them. In other words, the model of parentalism applies across the life span—to all of our interactions with others, both personal and professional.

The moral paradigm of parentalism is an ideal that most of us fall short of much of the time. With cases as complicated as those considered in this chapter, however, it serves as a reminder that ethics demands more than simplistic applications of rules or roles. From a parentalist as well as an egalitarian perspective, the need to balance the verities while applying them to the variables of each situation is ongoing.

9

Preventing Pregnancy and Birth

The use of medical technologies for fertility curtailment are often more troubling than those used for fertility enhancement. Presumably, this has to do with the contrasting goals of the interventions: to end or prevent new lives, as opposed to initiating or facilitating their development. Some variables may make curtailment more desirable than enhancement for some individuals, and some methods of curtailment (abortion) are highly controversial while others (contraception) are widely viewed as morally responsible. If health care practitioners are trained and obligated to save lives, termination of fetal life may be at odds with that commitment even if the fetus or embryo is not regarded as a person. It is not surprising, therefore, that abortion as commonly understood (i.e., as deliberately ending the life of a developing fetus) is psychologically disturbing even for some who do not object to the procedure on religious or moral grounds. Some, for example, worry that abortions are sought as a substitute for contraception; others find them emotionally distressing. Many practitioners prefer to refer patients who request abortions to others, especially when they are requested late in gestation.[1]

In chapter 3 I identify and examine a range of positions about moral status. Although that discussion is not repeated here, it underlies all of the topics addressed in this chapter. Different starting points or positions on this issue lead to different conclusions, not only about the disposition of embryos and fetuses but also about the capacity of men and women to become biological parents. Contraception and sterilization are means by which men and women can suspend or end this capacity.

Because of its relative irreversibility, sterilization is more ethically problematic than contraception. From the standpoint of women whose gender identity depends on their capacity for childbearing, sterilization may involve a significant psychological burden; for others, the irreversibility may be welcome. Similarly, some men may resist sterilization because they define their gender identity by their ability to become genetic fathers; others may prefer sterilization to condom use for contraception. From an egalitarian perspective, the fact that sterilization of men is less invasive and less costly than it is for women is ethically relevant.[2] On grounds of that difference and the verity of nonmaleficence, sterilization of men is more defensible than sterilization of women unless other variables shift the balance so that the procedure is more burdensome to men.

This chapter illustrates only some of the ethically relevant variables of situations involving sterilization, contraception, and abortion. As with previous chapters, actual cases are more complex and morally nuanced than mere narrations or discussions of them can capture.

Contraception and sterilization

Cases

1. Katrina Roberts, a 17-year-old with Williams syndrome, lives at home with her parents. Recently, she was sexually assaulted while returning from her special school. While she was recovering, her parents asked their pediatrician to recommend an obstetrician who would perform a tubal ligation on Katrina. They based their request, they said, on their belief that the demands of pregnancy and childbirth were not justified in someone who would not have the ability to raise the child. The obstetrician met with Katrina and asked her what she understood by the procedure she might undergo. Katrina said she knew that it would "hurt a little" and that after it was done she "couldn't ever have babies." Katrina's sterilization could be legally performed on grounds of the parents' request and their daughter's welfare. Nonetheless, the obstetrician questioned whether such a relatively permanent procedure could ethically be done on someone so young, or anyone whose decisional capacity was in doubt. He knew that when Katrina turned 18, her parents' consent would not legally suffice unless they had been adjudicated to be her legal guardians; even then, they might be required to obtain the court's permission for the sterilization. On grounds that such an irreversible decision deserved fuller and more careful examination than his expertise and time allowed, the obstetrician recommended Norplant as a contraceptive that would prevent pregnancy for several more years.

2. As a child, Sheila Paulson, now 26 years old, was diagnosed as "mildly retarded, of no known genetic etiology." When she was 16 years old, she underwent sterilization through tubal ligation at the request of her parents. For the past four years, Sheila has lived in an assisted-living facility with other adults who are developmentally disabled. Two years ago, she married another resident of the facility and moved with him to an apartment nearby, where they support themselves through part-time work at a local factory. Family members of both are attentive to their needs and willing to contribute financially, albeit modestly, if necessary. Sheila recently visited the women's health clinic and asked to have her sterilization reversed so that she and her husband could have a child together. After taking her history, the obstetrician referred her to the genetics clinic for a recommendation on whether the reversal should be attempted. The geneticist discussed the matter with colleagues and subsequently advised the obstetrician not to attempt the reversal because Sheila was "probably unable to fulfill the responsibilities of motherhood, whatever that means."

Empirical considerations

Methods of contraception vary not only in terms of their effectiveness, convenience, and cost but also in terms of which partner practices the method. The major methods available to women without partner involvement are birth control pills, intrauterine devices, diaphragms, Depo-Provera, and Norplant.[3] Condoms, the only method that offers protection against HIV infection, are used by men, but women are often the ones who ensure that men use them. Spermicides are used by both sexes but with limited effectiveness. That women assume most of the burden of contraceptive practice is not surprising because it is in their bodies that conception may occur. This is also true of sterilization methods. The major method available to men, vasectomy, is much less frequently pursued by them even though it is less costly and invasive than is the main means of sterilization for women, tubal ligation.

Worldwide, tubal ligation is the most common method of contraception. It is a fairly simple, effective operation on women, in which her fallopian tubes are severed and tied off, preventing fertilization. In the United States, the cost is generally covered by Medicaid. In contrast, reversal of tubal ligation is a complex, expensive, and less effective procedure, rarely covered by private insurance or Medicaid. Although pregnancy is achievable in many cases after reversal, the risk of ectopic pregnancy is increased through the presence of scar tissue in the fallopian tube.[4] Because of the relative irreversibility of tubal ligation, various methods of birth control are usually recommended instead for young women and those who have not yet had children. Norplant, a highly effective method, is also less expensive and less invasive than tubal ligation. It consists of six small capsules filled with a birth-control substance (synthetic progestin), inserted under the skin in the upper arm for as long as five years. To be safe as well as effective, the capsules must be inserted or removed by an experienced practitioner. The principal side effect of Norplant is irregular menstrual periods during the first few months; less common side effects are weight gain or loss, headache, acne, ovarian cysts, and excess hair growth.[5]

Williams syndrome is a congenital disorder characterized by cognitive impairment, physical abnormalities, and impulsive, excessive sociability. Despite their intellectual deficits, affected individuals are often quite competent verbally. The combination of an outgoing personality and cognitive impairment makes them particularly vulnerable to sexual overtures from anyone interested in taking advantage of them. Consequently, a potential offender would probably not need to force Katrina to have sex with him. In such circumstances, it is highly improbable that she is capable of providing ethically or legally adequate consent. This would be true for Katrina even if she were beyond the age of legal majority.

A significant variable in case 1 is the rationale for the parents' request. Apparently, they were spurred to seek tubal ligation for their daughter because she had been sexually assaulted. Although their worry that she might become pregnant could be assuaged through sterilization, the risk of being assaulted would remain; in fact, if a potential assailant were concerned about being tracked or identified through a pregnancy, he might be more prone to assault Katrina if he knew she had been sterilized. The risk of assault must therefore be addressed regardless of the decision about sterilization. Concern about this issue also requires attention to the possibility of incest or sexual molestation by relatives and family members. Depending on other variables, the physiological and psychological risks of further assault may be graver than the risk of pregnancy.

Cognitive impairment (cf. mental retardation[6]) covers a wide range of intellectual deficits, both qualitatively and quantitatively. Some people with Williams syndrome are more musically talented than individuals with a normal or superior IQ, but quantitative thinking is severely limited. Depending on the complexity of the information required for competent decision-making, mildly or moderately impaired individuals may fulfill the cognitive capability required for informed consent. Sheila has apparently satisfied this requirement, and Katrina may be close to satisfying it. Even if Katrina were not cognitively impaired, however, parental consent would be legally required for her sterilization because she is a minor. In the United States, when Katrina reaches 18, she will be assumed competent for decision-making unless a guardian is appointed to act in her behalf. As the obstetrician apparently recognizes, specific authorization for sterilization may still be required because guardianship alone does not obviate the need to determine whether a procedure as significant and invasive as sterilization should be performed on someone lacking decisional capacity.

Case 2 does not stipulate whether Sheila has a legal guardian. Since she is married and living relatively independently, this is unlikely. If she does have a guardian, however, the guardian is legally and morally obliged to make decisions that respect her wishes as well as her welfare. In other words, her standpoint should be the guardian's guide. An attempt to reverse her sterilization entails some risk to Sheila's health, as it would for any woman, but her cognitive impairment rather than her health was apparently the provocation for referral to the genetics clinic. Geneticists and genetic counselors are trained to educate clients about genetic risks and conditions. Assessing competence for parenthood is not an expertise for which they have any special qualifications. The obstetrician in this case realizes that he lacks adequate expertise and time to determine whether the procedure should be done. In other words, he recognizes the limitations of his own standpoint.

Theoretical considerations

As already suggested, for some women, sterilization is preferable to contraception because of its relative permanence, effectiveness, and long-term economic advantage. For others, its relative permanence is viewed as a limitation, thereby raising the threshold of justification. The younger the patient, the higher the threshold, because this implies a longer future in which the option of childbearing is foregone.

From the practitioner's standpoint, if the woman already has children, age is less problematic because the decision is presumed to be better informed than it would otherwise be. Even for older, childless women, practitioners are more reluctant about sterilization than about contraception because of its relative permanence. Distinguishing between cases on grounds of age or childbearing experience is based on recognition that autonomy is more complex than immediate, literal expressions of preferences sometimes convey. Moreover, respect for autonomy involves respect for the autonomous individual's wishes for the future, as well as present circumstances.

In most parts of the United States, contraception may legally be provided to adolescents who are not cognitively impaired without their parents' consent, but sterilization is not similarly available to them. For both types of procedure, respect for the teenager's autonomy may lead to different positions. Sterilization is avoided to preserve her autonomy for choosing pregnancy in the future; contraception may be encouraged as a means of respecting her developing autonomy and right to privacy. In both situations nonmaleficence is also relevant. Contraception is a means of temporarily preventing the physiological and psychosocial risks of pregnancy; sterilization may eliminate this risk more permanently or reliably but may be more harmful because of its invasiveness and relative irreversibility. It is doubtful that sterilization based on parental request would ever be legally or morally sanctioned for a teenager who is not cognitively impaired; this is a decision that an individual should make for herself when she is mature enough to consider its long-term ramifications.

Legally and morally, surrogates are expected to make decisions for others from the standpoint of those in whose behalf their are deciding—that is, in their "best interests." According to maxim 1, "interests" include preferences (cf. autonomy) as well as welfare, but these are occasionally at odds because people are free to choose what is not good for them. To the extent that someone's capacity for decision-making is compromised, respect for autonomy may be subordinated to beneficence and nonmaleficence toward her. However, only for those whose decisional capacity is totally lacking, such as those who are profoundly mentally impaired, is respect for autonomy irrelevant to the surrogate's decision in their behalf. Neither Katrina nor Sheila falls into this category. Sheila's sterilization at age 16, albeit legal, may thus be questioned on moral grounds.

These cases illustrate both sides of "reproductive rights": the right to curtail fertility and the right to enhance or promote it. On egalitarian grounds, these rights are supportable for people with disabilities, as well as those who are currently able, and as supportable for people with cognitive impairments as for those who have physical impairments.[7] Concerns about the impact of parental limitations on a potential child are also ethically relevant; these probably figure, whether justifiably or not, in the tendency of practitioners and others to view fertility enhancement as more problematic than fertility curtailment in people with physical or intellectual impairments.

The physician in case 1 may have been attempting to avoid the morally complex issue of sterilization for a young woman whose competence was compromised, but his recommendation may also have been based on an egalitarian desire for consistency between treatment of cognitively unimpaired patients and treatment of those who are cognitively impaired. By recommending Norplant instead of sterilization, the physician managed to treat Katrina as any 17-year-old might be treated. He also avoided the legal difficulties associated with sterilization of a cognitively impaired minor.

Although concerns about potential discrimination are always appropriate, treating patients differently does not imply that they are unequal or that they are treated unjustly. Every patient *should* be treated differently because each, no matter what her ability level, *is* different. An egalitarian perspective requires recognition of different needs and abilities, along with efforts to reduce inequalities associated with differences. In case 1, for example, while a decision about sterilization may legitimately be postponed, argument in its support is more compelling than it would be for a person who is clearly able to provide adequate care for a child.

Case 2 illustrates the dominant role that physicians play vis-à-vis infertility patients: they can curtail fertility by refusing to provide the treatment. Efforts to reverse tubal ligation are sometimes unsuccessful, but fertility is restored in a substantial number of cases. Interestingly, this case also demonstrates the tendency of some clinicians to "punt" messy problems that they could address themselves, and of others to overstep the bounds of their expertise. Since it was already known that Sheila's "mental retardation" was "of no known genetic origin," referral to the genetics clinic was inappropriate unless the main reason was to confirm this. Since the genetics team was unable to specify criteria required "to fulfill the responsibilities of motherhood," they lacked grounds for determining whether Sheila met those criteria.

Missing in the description of case 2 is any mention of the role and responsibilities of others in childrearing. Single as well as married couples who are currently able often need assistance in raising their offspring. The fact that both Sheila and her husband want to have a child, along with the fact that both have lived quasi-independently for several years, suggests that they may be capable of adequate parenthood, with similar assistance. People who are highly intelligent or professionally successful are sometimes less capable than intellectually or physically impaired, or economically disadvantaged, people of providing the nurturing environment crucial to the development of children. Accordingly, unless criteria for determining whether Sheila can fulfill the major responsibilities for motherhood are introduced and adequately defended, it hardly seems just to deprive her of that right.

Abortion

Cases

1. Ann Brown, a 32-year-old woman with multiple sclerosis (MS), became pregnant despite regular use of a diaphragm and spermicide. Following her last pregnancy, Ann was no longer able to walk unassisted, and her condition deteriorated since then. Although her husband is opposed to abortion on religious grounds, he is extremely concerned that continuation of the current pregnancy would further compromise his wife's health and her ability to care for their children, ages 4 and 6, while he supports the family through his job as a telephone repairman. She is 3 weeks pregnant when the couple meets with the obstetrician to discuss their options regarding the situation.

2. Carol Day is a 14-year-old whose parents work in the local factory. She and her 16-year-old brother both attend junior high school and spend much of their free time with their cousins, who live nearby. Although Carol's father had been accused of battering by his former wife, the charge was never substantiated. Carol became pregnant after her 19-year-old cousin convinced her to have sex with him, but she did not mention the incident to anyone because she was embarrassed and ashamed. About four and a half months into the pregnancy, she visited the women's clinic on her way home from school and told the nurse she would like an abortion because she is "pretty sure" she is pregnant. Carol also asks that her family not be informed about her pregnancy or her request for an abortion.

3. Eve Flynn is a pregnant, sexually active 16-year-old, who harbors an extremely hostile attitude toward her parents and other authority figures. She wanted to become pregnant because she thought that having a child would allow her to leave her parents' home and be "on her own." On learning of her pregnancy, her parents try to convince her to have an abortion.

4. Gail Hoy is a 28-year-old business executive who discovered she was pregnant despite her insistence that her partner use a condom. Because her periods tend to be irregular, Gail did not suspect the pregnancy until she was already in her second trimester. Her main reason for considering abortion is that motherhood would interfere with her lifestyle and with advancement in her profession. She says she doesn't particularly like children, never planned on having any, and doubts that she would be a "good mother" if she went forward with the pregnancy.

5. Jill Katz and her husband were overjoyed to learn of Jill's pregnancy. When her physician took her family history, she mentioned that her 21-year-old sister had had an infant with trisomy 21, who later died from a cardiac problem. Because her sister was apparently a carrier for the chromosomal translocation that causes Down syndrome, Jill is advised to undergo a test to determine if she is also a carrier. If so, she has a 15 percent chance of having a child with trisomy 21. The couple feel insecure about their ability to raise a child with Down syndrome and ambivalent on the issue of abortion.[8]

Empirical considerations

Crucial variables in the above cases are whether the pregnancy was begun voluntarily, the duration of gestation, the method of abortion, and the health status of the pregnant woman and potential child. By far, the majority of abortions are performed early in gestation through dilatation and curettage (D&C) of the uterus and vacuum aspiration of the embryo or fetus. Early abortions may also be performed through administration of drugs such as RU-486 (mifepristone).[9] Regardless of whether moral status is imputed to the fetus, late abortions of mature, economically able, healthy women with healthy fetuses are more troubling than early abortions by single, poor adolescents for whom pregnancy poses a threat and whose capacity or resources for parenting are apparently lacking. Many people who generally oppose abortion make an exception for situations in which the pregnancy was initiated by rape or incest or when the woman's life or health is threatened by continuation of pregnancy. In the United States, the health of the woman always provides legal grounds for abortion.

Abortion for fetal anomalies tends to be more costly, as well as physically and psychologically more burdensome for women, than abortion for other reasons. The physical risk is greater because the diagnosis and termination usually occur during the second trimester. The psychological risk is greater because the abortion usually occurs in a wanted pregnancy, accentuating the fact that the procedure involves rejection of a particular potential child rather than rejection of the pregnancy itself. In response to the woman's expectation, methods may be chosen to ensure fetal demise or reduce pain in a possibly sentient fetus; because of their directness, these methods are emotionally difficult for some practitioners who do not oppose abortion on moral grounds.[10]

Depending on the duration of gestation and the condition of the woman or fetus, some methods of abortion are medically contraindicated. Different methods also have different impact on clinicians and patients. When performed by an experienced practitioner, dilatation and evacuation (D&E) is the safest and most common method of second-trimester abortion.[11] It involves dilatation of the cervix to allow suction curettage and manual evacuation of the fetus and placenta. Because the woman is anesthetized, she does not observe the dismemberment that removal of the fetus entails. Instillation methods involve induction of labor and delivery of a fetus considered nonviable; the agent used for the induction may or may not be toxic to the fetus (e.g., prostin vs. saline or urea). Nurses rather than doctors usually face the unpleasant task of disposing of fetal remains. Rare cases of survival after abortion performed through instillation have been reported.[12]

Occasionally, hysterotomy is performed for medical reasons (e.g., if instillation is unsuccessful). This is the most invasive and risky method of abortion for the woman; concomitantly, it increases the possibility of survival for the fetus. An abortus that shows signs of life is legally a newborn that clinicians are bound to treat as such. The living survivor of a legal abortion must therefore be treated as aggressively as any infant.[13] Through ultrasound-guided injection of potassium chloride (KCl) into the fetal heart prior to instillation or hysterotomy, a clinician may ensure fetal demise and confirm prenatal diagnosis through examination of an intact abortus. If D&E is performed, the abortion may be preceded by KCl injection to ensure that the fetus does not experience pain during the extraction. Intact dilatation and extraction (D&X), which its critics call partial birth abortion, is rarely performed and highly controversial.[14] Although some practitioners believe D&X is never necessary for health-related reasons, many oppose efforts to declare it illegal.[15]

As discussed in chapter 8, pregnancy in patients younger than 15 years of age, such as Carol Day, is more hazardous than pregnancy in older adolescents.[16] At 4.5 months gestation, however, abortion carries greater medical risks and discomfort than an early abortion. The psychological and social risks of having a child at so early an age, especially one conceived in such circumstances, are probably greater than the medical risks of an abortion to Carol. Social supports for abortion decisions are especially likely when the pregnancy is induced by rape or incest.

Legally, Carol's 19-year-old cousin is guilty of "statutory rape" because he had sex with a minor. Clinicians have a legal obligation to report such cases. As for the fetus, the obstetric risks to Carol heighten risks of prematurity and complications of delivery, but the potential child's risk of inheriting a genetic (recessive) disease because of first-cousin parentage is low (less than 1 percent).[17] Even if medical and social risks to the potential child were great, termination of the fetus is not convincingly defensible on grounds of its own interests.

The hazards of pregnancy for women with diseases such as diabetes, asthma, epilepsy, hypertension, and cystic fibrosis are supported by research studies. Data are lacking, however, with regard to comparable risks of pregnancy for women with MS, such as Ann Brown. MS affects the central nervous system through destruction of the myelin sheath that coats nerve fibers, slowing transmission of electrical impulses and impairing nerve conduction. Its symptoms appear sporadically, mainly in people between 20 and 40 years of age, but the disease is not associated with any known genetic predisposition. It is possible, therefore, that Ann's symptoms may worsen even if she terminates her current pregnancy. If she decides to go to term, however, weakness caused by her underlying disease may prevent adequate pushing, necessitating use of forceps or suction assistance during delivery. In other words, childbirth is likely to be more difficult for her than it would be if she did not have MS.

Two of the preceding cases involve contraceptive failure. Ann Brown is apparently among the 12 percent of women who become pregnant over the course of a year of sexual intercourse despite regular use of a diaphragm. Gail Hoy is apparently among the 14 percent who become pregnant despite their partner's use of a condom, which they may well have chosen as a means of avoiding infection as well as pregnancy through their partners.[18] But none of the usual methods of contraception is an absolute safeguard against pregnancy, and abstinence is the only certain safeguard against sexually transmitted diseases.[19] Presumably, Ann and Gail were both aware of the risk of contraceptive failure. For some women, however, lack of education and the unavailability of, or inability to pay for, contraception are deterrents to its use. Although most insurance plans cover maternity care, many plans do not cover contraception. Arguments for better coverage have mounted since insurance plans began to cover use of viagra for men. The verity of justice supports these arguments as a matter of gender justice.

Theoretical considerations

Abortion is clinically defined as spontaneous or elective termination of a nonviable pregnancy.[20] In popular and legal usage, the term commonly applies only to deliberate termination of the developing organism in vivo, which obviously ends the woman's pregnancy. The preceding cases illustrate this usage. But abortion is also definable as termination of an embryo in vitro, when conception and pregnancy have not yet taken place. This is the definition employed by those who impute personhood to the embryo from fertilization onward and condemn abortion as applicable to the destruction of embryonic life regardless of whether conception and pregnancy have occurred. Conception refers to the beginning of a pregnancy within a woman's body, when the embryo is implanted within the uterus, days after fertilization has occurred either in vitro or in vivo.

Whether or not abortion is legal, the end point or intended goal of the woman undergoing termination of a nonviable fetus is morally relevant. In general, a good end or intention may excuse or reduce culpability for an untoward action, whereas a bad intention may make a good act morally blameworthy. Spontaneous abortion is morally neutral because there is no intention of terminating the life of the embryo or fetus. From the standpoint of those who impute full moral status to the fetus, elective abortions are always wrong. Nonetheless, procedures that result in destruction of the embryo but are intended to save a woman's life (e.g., treatment of an ectopic pregnancy) may be acceptable because they do not directly end the embryo's potential for development. The rationale for permissibility in these cases is the rule of double effect, which distinguishes between what is foreseen and what is intended.[21] Only the good end of maternal health is intended; fetal loss or death is an unintended but foreseen consequence of the intervention.

From the standpoint of those who hold maximalist or intermediate positions about moral status, elective abortions may be more or less moral depending on the intentions associated with them. Preservation of maternal health is generally, but not always, more compelling than nonmedical reasons. In case 1, for example, the patient's apparent intention, if she chooses abortion, is to support lives already born, those of her two young children, her husband's, and her own. In contrast, the intention of the patient in case 4 is to facilitate professional advancement, a legitimate but, from an egalitarian perspective, less compelling rationale than that of Ann Brown. Gail Hoy's doubt that she would be a "good mother" shows concern about the welfare of her potential child. This concern could be assuaged by exercising her option to continue her pregnancy, give birth, and relinquish her newborn to a woman or couple whose desire and capacity for good parenting she did not doubt. By giving birth, however, Gail would still be a biological mother.

The adoption option is also available in the other cases. However, most women in such circumstances choose abortion rather than relinquishment through adoption.[22] Their standpoint apparently involves not only a desire to end their pregnancy but also a desire to avoid motherhood through the birth or a child who, while biologically related to them, would be raised by another or others. The abortion option provides them with an opportunity to accomplish both goals. Whereas adoption is not only morally defensible but commendable in some circumstances, moral justification for abortion crucially depends on the controversial premise that the fetus lacks moral status or sufficient moral status to override the woman's autonomy or welfare.

Intentionality is ethically and legally relevant to decisions in bioethics, not only for patients but also for practitioners and surrogate decision makers whose standpoints are different from one another's. Clinicians who perform elective abortions usually intend to respect the pregnant woman's autonomy and practice beneficence or nonmaleficence toward her. Occasionally, however, these verities are incompatible. In case 3, for example, the physician may agree with Eve Flynn's parents that abortion is best for her, despite her desire to continue the pregnancy.

Some physicians attempt to bypass the moral complexity of abortion and remain morally neutral by simply doing what the competent, informed patient requests, without judging the morality of her decision. The moral position they thus affirm, that respect for the patient's autonomy is paramount (maxim 2), is consistent with the informative or instrumentalist model discussed in chapter 2. But moral neutrality is unachievable by anyone who facilitates or impedes another's moral decision. A physician who performs or refuses to perform an abortion is therefore responsible for what she does or doesn't do, regardless of the woman's decision or rationale.

Cases 2 and 3 illustrate the questionable capacity of adolescents to consent to medical procedure for themselves. As discussed in chapter 8, parental consent is usually a legal requirement for treatment of minors, but contraception, drug treatment, and abortion are available to them without parental consent in many states. Because adolescents are prevalently recognized as having at least some degree of autonomy or competence for consent to their own treatment, respect for autonomy as well as beneficence is morally applicable to these exceptions. In case 2, nonmaleficence is applicable also because of the risks of late abortion and of pregnancy and childbirth at age 14. Further, the fact that pregnancy was induced by statutory rape not only has legal implications for practitioners; it also entails moral obligations to address the possibility of ongoing abuse. The clinician needs to weigh burdens and benefits to the patient, both medical and psychological, while also attempting to recognize and respect her developing capacity for autonomy in complex family circumstances.

Weighing the potential burdens and benefits involves concerns about confidentiality, which Carol Day has asked the nurse to practice by not informing her family of her pregnancy or abortion. Both legally and morally, confidentiality may be overridden on grounds of protection of others or, arguably, because disclosure to specific individuals may expand the patient's options. The ethical question faced by the practitioner is how to honor confidentiality while addressing the risk of possible harms to a minor. If the only way to protect her from these requires disclosure of confidential information to her family, maxims 1 and 4 support disclosure. Clinicians who are morally opposed to abortion may disclose the information on grounds of maxim 3, hoping that parental notification would serve as a deterrent to abortion. As in case 3, however, parents are not always opposed to abortions for their minor daughters; in fact, they sometimes advocate abortions that their daughters do not wish to undergo.[23]

Case 3 also illustrates the fact that decisions to become pregnant or to continue a pregnancy may be motivated by self-interest rather than affirmation of another's life. Because people's motives are often mixed, it is entirely possible that Eve Flynn is credibly committed to and capable of good parenting of the child she wants to have, even while undertaking her pregnancy as a means of achieving greater independence. Legally and morally, clinicians should give priority to her autonomy and welfare, and, while informing her as fully as possible of her options, ensure that her parents' efforts to persuade her to have an abortion are not coercive. Even for those who are maximalists regarding moral status, support for Eve's autonomy in this case is probably more compelling than support for her parents' decision on grounds of maxim 1: the interests of the patient count most. From the standpoint of those who are minimalists, Eve's decision is supportable solely on grounds of its consistency with their starting point. And from the standpoint of those who attribute partial moral status to the fetus, support for her wishes is demanded not only on grounds of respect for her autonomy but also on grounds of beneficence or nonmaleficence toward the potential child.

Case 5 involves a different rationale for abortion than the other cases because here the procedure is not intended primarily or only to end the pregnancy or avoid having a child, but to avoid having a particular child, one with characteristics that the woman or couple want to prevent in their offspring. Jill Katz was apparently happy about being pregnant until she learned that her fetus may have a 15 percent chance of Down syndrome. If her carrier test is negative, she and her husband will probably resume their positive attitude about this pregnancy. If she is a carrier, though, she will probably have her fetus tested for trisomy 21 and face the option of abortion if the result is positive. The couple's insecurity about their ability to raise an impaired child is an understandable and nondiscriminatory rationale for abortion. From an egalitarian perspective, however, this factor alone doesn't justify abortion if the impaired fetus has the same moral status as an unimpaired fetus or child.

With some prenatally diagnosed fetal conditions, termination in late pregnancy may be defended on grounds of beneficence or nonmaleficence toward the potential child. Direct termination in these cases may be considered "fetal euthanasia." In light of palliative possibilities, this argument is weak. Even if no moral status is attributed to the fetus, the possibility that the nervous system has developed sufficiently for the fetus to experience pain through a specific abortion procedure is morally relevant. If this possibility carries a moral onus applicable to fetuses destined to be aborted, intercardiac KCl injection prior to D&E is defensible as analogous to active euthanasia toward a sentient animal that is dying an otherwise painful death. Admittedly, this rationale is at odds with the legal prohibition of active euthanasia toward born human beings.

Applying the verities to the variables delineated for each of the five cases in this section, the strongest cases for abortion are the first two and the weakest case is the fourth. Respect for patient autonomy could be adequate grounds for abortion in all of the cases except the third, but concerns about beneficence and nonmaleficence strengthen the argument for acceding to the requests of Ann Brown and Carol Day. Although these concerns are present also for Jill Katz, continuation of pregnancy does not entail physical risks for her to the degree that the other cases do, nor do the other cases entail a decision to terminate a particular fetus because of its specific characteristics. An egalitarian perspective attributes the same value to human fetuses, regardless of their characteristics.

Termination of pregnancy before fetal viability has long been a controversial and volatile ethical issue, despite the relative clarity of its legality in a broad range of instances. Practitioners are as likely as pregnant women and the public to vary widely in their views on the morality of these abortions. Some support a woman's decision to terminate her pregnancy at any point during gestation for any reason because their starting point is that the embryo or fetus has no moral status. As long as they give priority to the pregnant woman's interests, particularly through support of her autonomous decision, they act consistently with this starting point. For those who impute moral status to the developing organism, however, the legal permissibility of abortion does not confer moral legitimacy for performing, facilitating, or undergoing it. Practitioners who reason from this starting point often refer women who request abortions to those who are willing to perform the procedure. However, the referral itself is morally problematic because it is inconsistent with their ongoing opposition to abortion, comparable to telling a would-be murderer where he might find his intended victim.

An egalitarian perspective alone cannot adjudicate between opposition to and support for termination of a human embryo or fetus. Its applicability depends crucially on whether the developing organism has some moral status or value with which to compare values that are relevant to the pregnant woman, whose moral status is clearly established. Moreover, respect for autonomy applies not only to patients but also to practitioners, and no practitioner may morally be compelled to violate her own moral principles by performing a procedure that is not medically necessary. Respect for the autonomy of the pregnant patient does not demand this.

Because elective abortions require the involvement of medical professionals,[24] the difference between the negative right to refuse and the positive right to obtain them is also relevant. Legally as well as morally, the former right is compelling, as long as it is exercised by a fully competent and informed person on her own behalf; interventions in these cases, regardless of whether they are medically appropriate and as long as they do not harm others, are considered assaults. In contrast, the right to obtain a medical intervention cannot be defended on grounds that others are bound to provide it unless the procedure is necessary for the patient's health. Only a small number of abortions fall into this category.

Except for the fact that an embryo or fetus is involved, the cases in this section may seem comparable to requests for other medical procedures that are sought and obtained for nonmedical reasons. From an egalitarian perspective, some nonmedical reasons, such as those of Ann Brown, are more morally compelling than others. However, an important difference between these cases and others based on nonmedical reasons is that termination of pregnancy is only undergone or forgone by women, whose standpoint with regard to policies about its availability thus deserves privileged status vis-à-vis that of men. The extent to which the woman's standpoint is privileged vis-à-vis that of the embryo or fetus depends on one's starting point regarding moral status.

As already mentioned, sterilization is less morally problematic and controversial than abortion, and contraception is hardly morally problematic for most people. However, women are generally more affected than men by decisions and policies about any of these means of preventing pregnancy and birth. This need not be the case for sterilization and contraception because both can be undergone or practiced by men instead of women, and a more egalitarian relationship between the sexes might prevail if sufficient numbers of them did so. A society committed to gender justice would encourage couples to choose methods that are least invasive for either partner. A society committed to justice for all of us would, in addition, reduce the number of instances in which some women desire and obtain abortions by supporting them and those they might otherwise care for more equitably. Regardless of one's starting point about the moral status of human embryos or fetuses, an egalitarian perspective clearly calls for that support.

10

Violence and Discrimination toward Women and Children

Violence involves physical, sexual, or emotional harm, or threats of harm, to another. Unlike the pain or suffering that may be inflicted on someone (e.g., through medical treatment) as a transient means through which to promote her welfare or health, violence has no balancing justification: it is *only* meant to harm. Beyond the domestic sphere, men are the predominant victims as well as perpetrators of violence. Within that sphere, women, children, and the elderly are the predominant victims, and men are the predominant perpetrators of violence toward women. Women are also the main victims of gender discrimination and sexual harassment. Typically, the perpetrators of violence and discrimination are dominant individuals, those who have power over others. The power discrepancies may be physical, psychological, economic, political, or social, and some of the factors that trigger the discrepancies are unchangeable (e.g., sex, race, age). An egalitarian perspective calls for efforts to minimize the harms associated with these differences.

Although the issues addressed in this chapter are seldom covered in clinical literature, domestic violence has been increasingly recognized not only as a serious public health problem but also as one that calls for recognition and response from clinicians.[1] Many of the ethical questions that arise in this context involve respect for privacy in family or personal matters and wide social endorsement of a dichotomy between "private" or "domestic" matters and "public" spheres of life. As Susan Moller Okin and Iris Young have argued, a stark dichotomy between these spheres is all too likely to obscure injustices that occur within the private or domestic realm.[2]

Clinicians are not specially trained to track or address the causes of domestic violence, which, like gender discrimination and sexual harassment, are mainly social in origin. Nonetheless, all three issues are relevant to clinical practice because they imperil the health and welfare of patients. To the extent that they threaten health or life, clinicians have responsibilities not only to identify and treat those affected who come to them as patients, and to report suspected abuse or neglect to appropriate authorities, but also to support the efforts of others in society to reduce the incidence of these harmful practices.

The cases that follow show that discrimination or violence is manifest in many different ways in the clinical setting.

Child abuse and neglect

Cases

1. Clara Harris, 21 years old, brought her 6-week-old daughter for a routine postpartum visit with the nurse practitioner. The full-term infant weighed 9 lb. 1 oz. at birth and had been discharged with her mother the day after delivery. Although Clara breast-fed the baby at first, she soon switched to bottle-feeding and returned to work, leaving the infant in the care of her unemployed boyfriend. To the practitioner, the child looked pale and emaciated. Asked about this, Clara said the baby didn't cry much but wasn't feeding or sleeping well and had a few sores that she noticed when she diapered her. On examining the infant, the practitioner observed bruises and redness around the vagina and wondered whether she should report this to anyone.

2. Sophie Wong is a 17-year-old who has a tumultuous relationship with her parents, based largely on their prohibition of dating. Unknown to them, she visits the women's clinic to ask for "emergency contraception." In conversation with the nurse, Sophie indicates that her father "would beat me if he knew," adding that she has been beaten many times in the past for "doing things he doesn't like that other kids do." When the nurse says she needs to report this to proper authorities, Sophie pleads with her not to do so because it would probably lead to more beatings.

3. Ruth Owens is an 11-year-old who lives with her parents and two older brothers. Her mother brings her to the pediatrician after finding blood on her underwear. Ruth's mother tells the doctor she thinks there "may be something wrong because Ruth hasn't started menstruating yet." On physical exam, in the presence of Ruth's mother, the physician observes sexual penetration but is uncertain how or to whom this information should be disclosed.

Empirical considerations

Child abuse involves acts or omissions leading to death, serious physical or emotional harm, risk of serious harm, or sexual abuse or exploitation of a child by a parent or caregiver. Child neglect occurs when the responsible person fails to provide for a child's basic needs.[3] At times, the neglect stems from the parents' poverty, lack of education, or cultural values; others may then be the culpably neglectful parties. Legally, however, actions or omissions that injure or endanger a child are considered abuse or neglect regardless of whether the responsible parties intended the injury or endangerment. Children may be removed from situations that jeopardize their welfare without their parents or caregivers being legally or morally responsible for the neglect.

Child abuse and neglect occurs at every socioeconomic level, in all cultures, and in diverse family or institutional arrangements. Many of the perpetrators had been victims of abuse or neglect themselves. Because mothers or female relatives tend to be the primary or only caregivers of children, the perpetrators are often female.[4] Children of single mothers, those whose parents abuse drugs, those in large families or in low-income brackets, and those who are impaired are more likely to be abused or neglected than other children. Although younger children are more likely to be neglected than older children, the risk of sexual abuse increases with age. Girls are significantly more likely than boys to be sexually abused, and their abusers are also more likely to be male.[5] Ruth Owens's father and older brothers, as well as her contacts at school, are possible perpetrators of the sexual abuse observed by the pediatrician in case 3.

The severity of physical abuse ranges from minor bruises to severe fractures or death. The National Clearinghouse on Child Abuse and Neglect Information in the United States reported a rate of 1.96 per 100,000 fatalities from child abuse or neglect in 2002, but 50 to 60 percent of deaths resulting from abuse or neglect are not recorded. Neglect, according to these studies, is the most under-recorded form of fatal maltreatment of children.[6] As in cases 1 and 3, practitioners are considerably more likely to observe child abuse or neglect than to have it reported to them. Reporting is most likely when the clinician notices and asks about the signs of abuse and when a trustful and encouraging relationship with the child or parent has been established.

Sexual abuse includes fondling a child's genitals, penetration, incest, rape, sodomy, indecent exposure, and exploitation through prostitution or the production of pornographic materials.[7] Emotional abuse includes behavior that may severely impair the child's emotional development or self-worth, for example, through constant criticism or threats.[8] Emotional abuse is often difficult to prove, but it is almost always present when other forms of abuse occur.

Theoretical considerations

Laws throughout the United States oblige all health care workers to report suspected cases of child neglect or abuse to the appropriate authorities. From a legal point of view, therefore, the question of whether to report the possibility of abuse or neglect is always answered affirmatively. Although the term "suspected" covers a range of possible interpretations, any level of doubt is legally sufficient not simply to justify but to demand reporting of suspected abuse to the appropriate authorities. The authority to whom the report is given is legally and morally responsible for determination of whether the suspected neglect or abuse has actually occurred and what is to be done about it.

Ethically, the legal obligation to report suspected child abuse or neglect is based on the priority of nonmaleficence toward a patient who is incapable of adequately informed or autonomous decision-making or of defending herself against possible harm. This is obviously the situation in case 1, where the apparent victim is the newborn. Even though the nurse practitioner is not a physician, she is legally and ethically bound to report her suspicion to the appropriate authorities. In the other cases, respect for patient autonomy is relevant but not necessarily adequate to determination of how to respond to the allegation or observation of abuse. As maxim 3 puts it, the interests of others may outweigh respect for an individual's autonomy.

For clinicians, an ethically relevant variable is whether harms to the apparent victim are directly observed or only reported to have occurred. In cases 1 and 3, for example, the practitioner actually observes the injury. If an accidental cause is ascertained, the harm is not abuse (although it may be an indication of neglect), but this is hardly the situation in either of these cases. In case 2, the grounds for suspecting abuse are not as clear because the patient may be misrepresenting what has happened, whether deliberately or not. Sophie may have alleged abuse by her father not because she had actually been beaten but because she thought (wrongfully) that the nurse would otherwise disclose to him the reason for her visit to the clinic, and she might then be curtailed from engaging in the sexual activity that led to her visit. Given the possibility that Sophie's report of abuse is inaccurate, the nurse should attempt to determine whether it actually happened or is likely to happen, for example, by facilitating honest disclosure through explicit assurance of confidentiality. If Sophie's allegation persists, the nurse must report not only her suspicion but also the probable risk of more beatings if her father learns of her disclosure. The verity of nonmaleficence demands practical efforts by both clinicians and those to whom such risks are reported to avoid potential harms to patients.

Case 3 raises the question of confidentiality with regard to gynecological examination of a minor and discussion of the results in the presence of her parent. These are separable events. A clinician may reasonably assume that an 11-year-old would prefer to have her mother present for such an exam, and Ruth Owens's mother is legally entitled to be present. From the standpoint of an 11-year-old, a gynecological exam may be emotionally disturbing, even frightening. At this age, however, Ruth's developing autonomy should be respected and fostered by adults. The physician may facilitate this respect, as well as the exam itself, and disclosure of matters pertinent to interpretation of findings, by offering Ruth and her mother options regarding how the exam is conducted. Her mother should be encouraged to abide by her daughter's preferences. As with older patients, if staffing permits, respect for Ruth's autonomy may also be promoted by allowing her to choose the gender of the practitioner examining her.

Beyond the ethical challenge of maximizing respect for an 11-year-old's autonomy and minimizing the risks or harms to her of the exam itself, the pediatrician in case 3 faces the daunting challenge of whether, how, and by whom Ruth should be questioned about the circumstances in which the observed sexual penetration occurred. To answer these questions, she needs to consider variables such as her own relationship with the patient, the patient's relationship with her mother, the maturity of the patient, and the past history of and home situation of the patient.

After considering as many of the relevant variables as she can ascertain, the pediatrician must make a judgment call based on the priority of Ruth's welfare and respect for her autonomy (maxim 1). Even if Ruth's mother is also her patient, this priority should be observed because Ruth, not her mother, is the patient for whom the practitioner is immediately responsible.

Clinicians in the above cases either observed possible neglect or abuse, or had it reported to them. Unfortunately, many if not most instances are neither observed nor reported by the child or the child's caregiver, and laws requiring health care workers to report them cannot cover all of the cases that occur. Nevertheless, nonmaleficence and beneficence make it incumbent on all practitioners, in every setting, to be attentive to the possibility and to encourage disclosure of abuse or neglect through respectful and supportive interactions with the child and those who care for her. From an egalitarian perspective, measures to reduce the factors that trigger child abuse or neglect should be supported by all segments of society.

Elderly abuse and neglect

Cases

1. Cathleen McCarthy is an 85-year-old widow with five children, four of whom live in other states and seldom visit or inquire about her. A daughter, Ellie Smith, lives nearby. Although Ms. McCarthy's memory "is not as good as it used to be," and she hasn't the physical energy to prepare her own meals or clean her home, she is unwilling to enter a nursing home, move in with Ellie, or allow an outsider to clean or prepare meals. Ellie usually stops in after work, brings her mother food, and occasionally cleans and clears some of the clutter. Exhausted from doing this for the last decade, with no siblings or other relatives willing or able to relieve her, Ellie asks her physician to write a letter indicating that her mother is decisionally incompetent, so that she can arrange for her placement in a nursing home.

2. Brigid Sheldon, 78 years old, has severe dementia, probably due to Alzheimer disease. She lives with her son, Andrew, who was legally appointed "guardian of the estate" and "guardian of the person" when his mother was judged decisionally incapacitated four years ago. Since then, he has been using Brigid's social security check to pay for living expenses for both of them. Andrew has no other regular source of income. When he brought his mother to the clinic, the nurse noted that she seemed frightened, dazed, confused, and considerably more frail and fragile than she had appeared at her previous visit. She was unable to explain some welts on her arms and bruising on her back. The nurse told the physician she wondered whether Andrew had abused his mother.

3. Same as above, but there are no indications of physical neglect or abuse, and the nurse, who has observed Andrew at the race track, looking "high," suspects he is a drug user and "bets on the ponies." The nurse tells the doctor she thinks he is using his mother's money to pay for drugs and gambling debts.

4. Noreen Zink is an 80-year-old whose only son and legal guardian, Fred, lives in another state. Although state law requires guardians to ensure the welfare of their appointed wards, Fred only visits his mother once a year for several hours. He has arranged for a minimum wage worker to look in on her each morning, set out meals, and do light housework. When Noreen is hospitalized for a minor stroke, a social worker is asked to determine whether the patient's home is equipped for her to continue her recovery there. With Fred's permission, she visits the home and finds it dirty, in need of electrical and plumbing repairs, and ill equipped for healthy living. She tells Noreen's doctor that the patient needs to be discharged elsewhere because her son and legal guardian "isn't doing his job."

Empirical considerations

As the average life span has been extended through advances in health care and increases in health-promoting behaviors, so has the incidence of abuse, economic exploitation, and neglect of older people. Each year, approximately 2.1 million older Americans are victims of abuse or neglect, and experts estimate that for every reported case there may be as many as five unreported cases.[9] Some incidents occur in nursing homes, but most are in noninstitutional settings, where the abuser is either a family member or an unrelated caregiver. Abuse leads to earlier death even in the absence of chronic conditions or life-threatening disease.[10]

As with children, abuse and neglect of the elderly may be physical, emotional, or sexual, but it may also involve affronts to their autonomy through improper use of legal guardianships or powers of attorney and exploitation of economic assets. Forms of economic exploitation include fraudulent schemes, taking money under false pretenses, forgery, forced property transfers, and denying the elderly access to their own funds.[11]

Neglect occurs when the elderly person is deprived of services necessary to facilitate the basic activities of daily living (ADLs)—for example, proper nourishment, cleanliness, and basic health care. Isolation that prevents the elderly person from having normal human contacts or companionship is another form of neglect. As with children, suspected abuse or neglect of any elderly person should be reported by health care workers to the appropriate authorities, regardless of the circumstances that triggered the behavior.

Caregivers of the elderly, who are often elderly themselves, and mainly women, are sometimes abused by their charges, especially when neurologically debilitating diseases such as Alzheimer's trigger the abusive behavior. Family dynamics as well as caregiver stress may exacerbate the risk of elderly abuse or neglect. Aging usually entails increasing physical vulnerability and occasional loss of mental acuity, both of which enable the caregiver to inflict harm that might not otherwise occur. Cultural stereotypes, by which elderly individuals are seen or see themselves as less deserving of the respect they enjoyed at an earlier age, also contribute to the incidence of abuse or neglect. In some quarters, these involve the erroneous assumption that old age implies an incapacity for decision-making or that physical weakness connotes this incapacity.

Theoretical considerations

Case 1 illustrates the fact that neither aging nor physical weakness necessarily indicates lack of decisional capacity, even though it generally involves gradual diminishment of one's physical powers. Even then, many elderly people are more physically and mentally able than some of their younger counterparts. These differences across age groups need to be identified and addressed in order to reduce a tendency toward unjust and empirically unsupportable stereotyping.

Although the alternatives she has refused (nursing home placement, moving in with her daughter, etc.) would probably promote her health, Cathleen McCarthy is apparently as capable of autonomous refusal of health-promoting behaviors as are young adults who jeopardize their health or welfare through their autonomous decisions. From an egalitarian perspective, her autonomy should be respected to the same extent that it would be respected in a younger person: that is, as long as the burdens it entails for others do not outweigh respect for their autonomy (maxim 3). Even when others find their chosen behaviors objectionable, the standpoints of competent individuals of any age have privileged status with regard to decisions that mainly affect them.

Case 1 also illustrates the fact that women predominate not only among the elderly but also among caregivers of the elderly. Here, too, the standpoint of those who are nondominant should be granted privileged status. Caregivers in informal settings are often inadequately remunerated financially or psychologically, or both, and they are often subject to physical exhaustion and depression.[12] Ellie Smith is like many daughters and daughters-in-law whose own health is at risk from long-term, arduous caring for elderly parents.[13] Ethically, the physician asked to help her obtain nursing home placement for her mother should be guided by beneficence and nonmaleficence toward Ellie also. Although this does not imply that it is morally permissible to lie about Cathleen's decisional capacity, it does imply an obligation, on egalitarian grounds, to relieve the burden of caregiving for Ellie. If the burden to the caregiver poses a significant health risk that is unrelievable by other means, Cathleen McCarthy's refusal may be overridden on grounds of maxim 3.

The remaining cases involve patients who have legal guardians, the appointment of whom requires court proceedings in which medical documentation of the person's decisional incapacity is provided. Regardless of physical impairment or weakness, patients have decisional capacity as long as, and to the extent that, they are able to make and communicate informed and autonomous decisions.[14] When this ability is lacking, different forms of guardianship, conservatorships, and powers of attorney are legal mechanisms for decision-making. A guardian of the estate, for example, may decide about disposition of the patient's assets, and a guardian of the person or power of attorney for health care may make medical decisions for the patient. As both guardian of the estate and guardian of the person, Andrew Sheldon is responsible for his mother's financial and medical welfare. However, the grounds on which he is bound to make decisions for her are his mother's own interests, not his, giving priority to autonomous wishes that she may have previously expressed.[15] In other words, the standpoint of the patient has privileged status both legally and ethically.

In case 4, Fred Zink has apparently neglected his responsibilities as legal guardian of his mother, and the social worker is therefore correct that something should be done to remedy the situation. Presumably, this could be accomplished either by enforcing the son's fulfillment of his legal responsibilities as his mother's guardian or by replacing him in that role with someone who will reliably fulfill these responsibilities. Noreen Zink's physician should certainly support the social worker's efforts to effect such a change, and she should ensure, to the extent that she is able, that the patient is not returned to an environment in which her health is endangered.

Violence against women

Cases

1. Yvonne Stokes, 26 weeks pregnant, arrives at the prenatal clinic with concerns about her fetus. She tells the medical resident that she was injured when she fell down the stairs at home. Although she "feels OK," she is fearful that "my baby is hurt." On physical exam, the resident notices bruises and swelling inconsistent with the patient's report of how her fall occurred. Asked if anyone may have hit her, Yvonne replies: "No, I'm just clumsy."

2. Cassie Cowan has been supporting her drug addiction by prostitution for the past three years. Looking tearful and unkempt, she comes to the emergency department and tells the nurse she was raped by her pimp after he discovered she had not given him all her "earnings." Police are called and ask for a rape kit exam, but the nurse questions whether the evidence obtained would be useful to investigators; if not, she says, the exam should not be done.

3. Anita Muldoon, 46 years old, was mugged at gunpoint and sexually assaulted after leaving work. Before reporting the incident, she went home and took a shower because she "felt so dirty," then went to the emergency center of the local hospital to be "checked out." After telling the nurse what happened, she was asked if she wanted to report the incident to police. She said she was unwilling to talk more about it with anyone. She just wanted "to forget about" what happened, and reporting the incident would make that impossible.

Empirical considerations

Violence occurs toward women of all ages. With many women, it takes the form of "intimate partner violence"—violence in which the perpetrator is a current or former spouse, partner, boyfriend, or girlfriend of the victim. The National Center for Injury Prevention and Control estimates that roughly 1 in 5 women in the United States is physically assaulted each year by an intimate partner.[16] Women are less likely to report abuse or press charges by intimate partners than to do so when the violence is inflicted by strangers.

Although there is no single profile of an abused woman or of a perpetrator, pregnancy increases the risk of violence toward women by their partners. According to some studies, violence toward pregnant women is 60 percent more likely than violence toward nonpregnant women.[17] Some authors suggest that violence is more common for pregnant women than is preeclampsia, gestational diabetes, or placenta previa, all of which are routinely addressed during prenatal care.[18] Factors that exacerbate the risk of violence toward them are the unintentionality of the pregnancy, unmarried status, younger age, delayed prenatal care, and smoking, alcohol abuse, or drug abuse.

Prostitution involves an extremely high risk of physical, sexual, psychological, and economic violence toward women. Studies report that 70 to 80 percent of prostitutes are victims of rape, and 85 percent of these are raped by their pimps.[19] Typically, the perpetrators target girls or women who are naive, lonely, homeless, or rebellious, and they recruit them by feigning affection and support; once recruited, they keep them in virtual captivity by maintaining and reinforcing a sense of worthlessness and dependence. As with women who stay with domestic partners who batter them, prostitutes often stay with their pimps because they bond emotionally with them as a psychological and economic means of survival.[20]

The majority of victims know their assailants, but some don't, as in case 3. Victims are advised to go to an emergency department after an assault to check for injuries, especially those that may not be immediately detectable. Antibiotics are offered prophylactically, and baseline tests for pregnancy and sexually transmitted diseases are usually performed to determine whether the victim was infected or pregnant before the assault. If the assault took place during a high-risk time for pregnancy, the victim may be offered the "morning after pill," a high dose of estrogen intended to prevent conception.

Another important reason for immediate medical attention after sexual assault is to collect physical evidence for a criminal investigation. If the incident happened within the previous 72 hours, emergency departments are required to offer victims a rape kit exam. To be useful in determining the guilt or innocence of alleged assailants, the evidence obtained through the rape kit must be tested by DNA experts. However, funding shortages throughout the United States have left thousands of untested kits in storage, rendering futile the victims' endurance of invasive and uncomfortable exams that may revisit in them the trauma of the rape itself.[21] Showering prior to physical exam, as in case 3, may preclude the possibility of obtaining useful evidence, but the crime itself is still reportable and prosecutable.

Theoretical considerations

Suspicion of abuse or neglect is obviously different from verification of abuse or neglect. For health care workers, the term "suspicion" is well chosen because their role vis-à-vis possible victims generally precludes verification that the violence has occurred. Recognizing how psychologically difficult, sometimes even impossible, it is for women to acknowledge intimate partner violence (as in case 1), practitioners can fulfill their legal obligation of mandatory reporting without having to press their patients beyond their ability or willingness to talk about the matter with others. To the extent that others, such as social workers, facilitate a patient's autonomous involvement in efforts to prevent abuse or neglect, physicians and nurses should enlist their assistance.

The legal obligation of health care workers to report suspected abuse or neglect is clear in all three cases. In cases 1 and 3, this obligation is at odds with respect for the woman's autonomy but justifiable on grounds of nonmaleficence toward others—those whose risk of harm may be reduced through follow-up by appropriate authorities to the reports of neglect or abuse. When the woman is already pregnant, as in case 1, the suspicion of harm is applicable to the potential child as well as the woman. Maxim 3 and the verity of justice also support mandatory reporting of suspected abuse or neglect, but when follow-up does not occur, this rationale is inadequate. Moreover, if a rape kit exam is performed but the semen obtained is not tested, maxim 1 is violated because the interests of the person whose standpoint is privileged, the patient and victim, are subordinated to the less weighty (if any) interests of others. To the extent that practitioners as such may further efforts to ensure that evidence obtained through rape kit exams is used, justice requires that they do so.

Although the legal obligation to report suspected abuse or neglect is ethically justifiable, no clinician may legally or morally perform a rape kit exam without the victim's (or her proxy's) consent. This is consistent with the general prohibition against intrusive physical interventions without the patient's (or proxy's) consent, even if these are intended solely for diagnostic or treatment purposes (maxim 2). Even with consent, if a rape kit exam offers no realistic expectation that it will produce useful evidence, a clinician may morally decline to perform it, as in case 2, on grounds that neither the woman's welfare nor social interests are thereby served. Refusal to perform the exam may be defended on grounds of respect for the clinician's autonomy in circumstances in which the procedure apparently serves no therapeutic purpose for the woman or others. It is possible, however, that respect for the victim's autonomy serves a psychologically therapeutic purpose for her also, in which case her interests ought to supersede those of the practitioner (maxim 1).

The woman's refusal to talk about the incident, as in case 3, should also be respected on grounds of respect for her autonomy and her privileged standpoint. However, this rationale applies not only to the current decisions of patients, whether these involve acceptance or rejection of medical recommendations, but also to different decisions they may make as circumstances change. Anita, for example, like many victims of sexual assault, may not want to talk about what happened to her when she visits the emergency center, and she may decline to give further details to clinicians or to the police to whom the incident is reported. Later on she may be willing, possibly even eager, to divulge the details of what happened to appropriate authorities. Accordingly, she should be *offered* the rape kit exam, informed about the discomfort it involves, and told that undergoing the exam now would preserve evidence she might subsequently wish to act on. If she still refuses, maxim 2 remains morally as well as legally applicable.

It is possible that the victims in cases 2 and 3 were both impregnated through their rapists.[22] In light of that possibility, the woman's own perspective regarding the morning after pill is highly relevant to decisions about its administration. Most women would choose this means of avoiding pregnancy after rape. However, the distinction between "conception" and "fertilization" may be relevant to some, as well as to some clinicians, because the morning-after pill prevents the former but not the latter. Standpoint theory calls for attribution of privileged status to the woman's decision regarding this as well as other issues; practitioners who disagree with her decision on moral grounds are not obliged to provide the treatment but they may not abandon her, and they should disclose their moral position on the matter to the patient.

Gender discrimination and sexual harassment

Cases

1. Two medical students met with Sharon Bushey, dean of students, to complain about an experience that had offended them in their anatomy class. At the start of a scheduled lecture, a woman dressed in a white nursing cap, white shoes and stockings, and a white uniform under her buttoned coat, walked into the lecture hall and, as the professor looked on without surprise, proceeded to sing happy birthday while slinking toward the student who apparently was "the birthday boy." Continuing to sing and sway in a seductive manner, she removed each article of clothing down to her underwear and dangled it in front of the student. Finally, she kissed the student with a loud smack and exited the lecture hall as many of the students erupted in applause. On report of the incident to the dean, the complaining students were told that they were oversensitive and should let the matter rest because "boys will be boys."

2. Celia Downs, 50 years old, fell down a flight of stairs and was taken to the nearest medical center for emergency care. On arrival, she told the female physician who attempted to examine her that she wanted a male doctor instead. She said she didn't trust female doctors because "they're not as smart as men. They don't think as clearly because they're too emotional." Only women were on duty at the time.

3. Same as above, but only men are on duty, and Celia insists on examination by a woman, saying "I don't trust men."

4. Penny Zawicki and Ann Burke have lived together for five years and would like to have a child together. In order to allow both to be biologically related to the child, they would like Penny to undergo ovulation stimulation so that her eggs can be retrieved, fertilized with sperm from an anonymous donor, and transferred to Ann, who would then gestate and give birth to the child they would like to raise. The first reproductive endocrinologist they visit refuses to assist them; her colleague, however, is happy to do so.

5. Florence Dixon is completing a fellowship in high-risk obstetrics. The fellowship director has complimented her several times for "how good she looks in her scrubs" and has suggested that it would be "fun to see her without them."

Empirical considerations

Although the terms "sexual harassment" and "gender discrimination" are comparatively new, the practices to which they apply have occurred throughout history. Decades ago, Susan Brownmiller, along with Andrea Dworkin and Catherine MacKinnon, identified sexual harassment as an issue of power rather than sex: one based on the fact that women in general can be dominated by men because women occupy less powerful positions in society.[23] Their work challenged a rather prevalent view, apparently held by the dean in case 1, that sexual harassment is a normal expression of male sexuality. Gender discrimination also involves a power discrepancy between the sexes, and both practices occur in same-sex as well as opposite-sex interactions.

Many studies indicate that sexual harassment is widespread but underreported and that it takes a serious toll on women's lives and careers. Reasons offered for the underreporting include lack of confidence that supervisors will "do anything about it," fear of being blamed for provoking the harassment, and "not wanting to hurt the harasser."[24] Studies also show that women and men interpret sexualized behavior differently: men report that they would be flattered by sexual attention at work; women report that they are annoyed by similar behavior.[25]

At times, sexual harassment takes the form of a "quid pro quo," for example, when its acceptance is, or appears to be, a condition for maintaining or evaluating one's status as a student or employee. Stereotypic construals of gender and professional power differentials contribute to the incidence of quid pro quo harassment. In a study of residents in internal medicine, for example, 73 percent of the women and 22 percent of the men reported that they had been sexually harassed at least once during their training, usually by supervisors or evaluators of their work.[26] As more women enter the field while continuing to predominate at lower levels of power, the incidence of harassment may increase unless preventive or corrective measures are introduced.

Victims of harassment include those who may be insulted or demeaned by the offensive conduct, such as the students in case 1. Moreover, despite the usual power differential between patients and caregivers, female practitioners may be harassed by their patients, as in case 5, as well as their supervisors. In a study of family physicians, 75 percent of the female respondents reported having been sexually harassed by a patient at some point in their careers.[27] Whatever its source or target, sexual harassment of practitioners creates a hostile environment that impedes their work performance.

Theoretical considerations

Although the term "discrimination" may have a commendable as well as a condemnable connotation, it is most often used in the latter sense, as associated with unjust or unfair practices. Unjust discrimination involves differential treatment of individuals based on irrelevant characteristics, leading to or exacerbating disadvantages in those individuals. Typically, these characteristics are defined by membership in a particular group. As illustrated by cases 2, 3, and 4, unjust gender discrimination occurs when individuals are disadvantaged solely on grounds of their gender identity (as male, female, bisexual, homosexual, transsexual, or lesbian) but the discriminatory practice is not of a sexual nature. Sexual harassment is a form of unjust discrimination that involves unwelcome sexual advances, requests for sexual favors, and other verbal or physical conduct of a sexual nature that interferes with someone's work performance or creates an intimidating, hostile, or offensive environment.[28]

Implementation of standpoint theory serves as a corrective to unjust discrimination of any kind. In case 1, for example, it might have led the anatomy professor to prevent the offending event or the dean to support those whom it offended rather than the offenders. In case 5, it would (and should) have led the fellowship director to avoid sexually suggestive comments to Florence Dixon. In neither of these cases was the rationale that men are naturally prone to sexual harassment ("boys will be boys") an adequate ethical justification for the behavior. Nor is gender discrimination justified on grounds that it has been practiced throughout history. As philosophers put it, "*is* does not imply *ought.*"

Cases 2, 3, and 4 all illustrate the complexity that arises from the fact that nearsightedness is not limited to those who are dominant, and nondominant perspectives sometimes mingle with dominant ones. Cases 2 and 3 also involve patients whose judgments about unknown individuals are based on gender stereotypes. In general, respect for patient autonomy should be maximized even in matters unrelated to clinical care, not only because the patient's interests are primary (maxim 1) but also because compliance with their wishes often contributes to successful treatment.

Another variable relevant to cases 2 and 3 is the difficulty or possibility of compliance with patient requests involving nonclinical matters in emergency situations. In both cases, staff limitations evidently preclude compliance with the patient's gender-based request if optimal medical treatment is to be provided. A competent patient should be informed of this limitation and allowed to determine whether she nonetheless prefers to refuse or postpone treatment. If she is not competent to decide, beneficence and nonmaleficence have priority because respect for her autonomy is not possible.

Gender-based preferences for practitioners sometimes stem from cultural or religious traditions that require women to be examined or treated only by other women. From an egalitarian perspective, efforts (whether successful or not) to respect these traditions are required, whereas compliance with requests based on unjust gender, racial, or ethnic stereotypes is not. An argument that a patient's request should be honored even if it arises from prejudice in order to promote her emotional welfare or facilitate healing is valid but inadequate unless the patient is not otherwise treatable effectively. Even then, the practitioner should avoid complicity in the patient's prejudice by informing her that compliance with her request is not based on agreement with her standpoint.[29]

Clinicians are always obliged to treat patients in need of emergency care, but they are not obliged to accept patients for elective treatment. In most if not all cases, infertility treatment is elective. Accordingly, when Penny Zawicki and Ann Burke request infertility treatment, their request need not be honored. The different positions of the two reproductive endocrinologists in this case may stem from different religious or moral standpoints. Possibly, the first physician considers reproductive assistance morally acceptable only for married heterosexual couples. Ordinarily, such commitments should be respected on grounds that respect for autonomy applies to clinicians as well as patients. Exceptions to this prima facie obligation may arise from the primacy of justice, which is more likely to be violated if the refusal to treat is based on gender stereotypes or prejudice toward lesbians and homosexuals.

As already indicated, once a practitioner undertakes care of a particular patient, she may not abandon her. Apparently, the first physician in case 4 did not reach this point, and a colleague was able to provide the requested care without violating her moral integrity. Not only different moral values but also personality clashes may prompt clinicians to refuse elective care for particular patients; in such cases, the patient's interests may be best served through referral. However, if the reason for refusal is to preserve the practitioner's own moral integrity, referral to someone whose practice is at odds with the reason for refusal is morally questionable because it constitutes complicity in the behavior judged immoral.

The issues examined in this chapter have been increasingly addressed in clinical literature and in statements or guidelines of medical organizations. It is still true, however, that medical students and other health professionals in training hear little about the significant impact of these issues on their future patients' health, let alone instruction about ways through which to detect and address that impact. From an egalitarian perspective, recognition of the inevitable connection between public and private spheres of life, as well as the connection between needs that are not strictly medical (e.g., safety, social nurturance, and respect) and human health, is incumbent on practitioners whose goal is to optimize care for their patients. Those who recognize these connections but lack expertise for remedying the circumstances in which violence, discrimination, or harassment occurs seek ways by which to enlist the expertise of those who do.

11

Nonreproductive Health Issues

Many bioethicists examine cases related to women's health only in conjunction with women's reproductive capacity. This is true even when the woman herself is unconcerned about the implications of her condition for reproduction. But ethical issues in women's health care occur across the entire life span, and many of these have nothing to do with reproduction, either directly or indirectly. An adequate bioethics for women must consider these also. Accordingly, in chapter 10 health issues raised by the social environment and by the nondominant status in which women often find themselves, regardless of their reproductive role, are discussed. This chapter is focused on conditions that have particular impact on women because of gender-specific expectations and implications, regardless of whether the issues are also related to reproduction. The remaining chapters consider bioethical issues of health care for elderly women and research issues involving women of any age.

Some nonreproductive issues have special relevance to women because of biological differences as well as gender-based differences in the impact of the conditions addressed. The great majority of women who are HIV positive, for example, were infected with the virus by men, often their husbands. Breast cancer mainly affects women, and its treatment is made more onerous for them because of social expectations about feminine appearance. Menopause, a normal stage in a woman's life, may also be more onerous because of social attitudes that define women and their worth by their reproductive role. From an egalitarian perspective, efforts to minimize whatever injustice occurs because of these sex-based or gender-based differences are indispensable.

The cases that follow illustrate variables that are ethically relevant throughout the life span.

HIV testing and AIDS

Cases

1. Serena Kao, 32 years old, was rushed by helicopter to the nearest medical center after being severely burned in an apartment fire. Prior to losing consciousness, she asked the nurse to contact her boyfriend, who, on his arrival, told the staff that Serena had been estranged from her parents for the last decade. Routine tests revealed that she was HIV positive, and physical exam showed signs of AIDS. Although the staff considered this information pertinent to decisions about treatment, they wondered whether it should be shared with either her parents or her boyfriend.

2. Noah Spitzer is an attending physician in obstetrics. Over the years his residents have observed a pattern of avoidance of cases of scheduled cesarean sections when the patient is known to be HIV positive or symptomatic for AIDS. Because of their more limited experience, the residents believe his behavior unjustly deprives women of medically optimal care. They are reluctant, however, to report his behavior to the department chair.

3. Jessie Blair, age 20, tested positive for the HIV virus two years ago. Although she has been warned about the risk her sexual activities pose for her partners, she says she doesn't want to tell them because "that would really ruin the sex." She apparently understands the risks of becoming symptomatic if she doesn't comply with the recommended drug regimen, but persistently misses clinic appointments and fails to take her medications. Her physician decides not to prescribe a protease inhibitor combination drug therapy because she doesn't trust Jessie to comply with the regimen, and noncompliance would probably reduce the effectiveness of therapy later on. The physician thinks use of public funds for her drug therapy is unwarranted, and that Jessie's partners should be told about her HIV status.

4. Carrie Simons, a successful and popular obstetrician, became HIV positive from a needle stick in the delivery room. She was told by her department chair that her status would be kept confidential, and she could go on operating as long as she diligently observed the recommended precautions. Three months later, the department chair received an anonymous letter asking that Carrie be barred from performing any procedures because of her HIV status. Over the objection of Carrie's colleagues, the department chair complied with the request.

Empirical considerations

HIV (human immunodeficicency virus) reduces the body's capacity to fight infections. Exposure to bodily fluids of affected individuals places others at risk of transmission, but whether this has occurred is not determinable for several months after exposure. Although a positive test for HIV does not imply that an individual has AIDS (autoimmune deficiency syndrome), it is an indicator that the body's immune system is being gradually depleted, increasing the risk of "opportunistic infections" that affect the lungs (pneumocystic pneumonia), skin (Kaposi's sarcoma), eyes (cytomegalogvirus), throat (thrush), or vagina (candidiasis). If symptoms of any of these infections are manifest, the HIV-positive person has AIDS. Without treatment, she is highly likely to die from the infection or from other related health problems, such as brain tumor.

Medications can slow damage to the immune system, but they cannot totally eliminate the suppression of the immune system caused by the virus. Other drugs can effectively prevent or treat opportunistic infections, allowing some HIV-positive individuals to live healthy lives for many years and some who have AIDS to live longer with less morbidity than they would otherwise experience. A few people who are HIV positive have escaped infections without anti-HIV medications. The course of HIV and AIDS is thus different for each infected person.

Across the globe, the number of women with HIV and AIDS has steadily increased. In 2005, roughly half of the 40 million adults living with HIV/AIDS were women.[1] In the United States, the proportion of AIDS cases in women rose from 7 to 26 percent between 1985 and 2002, and the majority of the affected women belonged to nondominant minorities.[2] Women are generally infected from their male partners, but infection also occurs through use of contaminated needles.

Women are subject to the same complications of AIDS and antiretroviral therapy as men. However, they also suffer gender-specific manifestations such as recurrent vaginal yeast infections and severe pelvic inflammatory disease, both of which increase the risk of cervical cancer and metabolic abnormalities. Lack of social and economic support frequently interferes with the ability to adhere to the demanding treatment regimens of AIDS and HIV medications.[3] Women who are HIV positive tend to have greater difficulty accessing health care and carry a heavier burden of caring for children than do their male counterparts.

Although health professionals risk exposure to HIV/AIDS through their patients, their risk of being infected is still low, about 0.3 percent.[4] Clinicians such as Noah Spitzer are usually well aware that the risk is higher in surgical suites and delivery rooms than in other clinical settings. Estimates of the risk in these settings range from 1 in 40,000 to 1 in 400,000. (Comparatively, the risk of a fatal reaction to anesthesia during surgery is 1 in 10,000.[5]) As case 1 illustrates, patients themselves do not always know or reveal their HIV status to those who care for them. Practitioners are therefore required to observe "universal precautions" that include protective gloves, gowns, aprons, masks, and eyewear. If accidents such as needlesticks or scalpel wounds occur, they are expected to obtain immediate prophylactic treatment.

While it is possible for physicians who are HIV positive to infect patients, no such case has ever been reported in the United States. HIV transmission from a dentist to his patient has been alleged but not demonstrated. Citing the lack of data showing HIV transmission from physicians to patients, the American College of Surgeons maintains that "HIV-infected surgeons may continue to practice and perform invasive procedures and surgical operations unless there is clear evidence that a significant risk of transmission of infection exists through an inability to meet basic infection control procedures, or the surgeon is functionally unable to care for patients."[6]

Theoretical considerations

Probably the most complicated ethical issue surrounding HIV/AIDS is that of confidentiality. As discussed in chapter 8, confidentiality facilitates full and honest disclosure as required by respect for patient autonomy. However, this is an a priori obligation which, as such, is occasionally overridable by nonmaleficence to others. Because disclosure of HIV status may lead to stigmatization, ostracization, and loss or denial of health insurance and job opportunities for those who test positive, the obligation of confidentiality about HIV status is more compelling than it would be with regard to other medical information. Nonetheless, because of the risk of HIV-positive status to those with whom an affected person is sexually intimate, the obligation to reduce the risk of so severe and still-not-curable disease in others is also compelling. From an egalitarian perspective, clinicians need to weigh these risks carefully and override confidentiality only if, after adequate counseling, the patient herself is unwilling or unable to warn those at risk. By these criteria, the physician in case 3 has grounds for seeing that Jessie Blair's sex partners are warned of their risk. This does not imply that she herself may or should reveal Jessie's HIV status to them. To preserve confidentiality as much as possible, the information should be communicated in a nonidentifying way, such as through health department personnel.

The physician's decision not to prescribe drug therapy for Jessie is supported by beneficence and nonmaleficence toward Jessie and respect for the physician's own autonomy—that is, her right to withhold treatment that threatens a patient's health. However, the physician's rationale that use of public funds in this case is unwarranted is problematic. If she believes that use of these funds to provide therapy for Jessie would deplete the resources necessary to treat others for whom therapy is likely to be effective, her rationale is consistent with an egalitarian perspective. If she believes that patients like Jessie should be denied funding for treatment because they are of lesser value than other patients, her belief is at odds with that perspective.

In case 1, the complexity raised by the obligation of confidentiality is exacerbated by the fact that Serena is unconscious, has come to the hospital for an emergency unrelated to AIDS, and knowledge of her AIDS status is pertinent to decisions others may be asked to make on her behalf. To the extent that a surrogate decision maker is expected to make decisions that the patient would make, the surrogate should be informed of whatever the patient herself would want to know. Because the surrogate stands in the place of the patient as decision maker, depriving the surrogate of this information is equivalent to denying information demanded by respect for the patient's own autonomy. Unfortunately, laws in the United States do not usually allow for this exception to the requirement of confidentiality about AIDS status; if they did, they would support the exception.

Determination of who should be the woman's surrogate is another complexity of case 1. Some state statutes prescribe an order of surrogates based solely on family or legally established relationships. Such stipulated ordering ignores the fact that someone not included in the order may be more likely than those included in it to know the patient's standpoint on the issue at hand. In this case, for example, Serena's boyfriend is probably the ethically preferable surrogate. Regardless of whether state statutes allow him rather than her parents to serve in this capacity, the ethical argument for doing so is compelling.

Case 4 raises the question of confidentiality from the standpoint of clinicians: whether those who are HIV positive are obliged to reveal this to patients on whom they may perform invasive procedures. Despite the restrictiveness of laws on disclosure of HIV status to people other than the affected person, some have argued that the same restrictiveness should not be applied to clinicians who are HIV positive. This argument is supportable on grounds of the increased risk to patients, but it is considerably weakened by the lack of evidence that a patient has ever contracted HIV from a physician.[7] From an egalitarian perspective, the mere fact that a patient wants to know her clinician's HIV status doesn't justify the disclosure. Neither does the anonymous request to have Carrie Simons barred from performing procedures provide adequate grounds for doing so.

Although reported cases are few, patient-to-physician transmission of HIV infection is well documented. Physicians are morally and legally bound to treat affected patients in emergency situations, but many surgeries and deliveries are not emergencies. If Noah Spitzer tends to avoid these cases, as his residents believe, he reduces his own risk but doesn't harm patients if other competent physicians then assume their care. He nonetheless places those who provide the care at greater risk, and this is not defensible from an egalitarian perspective unless other ethically relevant variables justify his avoidance. A possibility in this regard is that Noah is so nervous in performing procedures in these cases that he puts the patient at greater risk.

Legally, attending physicians rather than residents are generally responsible for patients. Unless the residents have performed procedures illegally, another experienced physician has therefore been responsible for the cases that Noah avoided. If that has not happened, the illegality should be reported because it risks harm to others. From the residents' standpoint, Noah has apparently failed to provide a model of how physicians fulfill their moral obligations to treat patients, regardless of risks to themselves. The attending physician's standpoint is also crucial to adequate analysis of whether his behavior is "morally wrong and unprofessional." The department chair to whom the residents may report their concerns should elicit that standpoint to learn of variables that the residents might have missed.

Breast and gynecological cancers

Cases

1. Beth Comiskey is a 39-year-old widow with two daughters, ages 12 and 14. Her grandmother died of ovarian cancer, and her mother had a mastectomy for breast cancer ten years ago. Recently, Beth's sister was diagnosed with breast cancer and treated with a lumpectomy. Responding to an offer of free testing for people with a strong family history of cancer, Beth had her blood drawn for the test at a cancer risk clinic near her workplace. On returning to work, she looked at her policy and learned that her health plan would not cover treatment of "preexisting conditions," conditions that had not been disclosed before being hired. The document did not distinguish between conditions that the employee knew about and those she was unaware of prior to her employment.

Beth called the clinic to ask that her drawn blood not be tested or, if it had already been tested, that the result be withheld from her and any documentation regarding the test be expunged from her medical record. The clerk who answered already knew that the test had been performed and that the result was negative. Aside from the question of whether the record of the visit could be ethically or legally deleted, the dilemma this introduced was whether to respect Beth's autonomy by refraining from disclosure of the result or to give her the good news that she had no identifiable genetic risk for breast cancer.

2. Leslie Peters, 45 years old, was treated successfully through lumpectomy for a small malignancy in her right breast. Six years later, she requests prophylactic oophorectomy (elective removal of ovaries) to reduce her risk of ovarian cancer. Her physician refuses to perform the procedure unless Leslie tests positive for a specific genetic mutation, BRCA 1 or BRCA 2. Leslie refuses the genetic test but persists in her request for oophorectomy over the next few months. During this time she exhibits a great deal of anxiety—equivalent, from her physician's standpoint, to "cancer phobia." Eventually he agrees to perform the surgery on grounds that it is necessary for the patient's mental health.

3. Katrina Kaye, a 40-year-old mother of seven, was diagnosed with early-stage cervical cancer. Her physician advises her to undergo a radical hysterectomy with removal of pelvic lymph nodes. On learning that the surgery also entails loss of her uterus, Katrina refuses the treatment. "I don't want to have more children," she says, "but I wouldn't be a real woman any more if I don't have that."

Empirical considerations

Although heart disease is the leading cause of death in the United States, cancer is the leading cause of death in people under age 85. In the United States and in Europe, lung cancer is the leading cause of cancer deaths and, for women, the cause of more deaths than all gynecological cancers combined.[8] Of the three types of cancer illustrated in this section, ovarian is the most deadly because it usually progresses without becoming symptomatic, delaying diagnosis until treatment is likely to be ineffective. According to a 2006 report from the American Cancer Society, the five-year survival rate of ovarian cancer is 44.6 percent of those affected, whereas the five-year survival rates of breast cancer and cervical cancer are 88.2 percent and 73.3 percent respectively.[9] However, a woman is considerably more likely to have breast cancer during her lifetime than either of the other two cancers. The lifetime risk for breast cancer is 1 in 8 women, for ovarian the risk is 1 in 58 and for cervical cancer, the risk is 1 in 135.[10]

A minority of breast and ovarian cancers arise in women who have BRCA 1 or BRCA 2 mutations, and symptoms manifest themselves earlier and more aggressively in 60 to 85 percent of these women.[11] Other risk factors for breast and gynecological cancers include age, reproductive and menstrual history, hormone therapy, radiation exposure, and lifestyle factors. Women who begin having sex at an early age or who have multiple sex partners are at greater risk of infection with certain types of the human papilloma virus (HPV), which causes cervical cancer.[12] However, women whose history shows none of these risk factors may also develop breast or gynecological cancer.

Symptoms vary for different types of cancer and stages of the disease. Physical change in breast tissue is the most common symptom of breast cancer. Abnormal vaginal bleeding may be a sign of cervical cancer, and enlargement of the abdomen may indicate ovarian cancer. Mammograms and pap tests facilitate early detection of breast cancer and cervical cancer. Neither of these tests is totally reliable, but their regular use has enabled successful treatment in many cases.[13] Through regular examination of their breasts, women themselves discover abnormalities early enough for minimally invasive and successful treatment. Because early treatment has so dramatically improved survival rates, regular screening is encouraged and covered by insurance for most women.

As with other cancers, the available treatment modalities for breast and gynecological cancers are surgery, radiation, and chemotherapy. Depending on the stage at which the disease is diagnosed, different types or combinations of treatment are recommended (e.g., lumpectomy vs. mastectomy). When there is a strong family history of breast or ovarian cancer, prophylactic surgery may be recommended. Prophylactic oophorectomy in women who have BRCA 1 or BRCA 2 mutations decreases the risk of breast cancer as well as ovarian cancer.[14] For early-stage cervical cancer in women who no longer plan to have children, radical hysterectomy and removal of lymph nodes is routinely recommended, but radiation therapy may be just as effective.

Theoretical considerations

The term "cancer" often invokes fears that belie the reality of specific manifestations of the disease. Cases in which cancer is life-threatening or terminal are considered in chapter 12. In contrast, the cases of cancer considered above are not necessarily life-threatening if diagnosis occurs early enough for effective treatment. The burden of cancer and cancer treatment may be exacerbated by its impact on reproductive decisions, sexual performance, and gender-based expectations about appearance or identity. Breast and gynecological cancers are especially likely to entail these burdens, which cause greater anxiety in some women than other aspects of their treatment. In light of these variables, it is incumbent on health caregivers to impute privileged status to the different standpoints of women in decisions about their treatment.

Beth Comiskey's request not to reveal her test result didn't necessarily pose an ethical dilemma regarding disclosure. As often happens in human encounters, knowledge helpful to others can be facilitated without actual disclosure of information that one may be morally obliged to withhold. In this case, for example, Beth's request could be answered with a question such as, "Do you mean you wouldn't want to know even if the result is negative?" Most probably, this would prompt Beth to say she would like to know about a negative result. If she insisted otherwise, the result should be withheld from her on grounds of respect for her autonomy. On grounds of beneficence toward others, however, she should be reminded that the information is relevant to her daughters, whose risk of breast cancer is related to their mother's risk.

Because health insurance has been denied or terminated for some people with preexisting conditions, legislation has been introduced to avoid these discriminatory practices. Nonetheless, respect for the autonomy of those to be tested obliges practitioners to provide them with information regarding the possible impact of positive results on their employment and insurance coverage. From an egalitarian perspective, no person should be denied employment or health insurance because of mere susceptibility to a disease. In a free enterprise system, therefore, laws are needed to require private insurance companies to expand their customer base sufficiently to cover those who are susceptible to late-onset diseases.

Cases 2 and 3 illustrate very different attitudes about cancer risk in women: fear of loss of life versus fear of loss of a defining characteristic of womanhood. Apparently, the former fear predominates in Leslie Peters, while the latter fear predominates in Katrina Kaye. Although clinicians treating these patients should impute privileged status to their standpoints, the clinicians' standpoints are also ethically relevant. As mentioned elsewhere, clinicians are not morally compelled to respond to patient requests solely on grounds of respect for their autonomy. If Leslie's mental health is seriously threatened through her physician's refusal to perform oophorectomy, he has adequate grounds for performing it; it seems doubtful, however, that this is the case and more probable that this is a rationalization, not a justification. Moreover, if Leslie really has a "cancer phobia," it is much more likely to be treated successfully by psychiatrists or psychologists than by surgeons.

The burden of the recommended treatment for Katrina Kaye seems to rest on her valuing her uterus more than her life, which may be better preserved by removal of her uterus. Her refusal of treatment may be overly influenced by gender stereotypes that reduce her autonomy by impeding the acuity of her standpoint. An egalitarian perspective requires the clinician to acknowledge this possibility and attempt to reduce the impediments to genuine autonomy that distorted conceptions of womanhood may entail. In other words, the physician should offer the woman a lens that allows her to see her life and personhood as not necessarily linked to her uterus. This may be done by asking her to explain what she means by being a "real woman" and exploring with her how this relates to her desire to preserve her life. If she is mainly concerned about inducing menopause through surgery, she should be told that this need not occur because her ovaries can be retained. If keeping her uterus remains a priority, radiation should be offered as an alternative to surgery. Based on maxim 2, respect for her autonomy prevails over beneficence and nonmaleficence toward her. However, to ensure that her final decision about treatment is adequately autonomous, Katrina should be reminded that if her presently curable cancer is not treated, it will progress to a point where neither her "womanhood" nor her life is preservable.

Menopause and hormone replacement therapy

Cases

1. Emma Johnson, 49 years old, is an academic who has studied the relationship between language and social attitudes for many years. Recently, she scrutinized a half-dozen clinical texts in which developmental events in women's lives were identified and discussed. While reading sections on menstruation, pregnancy, and menopause, she noticed that the definitions of all three related the condition to women's reproductive capacity. Menstruation was defined in positive terms, as entailing the ability to become pregnant, which was also described in positive terms; in contrast, menopause was defined negatively, as failure in ovarian function, cessation of menses, and loss of reproductive capacity. To Emma, the negative definitions were consistent with what she had recently read in the popular press about the distress and discomfort associated with menopause, but they were at odds with her mother's account of the experience, as a relief or "liberation" from having to worry about menses and pregnancy. As an academic, Emma questions why the clinical definition is mainly negative. From the standpoint of her personal experience, she believes she is menopausal because her periods are not as regular or as heavy as they used to be. Although she feels healthy, she wonders whether this is abnormal.

2. Jamie Church, 32 years old, was taught throughout medical training that hormone replacement therapy (HRT) should be prescribed for the majority of women going through menopause because of its multiple therapeutic benefits. As a resident and as a young practitioner, she has dutifully done this, and most of her patients have happily complied with her advice. Jamie was greatly surprised, therefore, when she learned of studies demonstrating that HRT is not therapeutically helpful in many instances and that it even placed some women at greater health risk than they would otherwise be. Feeling remorseful about the many women who have taken HRT because of her strong recommendations, she wonders whether she has a moral obligation to contact them to suggest that they return to the clinic for evaluation of whether to continue taking HRT.

3. Jane Harris is a 55-year-old woman with a history of breast cancer, treated successfully with a lumpectomy two years ago. Her mother had severe osteoporosis before she died at the age of 80. Prior to her diagnosis of breast cancer, Jane had taken HRT to relieve hot flashes associated with menopause, but she discontinued the medication when the hot flashes subsided. Subsequently, she noticed a reduced level of energy, sex drive, and mental acuity, and she attributed these symptoms to the lack of estrogen replacement through HRT. During her bout with breast cancer, she did not mention these concerns to her physician. Now, however, Jane asks for a renewal of her prescription for HRT on grounds that curtailment of osteoporosis and promotion of her general well-being outweigh the risks of HRT. Consistent with recommendations from the breast surgeon and oncologist, her gynecologist declines to prescribe HRT and advises her to take a different medication for her osteoporosis.

Empirical considerations

Menopause refers to the time in a woman's life cycle when she ceases menstruating—having her monthly periods. Unless menopause is induced through cancer treatment or bilateral oophorectomy, the process through which menopause occurs is natural, gradual, and highly variable in its onset, duration, and symptoms. At about age 35, many women begin to experience slight changes in their reproductive cycles; these include unpredictability regarding the degree of blood loss, as well as the onset and duration of menses. Ovulation decreases gradually and periods become lighter and less frequent, but women retain their reproductive capacity until menstruation has completely ended during their fifties. Clinicians generally track the onset of menopause as one year from the date of the woman's last menstruation.

Symptoms associated with menopause include hot flashes, vaginal dryness, and reduction in bone density, all attributed to the decreased supply of estrogen that cessation of ovulation entails. Hot flashes are sudden, uncontrollable fluctuations of body temperatures, sometimes disrupting sleep. Vaginal dryness or atrophy can make sexual intercourse difficult and painful; bone loss makes women more susceptible to fractures and osteoporosis. Although mood swings and depression have been attributed to menopause, these are just as likely to be caused by midlife stresses such as marital strife, divorce, professional crises, and death of a parent. Most women experience mild symptoms caused by fluctuations in hormonal levels; a minority (10%–15%) find the symptoms emotionally or physically disabling, and about the same number of women experience no symptoms at all.[15] For women who seek medical care for menopause, the symptoms are relievable through lifestyle changes and medical therapies. Regardless of whether care is sought, the symptoms may be evoked or exacerbated by negative understandings of menopause.[16]

Until recently, HRT was routinely recommended for menopausal women to slow the rate of bone loss, some cancers, heart disease, and the frequency or severity of hot flashes and vaginal dryness. Current studies refute the earlier claims of reduced risk of cancer and heart disease, and nonhormonal treatments for bone loss have proved at least as effective as HRT. Although HRT is still recognized as more effective than other measures in providing relief for severe hot flashes and vaginal atrophy, some studies indicate that, on average, the health risks and side effects of HRT outweigh its benefits. Unwanted side effects are vaginal discharge, genital irritation, uterine bleeding, and, occasionally, painful engorgement of the breasts.[17]

Theoretical considerations

Etymologically, the term "menopause" comes from the Greek roots *men*, meaning "month" or "moon," and *pauein*, which means "to cease." Popularly, menopause is sometimes called "the change," presumably because it indicates that some aspects of a woman's life are not the same thereafter. Clinically and developmentally, menopause is as normal and natural in the life of healthy women as menstruation is at an earlier age. Both menstruation and menopause are related to the possibility of pregnancy, another normal, natural experience, but one triggered by a man's biological contribution to the process. All three processes involve certain inconveniences, discomforts, and sometimes pain, but each is also indicative of developmental normality. As Emma Johnson discovered, however, clinical definitions of menopause do not articulate its meaning in positive terms; instead, they define it as "loss" or "failure" (of ovarian or reproductive function) and even, in some instances, as a disease.

Because of advances in infertility treatment, a postmenopausal woman may gestate and give birth to children as long as she still has her uterus. The process through which she can become pregnant involves hormone stimulation, in vitro fertilization of another woman's eggs, and transfer to her of the resultant embryos. Children born through this process are not genetically related to the postmenopausal women who bear them. For women in whom menopause has been induced before it would normally occur (e.g., to maximize the effectiveness of cancer treatment), support for postmenopausal gestation is stronger than it is for women in whom infertility occurs in conjunction with natural menopause. From an egalitarian perspective, the younger woman does not have the same capability as her peers, while the older woman does. Arguably, other variables such as the ability to parent and whether the woman already has children may strengthen the case for treatment of one woman vis-à-vis another.

The cases described here do not address the possibility of gestation in postmenopausal women. Instead, they illustrate the far more pervasive issues of how patients and clinicians alike should view menopause and interact with each other regarding it. Emma Johnson's quandary, for example, is not unusual in a social climate that tends to represent normal developmental events in women's lives as conditions requiring medical treatment. Based on beneficence as well as nonmaleficence, clinicians who see the majority of patients for whom menopausal symptoms are only mildly problematic should facilitate recognition that this is a totally normal and natural condition. Based on those same verities, they need to identify the minority of women for whom the symptoms are severe and recommend whatever treatment is likely to provide relief with the least health risk and discomfort. The daunting challenge this entails for physicians like Jamie Church is to keep up with the best empirical studies on these treatments.

Whether Jamie is morally obliged to contact her HRT patients to suggest that they be evaluated to determine whether to continue with HRT depends on a number of variables, including the circumstances in which the HRT was recommended or taken, the possibility that these patients are already adequately informed (e.g., through widespread media coverage) about the desirability or option of reevaluation, and whether the physician has time to make such contacts while also fulfilling other obligations. From an egalitarian perspective, patients should be informed of the matter (if they are not aware of it already), but the information need not be imparted by the doctor directly. The information to which patients who have taken HRT are entitled may be communicated to previous patients by the clerical staff without requiring the practitioner's involvement.

Although no physician is morally or professionally bound to provide medical treatment that she considers, in proportion to its potential benefits, unjustifiably harmful or overly risky for a patient, neither may a physician abandon care of a patient for whom she has assumed responsibility. In case 3, therefore, transfer of care to a physician who agrees with the woman's request is possible and should be facilitated because different physicians, from different standpoints, are likely to weigh the burdens and benefits differently. If physicians all agreed that the burdens outweighed the benefits, this would not be possible unless respect for the woman's autonomy is given priority over beneficence and nonmaleficence toward her (maxim 2). From an egalitarian perspective, if the medical risks are small, treatment may still be permissible, based on respect for the woman's autonomy.

An egalitarian perspective does not impute absolute priority to decisions made by patients, even though it imputes privileged status to their input because they are nondominant in the health care setting. A standpoint strategy demands that those responsible for treatment or nontreatment of women seek and listen to women's voices regarding these decisions, to ensure that they are maximally informed and autonomous. In the cases discussed above, as in other cases, every autonomous individual, whether patient, practitioner, relative, friend, or surrogate decision maker, has a moral obligation to weigh the variables of each case and make decisions based on recognition that every person has the same value but a different standpoint. In cases of conflict, the priority of justice demands that the decisions of moral agents as well as policy makers attempt to reduce disadvantages or inequities among all of those affected.

12

Care of the Elderly and End-of-Life Care

The term "geriatrics" refers to the branch of medicine that focuses on diseases and problems specific to people who have lived past middle age. Terms commonly used to refer to this population are "old," "elderly," and "senior."[1] Just when an individual enters "old age" depends on the average life span, which differs through time and for different populations. Since women today generally live longer than men, their entry point could logically be set later, but health problems and ethical issues associated with aging may occur at the same age for them as for men. As a result of women's longer life span, women predominate not only as geriatric patients but also as caregivers of the elderly.

This chapter considers ethical issues in the health care of elderly women, some of whom require end-of-life care. By various criteria of what age counts as "old," numbers of the elderly have increased exponentially in developed countries, making geriatrics an important specialty in many locales. In the United States, it is estimated that by 2030, about 20 percent of the total population will be 65 or older, up 13 percent from 2000. People 85 or older, 60 percent of whom are women, comprise the most rapidly growing segment of this group.[2]

Family members usually attempt to care for their elderly kin, but this is not equivalent to the societal respect that some cultures attribute to the elderly. In western society, youth is generally valued and rewarded more than age. Because of an emphasis on youthful images of feminine beauty, ordinary signs of aging such as wrinkling skin or graying hair carry a greater psychological burden for many women than for men. Women's greater longevity leads to greater numbers of widows than widowers, and the loneliness that this often entails may be exacerbated by their having had smaller numbers of more transient children than in times past. As with many issues in bioethics, some of the ethically relevant variables in health care of the elderly are gender specific and some are not.[3]

Health-related issues

Cases

1. Joyce Dawson is a 75-year-old woman who has been fiercely independent all her life. Until last year, she had a perfect driving record, but since then she has had several minor accidents that others attributed to poor driving. Joyce believes these attributions stem from prejudice against her because of her age. Seeking support, she asks her doctor, also a 75-year-old driver, to conduct whatever clinical tests are necessary to show that she is still an excellent driver. On exam, her doctor finds that her visual deficits are adequately corrected through her glasses and her manipulative skills are good. He concludes that she is as capable of safe driving as most young adults, and probably more capable than some teenage drivers.

2. Mabel Brooks, 78 years old and single, is a retired math teacher who has been living on her pension and social security check for fifteen years. Joseph, a nephew who visits regularly, has noticed that she no longer seems to enjoy his visits or show interest in neighborhood or family affairs. While in the past Mabel was fairly fussy about her appearance, she now pays little attention to it, and the house is so cluttered and dusty that Joseph considers it a health hazard. Except for an emergency appendectomy in her youth, Mabel has never sought or required medical attention. She mainly eats snack food, smokes and drinks moderately, watches TV, and rarely leaves home. Joseph has offered to pay for housekeeping services or help her move to a retirement community where such services are provided, but Mabel persistently resists these suggestions. Citing his aunt's possible depression, Joseph asks her physician to help him obtain legal guardianship so that he can ensure her environment is more conducive to her health and welfare.

3. Elise Addison, an 85-year-old widow, has been living in the large house where she raised her three children. She has a fixed income, based on her pension benefit. Ten years ago, Elise invited her unemployed son Herman to move in with her. Aware of his tendency to gamble and drink excessively, she thought that the stability of her home might help him overcome these habits. Until he found a job for himself, she told Herman he could take on the job of caring for the house and managing her finances, drawing money for his own basic needs, but not for gambling or alcohol, from her bank account. At first, Elise regularly reviewed how Herman was managing the money, house repairs, and upkeep, and she was satisfied that he was doing his "job" honestly and reliably even though he never found regular employment. Gradually, however, Elise developed symptoms of dementia and became less and less aware of how her son was managing her affairs. Two years ago, Herman was appointed "guardian of the estate" and "guardian of the person" for his mother; the former designation enabled him to sign all bank transactions in her behalf; the latter meant that he was responsible for decisions related to his mother's personal well-being.

Elise's daughter Charlotte visits each week to assist her mother in shampooing and bathing. She rarely finds her brother at home. Over the last six months, Charlotte has observed a lack of household cleanliness and basic upkeep (dirty dishes, dripping faucets, cracked window panes, missing doorknobs, stained rugs, etc.). Although she has written notes to her brother about these matters, none of the problems identified has been addressed, and she lacks the means for addressing them herself. Because she has seen numerous unopened letters from credit card and utility companies on the hall table, Charlotte believes Herman has been exhausting his mother's income to pay for drinking or gambling debts. When she confronts her brother with her suspicion, he denies the alleged behavior. Charlotte wonders what, if anything, she should do about the situation.

Empirical considerations

On statistical grounds, each of the elderly women in the above cases is likely to be less physically or mentally adept than she was in her younger years. Collectively, the cases illustrate different levels of competence for decision-making. In case 1, Joyce Dawson and her physician may both be outliers to the statistical probability of physical or mental impairment associated with aging. However, the fact that Joyce has had several recent accidents suggests that she may have lost some of her earlier driving skills. As a group, older drivers are involved in accidents at a rate equal to or less than middle-aged drivers, but the rate of older people involved in fatal crashes rises after age 70 to nine times higher than that of drivers aged 25 to 69. For drivers over 85, the fatality rate exceeds that of all other age groups, including that of teenagers.[4] Moreover, unlike teenagers, whose driving skills tend to improve as they mature, the driving skills of the elderly are more likely to decline as they age.

Physicians are not necessarily the best evaluators of the driving ability of the elderly. According to one study, the predictability of driving performance in people with early Alzheimer's is five times more accurate when the assessment is made by driving instructors rather than by physicians who are dementia experts.[5] Regardless of this assessment, however, the variables relevant to ethical decisions about elderly drivers include not only the possible impairment of the driver and risk to others but also the degree to which her welfare or others' welfare depends on her driving for necessities such as grocery shopping or medical care. Losing one's ability to drive can trigger depression because driving is linked to a sense of independence and self-esteem. Although dementia and depression are distinct conditions, dementia, even in its early stage, is often accompanied by depression.[6]

Loss of loved ones, fear of death, isolation, and deployment to the ranks of the "retired" are additional risk factors for depression in the elderly. Although depression increases risks of other ills and may impede decisional capacity, depression itself is not a normal part of aging.[7] The type of behavior that Mabel Brooks's nephew has observed in his aunt (decline in concern about her appearance or surroundings, and general withdrawal from interaction with others) may be symptomatic of depression. However, the extent to which this impairs cognitive function or autonomy may be impossible to assess. Situations that are unalterably miserable may induce depression that is appropriate in healthy individuals. From a mental health perspective, lack of depression may be more troublesome in these situations.

Case 3 clearly exemplifies a lack of decisional capacity. Senile dementia, which involves progressive deterioration of mental faculties and emotional stability, occurs not only in patients with Alzheimer disease but also in other elderly people. Physiologically, the dementia is caused by changes in brain tissue.[8] According to one study, about 12 in 1000 men and 30 in 1000 women have an Alzheimer type of senile dementia.[9] Some of those affected have an inherited predisposition to the disorder, but its expression cannot be definitively predicted before the onset of symptoms. Alzheimer's is neither preventable nor curable. Some of its symptoms are relievable through therapies and behavior modification techniques, but gradually the symptoms become more severe, usually reaching a point at which the patient is profoundly and irreversibly impaired. Death from infection or failure of other bodily systems typically occurs within fifteen years after the onset of symptoms.

Theoretical considerations

From an egalitarian perspective, the above cases illustrate the possibility of ageism: using age as the determinant of a practice, policy, or attitude in situations where age is irrelevant. Statistical probabilities provide data relevant to social policies or laws intended to maximize benefits or minimize harms to the majority, who are the dominant members of a particular group. However, because the majority does not include everyone, policies or laws based on age alone do not adequately address the needs or interests of a minority within the specified age group. Although Joyce Dawson and her doctor may belong to this minority, it is not certain that this is so for either one.

Case 1 raises not only the question of how to incorporate the standpoint of a minority into policies based on statistical probability or applicability to the majority but also the question of how to determine whether a specific individual falls within one or the other category. Policies and laws are more likely to take account of outliers if they enlist nondominant standpoints in their enactment. With regard to driving, for example, input by nondominant as well as dominant elderly individuals facilitates decisions that maximize respect for their different capacities for safe driving. The same strategy is applicable to Joyce's 75-year-old physician regarding his competence to practice medicine. Lest the nondominant party fail to recognize that her own standpoint is also limited, decisions affecting others should be made by incorporating their standpoints too. When the welfare of others is at stake, this may override the autonomy of an individual, no matter what her age (maxim 3).

Joyce may be as capable of safe driving as most teenagers, but this doesn't adequately support a recommendation that she continue to drive; to the extent that drivers in either age group place others disproportionately at risk, their driving may justifiably be restricted. Teenagers, however, are unlike many of the elderly in that they rarely depend on their own driving to provide for their basic needs. If these needs cannot be met for an elderly person who is prevented from driving, justice demands that they be adequately addressed through other means (e.g., publicly financed delivery services, Meals on Wheels). Although the other means cannot eliminate the psychological burden that loss of one's ability to drive sometimes entails, it can minimize its negative impact without placing others at risk.

Case 2 illustrates a recurrent ethical challenge for those who care for the elderly or for others whose behavior is at odds with their previous behavior. This challenge entails three separable questions: (1) Does someone's alteration of her previous pattern of behavior imply that her decision-making capacity has been diminished or lost? (2) Can behavior that threatens one's own welfare be autonomous? (3) Can respect for autonomy be justifiably overridden to benefit or prevent harm in the autonomous individual? The last of these questions is addressed in maxim 2: respect for autonomy outweighs beneficence and nonmaleficence toward the autonomous person. Not stated in this maxim, however, is that the autonomous decisions of individuals nearly always affect the welfare or autonomy of others, and duties toward them may supersede respect for their autonomy. Unless other risk factors are introduced, however, Mabel Brooks's behavior doesn't threaten the welfare or autonomy of others, even her nephew's, at least not to the degree that obstruction to her autonomy is justified.

With regard to the second question, maxim 2 implies an affirmative answer to which most of us can attest, regardless of our age: we sometimes behave autonomously in ways that are bad for us. Nonetheless, the greater the risk of someone's behavior to her own welfare, the more compelling the argument that her behavior is not autonomous. Presumption that a suicide attempt is not voluntary is usually based on this rationale. When a legal guardian is appointed, the justification for doing so is convincing evidence that the potential ward—the individual who may need a guardian—is incapable of autonomous decision-making. Mabel's behavior doesn't rise to this level of evidence against her decision-making capacity.

Answering the first question depends on whether autonomy is expressed in particular decisions or in one's overall pattern of decision-making. Consistency with an established pattern of behavior, by which one's values are discerned by others is sometimes referred to as "authenticity"; this is a more demanding notion of autonomy than the former because it implies that an immediate yes or no answer to a specific question is not necessarily a genuine expression of one's autonomy.[10] At times, individuals make decisions at odds with their usual set of values or overall life orientation, without thinking of their implications; such decisions may be triggered by anger or emotion that, in a more deliberate frame of mind, they would not make. Those who know them well rightly question whether such decisions are truly autonomous. But respect for autonomy requires openness to the possibility that an individual may radically change her behavior or lifestyle. If this were not true, religious conversion as well as rehabilitation of criminals would be impossible.

The fact that Mabel's decisions about herself and her home are at odds with her previous pattern of behavior suggests that these decisions are not fully or authentically autonomous. Her nephew's suspicion of depression is supported by his observation of these changes and her reduced interest in social interactions or family affairs. It is highly unlikely, however, that a judge would appoint him legal guardian of Mabel because to do so would require convincing demonstration of her incapacity for decision-making. Her ability to live independently, albeit in circumstances that are apparently not optimal for her health, suggests that she has not lost this capacity.

If Mabel is clinically depressed, she should be offered treatment to promote her autonomy, but refusal of treatment for depression does not imply lack of decisional capacity, and the persistence of her refusal of her nephew's suggestions argues otherwise. Although her welfare is apparently compromised by the decisions she is currently making, respect for autonomy requires support for behaviors that others would neither recommend nor choose and for behavior that may not serve the interests of the agent.

Case 3 illustrates the probability of a conflict of interest between a legal guardian and his ward, to whom the guardian may or may not be related. As Elise Addison's appointed guardian, Herman is legally obliged to make decisions that are in her best interests. Obviously, if he is using her income to support his gambling and drinking habits while neglecting her basic needs, he has failed to fulfill this obligation. Based on what she has observed, Charlotte is right to question her brother's conduct and, in the absence of any change, report the matter to appropriate authorities. If investigation verifies her suspicion, the state is obliged to appoint another guardian who will thereafter make decisions in her mother's best interests. Herman, presumably, would be held responsible for restitution and whatever legal penalties attach to his neglect of his mother and misuse of her income.

Caregiver issues

Cases

1. Ten years ago Mort Zimmer, 75 years old, was diagnosed with Parkinson disease. Since then, his wife Madlyn, also 75, has been caring for him at home. Currently, she bathes, feeds, places and empties the urinal or bedpan, gives him his medications, arranges for medical visits, and spends time with him watching TV. The couple has five children, all living out of state and apparently unable to assist their parents either financially or through direct involvement in their care. They cannot afford household help, and state support for home health care only covers four hours each day, five days a week. Although Madlyn stopped smoking five years ago, her lungs were so damaged from her long-term habit that she now requires supplementary oxygen intermittently. Through the years of caring for Mort, her mental and physical health has deteriorated to the point where her doctor has prescribed antidepressants, and her chronic pulmonary disease appears to be worsening.

2. Celia Halpern, 50 years old, is the only child of her 80-year-old mother. Her father, a policeman, died "in the line of duty" when she was 5 years old. After graduating from high school, Celia took a job at the local grocery store and worked her way up to a manager's position, where she has good benefits and job security. She never married and continues to live with her mother, who has become increasingly dependent on her emotionally and physically. Aside from work, Celia rarely goes anywhere without her mother, whose health is now severely compromised from arthritis, a heart condition, and obesity. Caring for her and for their home has become very difficult for Celia. Her employer, coworkers, and pastor all have urged her to get help to care for her mother, but her mother steadfastly refuses to allow anyone else into their home. Celia feels unable to fulfill her obligations to her mother, her employer, herself, and others and wonders how to sort them out.

3. Ella Baumgartner has worked as a health aide in nursing homes for three decades. Because she spends a great deal of time with her charges, she regularly observes interactions with their family members or friends who come to visit. Because Ella is warm and friendly, her clients, many of whom are lonely, sometimes share their personal concerns with her. Occasionally, a client tells Ella how she would like to be treated if she is no longer able to decide for herself. If the client subsequently loses decisional capacity and a family member fails to fulfill the client's previously expressed wishes, Ella is perplexed about what if anything she should do.

Empirical considerations

In home settings, the average caregiver of the elderly is a middle-aged married woman who is also employed outside the home.[11] When the elderly person is a married man, his usual caregiver is his elderly wife who, like Madlyn Zimmer, often has health problems of her own. In the United States and in much of the developed world, as marriage and childbearing have been increasingly delayed, the number of women who care for children and parents simultaneously (the "sandwich generation") has risen to about 2 million.[12] Longer life spans, lack of societal assistance, reduced family size, and more frequent divorce have all contributed to a reduced number of caregivers. Only children of single parents, such as Celia, are often the sole support of an aging parent who is psychologically as well as physically and economically dependent on them. When adult children move away from their parents, couples such as the Zimmers may be located too far from them to rely on their care.

In institutional settings, most health workers are women as well. Those who provide basic services such as housekeeping and washing and feeding patients often receive little or no prestige or economic reward for their labors in comparison with the respect and remuneration tendered to people in other types of work. Because of their consistent contact with elderly people, in their homes or in nursing care facilities, hired health care workers such as Ella Baumgartner may know more about their needs and wishes than family members who have much less contact.

Women have often been considered more naturally inclined and qualified than men to be caregivers because of their role in bearing and nurturing children. Socialization as well as higher earnings for men discourages this orientation in men while encouraging it in women, not only toward children but also toward people with impairments and the elderly. As a result, the principal caregiver of an elderly person is usually the wife, daughter, or daughter-in-law of the person in need of care. Health risks for caregivers include depression, stress, and chronic fatigue, and these are often compounded by the caregiver's own age or responsibilities for other family members.[13] Because men are usually older than their wives, they tend to need care earlier than their wives; women tend to need care longer because of their longer life span.[14]

With advancing age, disabilities are more prevalent and the need for chronic and acute care heightens. To cut costs, hospitals and rehabilitation facilities tend to discharge their patients earlier than in the past, placing greater demands on family members to provide for their needs at home. Like Celia's mother, most of the elderly prefer to remain at home rather than move to a retirement community or nursing home, where care is considerably more expensive. Increasing needs for care, coupled with the scarcity of able or willing home caregivers, have led to an escalating nursing home industry in the developed world. In 2002, about 72 percent of nursing home residents in the United States were women, whose average age on admission was 81.[15] This industry has proved highly profitable for its entrepreneurs but not for most of those who provide care in their facilities.

A minimal requirement of care is to ensure that the elderly person has personal contact with others. Although caregivers provide interpersonal contact, this does not mean that the elderly will respond in kind. Class or ethnic differences between a hired caregiver and the elderly person, or a history of dysfunctional family relationships, may trigger resistance, hostility, or prejudice toward the caregiver. Adult-onset senility sometimes evokes aggressive or insulting behavior even in those whose previous demeanor would have welcomed care from others. Regardless of how the elderly person responds to the caregiver, the tasks of basic care are as exhausting and sometimes as distasteful as cleaning someone after a bowel movement, as mundane as doing laundry or tying shoelaces, and as apparently superficial as trimming someone's nails or combing her hair. Unlike care of infants, which is also distasteful, exhausting, and stressful at times, care of the elderly is fraught with challenges that arise from the complexity of relationships between them and their caregivers. Adults of any age are not as manifestly lovable as babies.

Theoretical considerations

The caregiving considered in the above cases involves the provision of unpaid or underpaid assistance to an elderly person in the activities of daily living and in promotion of their physical or emotional health. Case 1 exemplifies the widespread and unjust tendency to ignore the informal caring that women routinely provide. As already mentioned, this poses health risks as well as economic risks to the caregiver. Through their personal and political decisions, however, practitioners, legislators, family members, and ordinary citizens can promote practices that reduce the burdens and risks of caregivers while ensuring that their charges are cared for appropriately. Legislators, for example, can introduce statutes that reduce caregiving expenses for those who need it, and they can encourage more and better caregivers by subsidizing their support. Clinicians can refer caregivers for respite care, and family members, including those unable to provide care themselves, can enlist the assistance of programs that provide such relief without cost. Although caregivers deserve care independently of their charges, caring for them is also a way of caring for those who depend on them.

Case 2 illustrates the fact that people in need of care are moral agents as long as they have decisional capacity. As such, they have moral responsibilities toward their caregivers. Not to recognize this responsibility in an elderly individual is disrespectful of her as a person. Parents such as Celia's mother may be particularly prone to disregard the interests of their caregiving daughters, thinking that they "owe" it to them to sacrifice themselves on their parents' behalf. In fact, however, regardless of their age, dependence, or relationship to the caregiver, moral agents are obliged to consider the interests of others as well as themselves. Moreover, caregivers such as Celia have obligations to others and to themselves that sometimes override the interests of the person for whom they care. Celia's mother seems to have had unreasonable and unjust expectations of her for many years. From an egalitarian perspective, if Celia can only fulfill her ongoing responsibilities to her employer, herself, and others through the recruitment of household or home care help, she is not obliged to comply with her mother's wishes to have no one but Celia care for her.

Nursing home caregivers such as Ella Baumgartner (case 3) are remunerated for their work, but rarely to the extent that they deserve. This is another illustration of the moral obligation of others to rectify the situation or at least do what they can to make it less inequitable. Clinicians who are well rewarded and respected, especially physicians and health administrators who determine staff salaries, may be particularly effective in proposing or supporting laws and practices that raise the income and prestige of basic caregivers. An egalitarian perspective also calls for them to show by their example that they regard these individuals as having the same value as themselves.

Case 3 introduces another ethical issue that societal and legal structures do not and perhaps cannot adequately address: the fact that some hired caregivers develop closer bonds with and know more than family members about the actual wishes or standpoint of the elderly. This is particularly likely to happen when relatives seldom visit and the caregiver spends a great deal of time with the elderly person. When someone becomes decisionally impaired and has not previously made her wishes known, family members have legal standing by which to make decisions on her behalf. A hired caregiver who disagrees with them is usually in a nondominant position vis-à-vis family members. Ella's puzzlement about what to do if she knows her charge wants something different than her family member chooses is therefore well grounded. Anticipating this potential problem, she should attempt to have her charge develop an advance directive about her wishes about her care. In the absence of a directive, if the elderly person loses decisional capacity, the caregiver should communicate her previously expressed wishes to the surrogate decision maker. On grounds of respect for the wishes of her client, Ella may challenge a surrogate's refusal to comply with her wishes. Sadly, however, if a surrogate persists in unwillingness to respect the elderly person's wishes, Ella has no remaining legal recourse.

End-of-life decisions

Cases

1. Nina Torres, 84 years old, had successful bypass surgery a decade ago. At the time, she composed an advance directive that designated her younger daughter, who lives nearby, as her durable power of attorney for health care. She told her daughter that she didn't want anything "heroic" done if she lost her ability to decide for herself. Two weeks ago, Nina suffered a stroke from which she appeared to be recovering when she suffered another stroke that left her completely unable to communicate either in words or signs. Because of her difficulty in swallowing, her doctor asks her daughter for consent to insert a feeding tube. The daughter wonders whether this procedure is "heroic."

2. Sue Chung, 80 years old, lost her zest for life about five years ago, after the death of her husband. Since then, she rarely leaves her apartment. When her children or grandchildren call or visit, she has little to say and seems somewhat annoyed. On more than one occasion, Sue has said she "just isn't interested in living longer." Two weeks ago, she suffered a stroke that left her immobile on the left side. While recovering in the hospital, she has been resistant to therapy and has refused to eat the meals provided, saying she has no appetite and wants no further treatment. A psychiatrist is called to evaluate her for clinical depression, but she refuses to speak with him. The attending physician is contemplating placement of a feeding tube. When Sue's children question the appropriateness of the procedure, he replies that he would be legally liable for allowing a patient to die for lack of nutrition.

3. Marguerite Torzinski, 76 years old, has resided for the past several years in a nursing home where she has many friends. In conjunction with surgery to remove her gall bladder, pancreatic cancer was discovered. The surgeon informed Marguerite's daughter of the diagnosis and recommended "comfort care only" because the cancer was "not effectively treatable." The daughter asked the doctor not to disclose the diagnosis to her mother. Her mother, she said, had been fearful of dying of cancer ever since her husband died ten years earlier from lung cancer. "Doctor," she explained, "I believe we owe it to her not to burden her during the time she has left with the anguish of knowing she has cancer."

4. Donna Friesl, 75 years old, has been summoned to the hospital because the staff caring for her 50-year-old son, Henry, wanted her consent to remove him from the ventilator. Henry, who lives with her, was diagnosed with end-stage chronic obstructive pulmonary disease (COPD) a year ago. Since then, he has been hospitalized several times for treatment of recurrent pneumonia. At home he has been dependent on supplementary oxygen around the clock. Henry is now unconscious and the health care team has no realistic expectation that he will recover; they believe the ventilator is only prolonging his dying. When Donna arrives at the bedside, the attending physician asks her permission to remove Henry from life support. Tearfully, she responds: "How can I say yes to that? I don't want my son to die."

5. Mara Mahmoud, 65 years old, visited her doctor because she thought she was experiencing early symptoms of Alzheimer disease. She reported that she was forgetting things she used to remember easily, and she felt frustrated or irritated in circumstances that had previously not bothered her at all. Twenty years earlier Mara had helped her mother care for her now-deceased father who had been clinically diagnosed with Alzheimer's. Over the last five years, her older sister has shown signs of senile dementia. After informing her doctor of her family history, Mara asks him to tell her what dosage of a medication she is presently taking would be definitively fatal. "Right now," she says, "I'm OK, but when my symptoms worsen I want to be able to end my life before I become a huge burden to my family and unable to enjoy life as it should be enjoyed."

Empirical considerations

Aging inevitably brings us closer to death. This fact, along with gradual diminishment of physical energy and more frequent disease or disability, evokes in the elderly thoughts about their death and dying that seldom occur to younger individuals. Although women in general live longer than men, the major causes of death and disability are the same for both sexes as they age.[16] Heart attacks are most likely to be fatal and strokes are most likely to be severely disabling, but the mortality and morbidity of cancer depends on the kind and stage of cancer diagnosed. In the United States, the average life expectancy after diagnosis of pancreatic cancer is three to six months.[17]

Strokes occur when the brain is deprived of oxygen and nutrients because a blood vessel is clogged or, occasionally, bursts. If nerve cells within the affected area of the brain are deprived of oxygen, they die within minutes, causing loss of whatever abilities that portion of the brain had controlled, such as speech, memory, or movement.[18] Depression, incited at times by the inability to communicate effectively, is a common sequel. According to one study, 25 percent of adults develop major depression after a stroke.[19] Its symptoms, all of which are present in Sue Chung, include persistent sadness, loss of appetite or energy, lack of interest in activities once enjoyed, and recurrent thoughts of death. Depression also plays a part in the recurrence of strokes. For those over 75 such as Sue, the recurrence risk is 50 to 70 percent.[20]

Although some types of cancer and cancers diagnosed at an early stage are curable, the word "cancer' suggests a terminal condition to many people. Most cancer patients want to know their diagnoses and prognoses, and clinicians generally inform them of "bad news" as well as "good news" regarding their condition. Some patients, especially those who have interacted with a friend or relative who struggled with cancer, develop such fear of the disease that this presents an additional health risk.[21] According to her daughter, Marguerite Torzinski has this type of "cancer phobia." Like the lung cancer from which her husband died, pancreatic cancer is often nonsymptomatic until the diagnosis is made. Given the poor survival rate of both conditions, patients with these diagnoses are legitimately concerned about dying. However, whether Marguerite's fear of the disease is associated with concerns about dying, pain and suffering is unclear.

Chronic obstructive pulmonary disease involves persistent blockage of the airway and occurs more prevalently in men than in women. It is typically associated with a history of smoking.[22] In its advanced stages, treatment of COPD often requires mechanical ventilation that leads to ventilator dependence. If a patient has decisional capacity and is adequately informed, she may forego ventilator support or ask that it be withdrawn; if she has permanently lost decisional capacity, clinicians may ascertain her previous wishes in the matter through an "advance directive," that is, written instructions about treatment or nontreatment formulated prior to loss of decisional capacity. The main forms of advance directive are a living will and a durable power of attorney for health care. Living wills are documents through which a competent person indicates the circumstances in which she would or would not want particular forms of treatment if she becomes decisionally incapacitated. A durable power of attorney for health care is someone designated by a competent person as her surrogate decision maker if she becomes unable to decide for herself about her treatment.

Some state statutes limit the circumstances in which the directives of a living will are to be followed. They may be ruled inoperable—for example, if the person is pregnant or capable of recovery. Because it is impossible to know or articulate in advance all of the circumstances that may arise for someone when she is no longer competent, designation of a durable power of attorney for health care is a more effective instrument of ensuring respect for the patient's previously expressed wishes than a living will. However, whether this designation accomplishes its goal depends on whether the surrogate adequately understands and articulates the patient's own standpoint when a decision must be made. Obviously, this requires adequate communication between the parties involved prior to the patient's loss of decisional capacity. The surrogate is expected to provide "substitute judgment" on behalf of the patient, and this may be at odds with the surrogate's own judgment about what should or should not be done.[23]

The family history of Alzheimer disease and senile dementia, coupled with increased irritability and possible short-term memory loss, supports Mara Mahmoud's suspicion that she is experiencing early stages of Alzheimer disease. Having assisted her mother in caring for her father, she probably has a much keener sense of how the disease progresses and what it requires of caregivers than others have. That this experience motivates her to avoid advanced stages of Alzheimer's is not surprising because it is often psychologically more difficult to accept care than to provide it. The ability to end one's own life to avoid the burden of caregiving for others may then be seen as a benefit.[24]

Assisting someone to commit suicide, whether the assistance is provided deliberately or not, is different from ending one's own life, and both are different from euthanasia, which entails deliberate killing of another person. Of different modalities that may be used to end or assist in ending a life, some (medications) are also prevalently used to prolong or improve lives. Ethically relevant variables in the means by which death is induced include their empirical and legal availability, cost, and effectiveness. Laws in most jurisdictions prohibit direct killing of another, regardless of whether the other requests it and regardless of whether prolongation of life is viewed as worse for the patient than death. However, laws in most jurisdictions permit the termination of life-sustaining treatment or withholding of life-saving treatment if a competent patient requests it or when treatment of an incompetent patient is judged futile or inhumane because there is no countermanding benefit to her.

Theoretical considerations

As we've seen before, people often attach different meanings to the same words or the same meanings to different words. Ongoing discussion can bridge gaps in understanding, but mistakes and misunderstandings still occur, especially in exchanges between people who scarcely know one another or rarely communicate. These mistakes and misunderstandings can have momentous and tragic consequences in end-of-life care, where decisions may be irreversible. Because people are often loathe to discuss the imminence of death and the process of dying, they are prone to use ambiguous expressions to convey their meaning. "No aggressive treatment," "No heroics," "Nothing extraordinary," "Let nature takes its course," and "Do not resuscitate" are commonly heard in this context. Each of these expressions may have different meanings for those who use or hear the words.[25] Moreover, what each expression means may change as the patient's condition changes, or when different treatment alternatives are introduced.

Nina Torres's daughter is more likely than the doctor to know what her mother meant when she said she didn't want "heroic" measures, and this may be different from what she herself would consider heroic. From the standpoint of some, ventilator support is "heroic" but a feeding tube is "natural"; the former is therefore permissible while the latter is not. Another variable associated with different forms of treatment is that patients occasionally survive after removal of a respirator, while deprivation of nutrition inevitably leads to death.[26] In light of that inevitability, uncertainty about whether Nina would want the feeding tube should be resolved by inserting it—at least temporarily. As a clinical cliché puts it, "When in doubt, treat." The defeasible presumption to treat is supported not only by beneficence but also by the probability that a person who has not clearly indicated otherwise prefers to live rather than die, even if she has been permanently impaired.

The possibility that depression has compromised Sue Chung's decisional capacity is an important variable in case 2. An ethically justifiable judgment to place the feeding tube should be based on the probability that depression has in fact impaired her autonomy and the likelihood that, if she were autonomous, she would not refuse any treatment necessary to prolong her life. If depression is ruled out through clinical assessment and there are no further reasons for doubting her autonomy, the physician is legally as well as morally bound to respect her refusal to eat and her refusal of medical interventions. Although he would be legally liable for treating Sue coercively, the physician should not be required to continue caring for her if his standpoint is at odds with this requirement. In that case, responsibility for her care should be transferred to someone whose standpoint allows him to honor the patient's refusal of treatment. In making that judgment, family members are available to consult on whether Sue's refusals are consistent with her previously expressed wishes.

Case 3 illustrates the mistaken presumption that the condition of a competent patient may be revealed to a relative without having obtained, or legitimately presumed, the patient's permission for doing so. Such disclosure is appropriate if the patient is unconscious and a decision must be made on her behalf, but only to whoever is her proxy or surrogate decision maker, whether or not a relative. Although many competent patients have no objection to disclosure of their health information to relatives, some prefer to keep the information to themselves. Respect for their autonomy requires clinicians to act in accord with these preferences, even if the news is not good. It is understandable that Marguerite Torzinski's daughter wants to spare her mother the bad news of her diagnosis, but her standpoint is not as privileged as that of her mother. Moreover, nondisclosure wouldn't necessarily eliminate, or even mitigate, her mother's cancer phobia. Accordingly, unless the patient herself has indicated that she would not want to be told, the clinician cannot justifiably withhold disclosure of the diagnosis to the patient.

Case 4 illustrates the lamentable fact that few patients, even among those who have life-threatening illnesses, provide the advance directives through which the uncertainty and anxiety of clinicians and family members regarding care of an incompetent patient can be averted.[27] Had Henry executed a living will or designated his mother as his durable power of attorney for health care, the situation would surely have been clarified for the caregivers. This case also exemplifies the difference between a parent's standpoint regarding care of her child and the standpoint of her child as a competent adult. Clinicians who ask parents for consent to treat or not treat ignore this important ethical variable. Donna Friesl's response to the physician in this case is a predictable and appropriate articulation of her standpoint, but it is Henry's standpoint rather than her own that has priority. Accordingly, the physician needs to clarify that he is not asking Donna's permission to let her son die but, instead, needs to learn from her what she honestly believes he would want done in the present circumstances.

Case 5 raises the issue of physician-assisted suicide, which is importantly different from withholding or withdrawing life-saving treatment. Some have argued that physician-assisted suicide is morally different from assistance in suicide by nonphysicians because the latter do not have the special commitment that clinicians have to save and prolong lives.[28] Presumably, the same point is applicable to health caregivers who are not physicians. Although clinicians usually aim to alleviate pain as well as extend lives, these goals are occasionally incompatible with each other or with compliance with the patient's wishes. In such circumstances, those who refuse to assist in suicide give priority to sustaining life: that is, beneficence or nonmaleficence. In case 5, the patient's rationale for requesting her physician's assistance is not only to avoid the burden to her that her disease will probably entail as it progresses but also to remove the burden to others that care for her is likely to require. However, the standpoint of those others is different from hers, and it is possible that they would experience greater burden through her early death than through caring for her through the natural course of her disease.

The physician's own standpoint is also relevant to her response to Mara Mahmoud's request. That standpoint involves not only concerns about legal, professional, or other consequences of such assistance but also her own moral beliefs about the value of life and the value of autonomy. Arguably, if it is morally wrong for a patient to end her own life, it is wrong for anyone, whether physician or not, to assist her in doing so, and others may be morally bound to prevent her, if possible. But if respect for someone's autonomous decision to end her life is a more compelling ethical imperative than respect for her life, it may not only be permissible but obligatory to assist her in doing so. As with positions about the moral status of the fetus, different starting positions are incompatible and lead to different conclusions. However, there are ethically relevant differences between the two types of cases. Unlike people who request assistance in committing suicide, fetuses are neither legally persons and respect for autonomy is obviously inapplicable to them.

The means of assistance is another relevant variable. Legally, physicians may help patients to die[29] through the physical act of removing them from life support, but this is not physician-assisted suicide if the patient has requested the removal or if prolongation of support has been judged futile. In case 4, the assistance requested by the woman is merely verbal: advice about lethal dosage of a medication the patient already takes. This information could have been imparted without the physician's knowing the patient's desire to commit suicide—for example, as a warning about taking more than the recommended dosage. Knowing the woman's intent, the physician could still provide the information while urging her not to take the lethal dosage and exploring possible avenues by which she might change her mind about taking her life when her symptoms get worse.

An egalitarian perspective, one that imputes the same value to every person, does not attribute priority to respect for autonomy in all instances; instead, it calls for balancing different preferences, burdens, and benefits among those affected so that inequalities are minimized. However, an egalitarian ethic does not address how the value of the patient's life is to be balanced against the value of respect for her autonomy. Life is the more *basic* value because there is no autonomy without it, but this doesn't necessarily mean that life is the *greater* value. Accordingly, an egalitarian perspective alone cannot settle the ethical question posed to the physician in this case.

Neither does the strategy proposed by standpoint theory settle the issue; it only argues that both physician and patient, as moral agents, should reduce their inevitable nearsightedness by eliciting the standpoints of other affected individuals. Those whose standpoints deserve to be considered include Mara Mahmoud's family members, as well as the physician's other patients and colleagues. As a mediating principle, the verity of justice calls for efforts to minimize the disparity in burdens and benefits that occur because of each one's different circumstances and preferences, while maximizing respect for the autonomy of those affected. Considering their diverse standpoints will provide both the physician and the patient with a more informed basis for their individual decisions, which may nonetheless remain at odds.

As with other cases in this book, those that arise in care of the elderly or dying involve more ethically relevant variables than can possibly be captured in descriptions or discussions of them, or even by the participants in actual cases, whose starting points about moral status may be different. The standpoint of each participant in an ongoing case embodies a distinct set of abilities, disabilities, preferences, and responsibilities, and each is affected differently by decisions made. These unavoidable differences, coupled with fallibility or inadequacy in determination of the ethically relevant variables of particular cases, makes it impossible and perhaps arrogant to offer definitive answers to the ethical questions raised. In each case, however, the verity of justice demands efforts to balance benefits and harms while respecting autonomy as much as possible, and this can only be done by incorporating and privileging the standpoints of those who are nondominant and most affected by decisions and policies. Elderly patients and their caregivers, most of whom are women, are predominant in both groups.

13

Research Issues

It is often said that the profession of medicine is an art as well as a science. In the clinical setting it would be more accurate to describe it as an art built on science. The art is the clinician's skill in applying what she has learned to particular patients. The science is the knowledge acquired through specialized and ongoing formal education, coupled with the knowledge gleaned through clinical practice. Because each case is unique, practitioners are continually learning from one patient how to treat other patients more effectively. In a sense, each patient is thus a research subject.

Most of the issues addressed in this book occur in a clinical setting in which diagnoses, prognoses, and treatment options are relatively routinized. Some conditions are outliers to this routinization because their manifestations don't fit neatly into the usual generalizations or because effective treatment options are unknown. Research on these conditions may be conducted by investigators whose findings have reached a point where the treatment being studied *may* be successful in humans. In the early stages of its application to humans it is experimental treatment rather than "standard of care." As such, the treatment deserves greater legal and ethical scrutiny than treatment whose effectiveness has already been proved.

The cases in this chapter illustrate variables relevant to the inclusion and exclusion of women in medical research. Ethical issues that arise in this context are complicated by the possibility of conflicting interests for researchers and subjects and by the fact that research on women may involve risks to potential children. The last section addresses issues that have aroused worldwide debate and sharply divided positions, based on the different starting points, standpoints, and end points of those who support them.

Women as research subjects

Cases

1. Members of an institutional review board meet to discuss policies regarding participation of women in research protocols. One member argues that all women of reproductive age should be excluded from studies because of possible threats to fetuses if they become pregnant. "Women may be willing to take risks for themselves," she says, "but fetuses can't consent to research that may harm them." Another member believes women of reproductive age should be permitted to decide for themselves whether to participate in research pertinent to their health, even if they are pregnant. A third member wants to exclude women who are not provably sterile or menopausal from research on nonpregnant women unless they are willing to undergo regular pregnancy tests. "The worst thing that could happen," she says, "is that someone enrolled gets pregnant and won't have an abortion."[1]

2. Lucy Fiorenza is taking a psychology course to see if she might like to choose this field as her major. Her professor is pursuing research to determine the percentage of college-age students who are sexually active before they start college. He distributes questionnaires asking for this information to everyone in the class, telling them not to put their names on their responses. The professor indicates he "is only looking for numbers, not names" and that participation is "a course requirement intended to provide students with a sense of what it means to do research in psychology." Lucy believes she should not be obliged to complete the questionnaire but does not want to risk getting a poor grade by not complying. If she returns the questionnaire without answering the questions, she thinks the professor will notice that she has not completed it.

3. The National Institutes of Health is currently funding a multicenter trial on adjuvant therapy for breast cancer. Dr. Keith Smythe is leading the study at his home institution. Melinda Bronson, one of his patients, was recently diagnosed with breast cancer, for which lumpectomy was recommended. Having learned of the multicenter trial in the medical center newsletter, she asks the doctor to enroll her in the study. Although she meets the criteria for enrollment, Keith honestly believes the experimental therapy carries more risks than benefits in Melinda's case, and he questions whether he should enroll her anyway.

4. Researchers at an infertility center have been attempting to develop a program for freezing human ova. The rationale for the project is to provide a means by which women who require chemotherapy for cancer may avoid its impact on their fertility by having their ova retrieved and frozen before the therapy. If the project is successful, the ova may subsequently be thawed, fertilized in vitro, and returned to them so that they can gestate and give birth to their own genetic progeny. Rita Young, unmarried and 30 years old, became a study subject before starting her therapy for cancer. She indicated that she hoped to use the ova herself someday, but if that were impossible, she would like them to be used for research. Following ovarian stimulation, the research team retrieved thirty of Rita's ova and attempted to freeze them. When she died before the research had been completed, the team wondered whether her consent to research with her ova implied consent to thaw the potentially frozen ova, fertilize them in vitro, and transfer them to another woman for possible gestation.

Empirical considerations

Throughout the world, nondominant populations such as racial minorities, mentally impaired individuals, and prisoners have been subjected to research without their consent and with no expected benefit to them. Recognizing these abuses, most countries have developed regulations regarding involvement of study subjects. In the United States, for example, federally funded studies involving human subjects must be reviewed at the local level through "institutional review boards" (IRBs). Members of IRBs include researchers from different disciplines and representatives of the public whose overall responsibility is to ensure that the research is scientifically and ethically justifiable. Explicit consent to participation in studies is usually crucial to the ethical justification. However, some populations, such as infants and incompetent adults, are unable to provide consent. Knowledge that can only be obtained through research on such individuals may be indispensable to development of optimal treatment of those within these populations.

Although women have at times been research subjects without their consent, they have also been excluded, without their consent, from research that might have benefited them. Reasons for the exclusion include (a) the presumption that data applicable to men are also applicable to women, (b) avoidance of the complexity introduced by inclusion of women (e.g., the unpredictability of menstruation), and (c) fears of liability associated with the possibility of pregnancy and damage to the fetus. Not only pregnant and potentially pregnant women but also those who are definitively infertile such as postmenopausal women and very young girls have been excluded. This has led to many women being treated unscientifically—that is, through means that have not yet been proved effective or safe.

Many protocols reviewed by IRBs involve experimental medications, drugs whose effectiveness has not been demonstrated. When the study subject is a pregnant woman, its impact on the potential child as well as the woman is at stake. However, perceptions of these risks are sometimes exaggerated. Although there are important exceptions, drugs taken during the first trimester tend to have graver impact on the developing fetus than those taken later; in many instances the likelihood is that a particular drug will harm neither the woman nor her potential child.

Research in which human subjects participate extends beyond the biomedical domain to social science, as in case 2. The risks encountered here are less obvious but can be even greater than those encountered in medical research. Questionnaire studies, for example, may entail psychological or social risks for respondents. Power discrepancies between researchers and nondominant subjects are exacerbated in the professor-student relationship, making the voluntariness of their consent highly questionable. Students such as Lucy Fiorenza have nonetheless been asked to participate in studies intended primarily to facilitate the research of their professors.

Research funding may come from multiple sources, both public and private. In the United States, research with human subjects is often supported by grants from the National Institutes of Health (NIH), which sometimes conducts multicenter projects such as the one described in case 3. Like Keith, researchers may also be physicians for patients who have agreed to be research subjects. The goal of research is to obtain knowledge that may be broadly applicable; the goal of the physician is to promote the health of a particular patient.

Case 4 illustrates the fact that women, unlike men, have a limited number of gametes, available for a limited period of their adult lives. Moreover, ova are retrievable only with risk and discomfort to women, and they are preservable only through a process that is highly experimental. Through sperm freezing, which is "standard of care" in infertility clinics, men who might otherwise be infertile after necessary therapy can preserve their procreative capacity, but women in similar circumstances cannot do this until and unless ova freezing is similarly successful. The option of retrieving, freezing, and storing ova for future use is also desired for and by women who want to postpone childbearing and wish to avoid the genetic risks associated with use of ova from older women.

Theoretical considerations

Although the primary goal of research is to obtain knowledge, biomedical research usually has a therapeutic aim also. The therapeutic aim is primarily to promote the health of future patients, but this aim may also be pursued with the hope of benefiting the patients being studied. When the therapeutic goal applies to participating subjects, the research may properly be called experimental therapy. The term "innovative therapy" refers to treatment or procedures implemented for the first time or without having yet been proved effective; it differs from "standard of care," which refers to treatment that is routinely administered because its effectiveness has been established. Innovative treatment may be considered experimental not only because its effectiveness has not yet been proved but also because those who practice it expect to acquire knowledge applicable to future patients.

In addition to the requirement of informed consent from research subjects or their surrogates, ethically justified medical research should also satisfy the requirement of "equipoise." Basically, this term refers to a balance between the potential benefits and risks of the alternatives being compared. For example, if two treatments (or treatment and nontreatment or placebo) are studied to determine which is more effective, researchers should be genuinely uncertain whether one arm of the study is more likely than the other to benefit the patient/subject. During the course of a study, if early results prove that one alternative is better than another for those involved, the study should be ended to allow those enrolled to be treated optimally. If early results show that an individual subject or group of subjects are more harmed than helped through the treatment being tested, or if they decide during the course of the study that they do not want to continue, their interests have priority over the goal of the research. From an egalitarian perspective, potential subjects may have a moral obligation to participate if risks are minimal and the anticipated benefit to others is great (maxim 4), but this does not imply that they may be coerced to participate.

Case 1 illustrates disagreement among IRB member about research on pregnant or potentially pregnant women. Their disagreement stems from different starting points on whether human fetuses or embryos should be considered human research subjects. Presumably, all of the IRB members recognize that research on women is necessary to ensure that their treatment is scientifically validated. Members who have different positions on the moral status of the embryo or fetus may support research on women who are unquestionably infertile. With regard to research on pregnant or possibly pregnant women, however, different starting points lead to different positions. From an egalitarian perspective, the welfare of future children is morally relevant even to those who impute no moral status to the fetus, but it is not as compelling as it is for those who believe fetuses have moral status.

Ethically relevant variables also occur within the purview of those who attribute moral status to embryos or fetuses. Some, for example, draw a line between in vitro and in vivo embryos and support research on the former but not the latter. Others approve research on pregnant women only if it is intended to benefit her embryo or fetus. Regardless of positions about moral status, however, an egalitarian criterion for research on pregnant women is that fetuses or embryos destined to be aborted should be treated in the same way as those destined to go to term. This criterion, first proposed by the National Commission for the Protection of Human Subjects in 1975,[2] facilitates respect for the pregnant woman's autonomy by allowing her to change her mind without jeopardizing the welfare of a potential child whose interests, at that point, she wants to promote.

All three of the comments by IRB members in case 1 are problematic. The first complaint, that women may take risks for themselves that fetuses are unable to assume for themselves, suggests a separateness between women and their fetuses that does not exist. The second claim, that pregnant women should be included in any research pertinent to their health, is supportable by those who subscribe to maximal criteria for personhood. From the standpoint of those who impute moral status to fetuses, restrictions on the research are justifiable. The third IRB member's comment is empirically misguided and untenable from the standpoint of those who oppose abortion. Fetuses and embryos may be damaged through the course of research on pregnant women, especially during the first trimester, but many drugs to be tested do not entail this risk. In fact, if nothing specific is yet known about the risks of a drug to be tested, the probability that it will harm a specific fetus is slight. Moreover, the third IRB member's comment suggests that a woman *should* have an abortion if there is risk to her potential child; this hardly indicates respect for the autonomy or standpoint of women who want to continue their pregnancies even if they are likely to give birth to a child with a disability.

Fully informed consent cannot be obtained if participation in a study is obligatory, as in case 2. The professor's assurance of confidentiality doesn't eliminate the coercive character of the requirement. Neither does the possible educational benefit, which is dubious. Lucy's judgment that participation should not be required is morally valid, but she still faces a personal moral challenge: whether to participate anyway for the sake of her grade. An egalitarian perspective supports her refusal unless the better grade is more likely to reduce injustice than nonparticipation. This is improbable because she may not get a better grade anyway and because the goal of the study does not appear morally compelling in its own right.

With regard to case 3, some scholars have argued that equipoise is impossible for investigators whose research subjects are also their patients; others contend that equipoise is required for the research community rather than for individual researchers.[3] By that logic, if the research community is uncertain whether breast cancer patients as a group will benefit more from the therapy being studied than from "standard of care" treatment, Keith may recruit Melinda Bronson for the multicenter trial at his institution even though he believes that participation carries more risks than benefits to her. However, if he believes that the criteria for enrollment in the study fail to identify a major risk factor in Melinda that he now recognizes, he cannot in good conscience enroll her solely on grounds of "community equipoise" or respect for her autonomy.

Medically assisted reproduction is an area of bioethics that is rife with complex and emotionally charged issues, including novel questions about beginning and ending human life. As case 4 shows, however, the research sometimes proceeds without anticipation or ethical analysis of its implications. Presumably, the researchers realized before starting the study that some of their cancer patient/subjects might die during the course of the research, but they had not anticipated the possibility that women's consent to research with their ova did not necessarily imply consent to making embryos with them that might then be transferred to another woman's uterus for gestation.

Quite possibly, it never dawned on Rita Young that consent "to use her ova for research" in the event of her death might be interpreted as consent to have the ova thawed after freezing, fertilized with someone's sperm, and have the resultant embryos transferred to another woman's uterus for possible gestation. The fact that Rita is no longer able to clarify her wishes in this regard does not imply that the researchers may presume her consent to "research" to encompass these uses. The situation calls instead for efforts to determine as faithfully as possible what Rita's wishes on the matter would be from those most likely to be acquainted with her standpoint: her family members or close friends. If, as is improbable, no one can be found who has a sense of whether Rita would consent to the proposed uses of her ova, her presumed consent may justify these uses. From an egalitarian perspective, however, neither in vitro fertilization nor transfer should be attempted without fully informed consent of the other participants, the sperm and gestation providers.

To promote gender equality, it may be argued that ova freezing should be developed and eventually available to fertile women who wish to postpone childbearing to an age when they would carry an increased genetic risk to their offspring and possibly have reached the normal age of menopause. This argument is valid on grounds of respect for the woman's autonomy and the benefit achieved by promoting health in one's offspring; it is less compelling on grounds that infertility and increased genetic risk are natural and normal for women as they age, whereas the choices available to women such as Rita are restricted by the occurrence of a disease process that is neither normal nor natural in a woman her age. From an egalitarian perspective, the standpoint of women whose infertility is caused by necessary treatment has priority over that of women for whom postponement of childbearing is not a medical necessity.

Maternal-fetal surgery

Cases

1. An obstetrician and a pediatric neurologist at a major research institution have developed a technique by which they hope to provide pregnant women with the opportunity to reduce the impairments of children born after prenatal diagnosis of myelomeningocele (MMC). The technique, which involves open uterine surgery on pregnant women, is based on the rationale that treatment of the disorder in utero may be more likely to be effective than treatment after birth. Before the procedure was offered to women, the protocol was reviewed and approved by the institution's IRB. When the number of procedures performed on the experimental protocol passed 100 and the physician researchers considered the results "promising," they told potential patients that the technique "was no longer experimental." The hospital's legal counsel challenged this description because the procedure was not "standard of care."

2. At 17 weeks gestation, Donna O'Donnell, 36 years old, learns that her fetus has normal chromosomes and MMC. She is counseled regarding the option of pregnancy termination and the implications of having a child with MMC. Donna and her husband are unwilling to consider abortion and are anxious to find any means by which to avoid or reduce impairment in their potential child. Through an internet search, they discover that a medical center in their state is enrolling patients in a randomized clinical trial of in utero repair versus postnatal repair for MMC.[4] The website for the center indicates that the procedure reduces hindbrain herniation and postpones the need for shunting in the newborn.[5] Thrilled with the possibility that they have discovered a means by which to avoid impairments in their potential child, the couple visit the center and ask to be enrolled in the study.

3. At 15 weeks gestation, Sally Trible learns that her fetus has "congenital cystic adenomatoid malformation of the lung, with hydrops." When she asks what this means, she is told that it is a lethal anomaly for which experimental treatment through "open uterine surgery" offers the only possible means of saving her future child's life. Sally's obstetrician discourages her from seeking the surgery because of its risks to her and the "extremely slim" chance that it will improve the outcome for her newborn. She decides to go ahead with the surgery because, she says, "I want to do whatever I can to give my child a chance."

4. Janice Caruthers learned during her fifth pregnancy, that her fetus had a "lethal condition" called "congenital diaphragmatic hernia." The obstetrician she had seen during her previous pregnancies explained the prognosis and her options regarding it: she could either terminate or continue the pregnancy, and if she chose the latter course physicians would be on hand to treat the newborn as effectively as possible. The possibility of maternal-fetal surgery was not mentioned by the doctor because (a) she realized that Janice could not afford to travel to the only center where it might be provided, and (b) she considered the surgery highly unlikely to be successful for the child and believed its risks to Janice were unwarranted.

Empirical considerations

In the 1980s, maternal-fetal surgery (i.e., surgery on pregnant women to correct problems in their fetuses) was performed mainly for conditions considered lethal or life threatening for the potential child. The procedure, also called "open uterine surgery," involves opening a woman's uterus to expose the fetus, operating on the fetus, and closing and returning the uterus to the woman's body. During the procedure the fetus remains attached to the woman through the umbilical cord. Among the life-threatening conditions treated through this method are congenital diaphragmatic hernia, sacrococcygeal teratoma, and congenital cystic adenomatoid malformation of the lung.[6]

Despite the potential effectiveness of intervention prior to birth, open uterine surgery introduces risks to the woman and her potential child that would not otherwise be present. For the woman, the risks include preterm labor (the "Achilles' heel" of prenatal surgical interventions), premature birth, pulmonary edema, infection, uterine rupture, placental abruption, extensive blood loss, and the mortality risk of general anesthesia and surgical complications. In newborns, chronic lung disease and neurodevelopmental disabilities are the major risks associated with their premature delivery. To deliver the fetus after the surgery, and to deliver any future children, the woman must undergo cesarean section. In light of these risks and poor outcomes in many cases, less-invasive methods of prenatal treatment have increasingly been attempted (e.g., endoscopic repair and laser surgery). All of these prenatal interventions are innovative or experimental.

Myelomeningocele, the most common and severe form of spina bifida, is a nonlethal congenital anomaly that occurs when the primitive neural tube fails to close at about the fourth week of pregnancy.[7] The major disabilities associated with this condition are permanent mobility impairment and lack of bladder control. Hydrocephalus (fluid in the brain) occurs through leakage of the spinal fluid. Other risks include bowel incontinence, developmental delay, and cognitive impairment. The standard of care for affected infants involves closure of the neural tube and shunting. Although the rationale for maternal-fetal surgery is that earlier intervention lessens the disabling impact of the condition, there is as yet no evidence that major impairments have been reduced through prenatal intervention. It has been shown, however, to reduce hindbrain herniation and postpone the need for shunting in the newborn.

Congenital cystic adematoid malformation of the lung (CCAM) involves the development of cysts that obstruct pulmonary function. The presence of hydrops (fluid retention) in an affected fetus makes the prognosis more dire. From the standpoint of some pediatric surgeons, CCAM with hydrops is lethal because of the high likelihood that the newborn will die even if treated optimally after birth.[8] According to other pediatric surgeons, however, some infants survive after postnatal surgery, and treatment decisions should not be based on "antenatal behavior."[9]

Congenital diaphragmatic hernia (CDH) is also called a lethal anomaly, but like CCAM, it does not always lead to death. This condition involves the absence of the diaphragm or an opening in the diaphragm that allows contents of the abdomen to protrude into the chest, cutting off lung development or function. The prognosis depends on when the condition is detected, the type of hernia, the extent of the opening, and whether other anomalies are present. One study cites 62 percent mortality in those born with CDH, and if an additional anomaly is present, a mortality of 79 percent.[10] Spontaneous loss and prenatal terminations apparently account for many losses prior to birth, and advances such as extracorporeal membrane oxygenation have improved outcomes for affected newborns.[11] Because open uterine surgery has not been successful, fetoscopic surgery, which is less invasive, is offered at some centers, but only for cases with the worst prognosis. The major risks of fetoscopic surgery include miscarriage, premature rupture of membranes, and premature delivery, along with slightly elevated risks of excessive bleeding, infection, and leakage of the amniotic fluid.[12]

Theoretical considerations

The term "maternal-fetal surgery" makes it clear that surgery on fetuses is impossible without surgery on the women on whom they depend for survival. Weighing risks and potential benefits of these interventions thus demands consideration of those applicable to both the pregnant woman and her potential child. How these are to be assessed if there is apparent conflict between her interests and those of the potential child depends on one's starting point regarding moral status. If the fetus has no moral status or only partial moral status, the woman's interests may outweigh those of the fetus or potential child even if the latter are considerable. If the fetus and the woman are each imputed to have full moral status, the conflict is only resolvable if the interests of one are clearly preponderant when compared with those of the other. Respect for autonomy is obviously only applicable to the woman, and the interests of others, including those of already-born children, are ethically relevant as well.

Because potential beneficiaries may never exist, research that is only intended to benefit future patients demands stronger ethical justification than research that also aims to benefit those who presently exist. As experimental therapy, maternal-fetal surgery exemplifies the latter if the fetus is considered apart from the pregnant woman but, as explained in chapter 2, fetuses as fetuses are neither separate nor separable from women. The woman herself may benefit from experimental therapy that improves the outcome for her potential child, since such improvement may accord with her wishes and reduce the burden of care for an impaired offspring. Even so, these benefits cannot be obtained without health risks to the woman that she would not otherwise face.

In case 1, IRB review, which is not legally required for innovative surgical procedures, brings other standpoints to the fore, reducing the myopia of individual researchers. Nonetheless, this particular IRB apparently failed to reduce the nearsightedness of physician researchers who considered their innovative procedures so "promising" that equipoise was impossible for them personally. Mere numbers of procedures performed, as cited on the website, did not demonstrate that the surgery produced a better outcome than the alternatives. Accordingly, the hospital's legal counsel was right to challenge the research team's claim that maternal-fetal surgery for treatment of MMC was no longer "experimental." Only when an experimental therapy has proved at least as successful as the alternatives should it be considered "standard of care" instead of "experimental."

Case 2 illustrates the myopia to which potential parents are also subject. Here, the limitation seems to arise from their focus on avoidance of disabilities associated with MMC while increasing the risk that their potential child may suffer other impairments from the earlier intervention. Ironically, despite their pro-life commitment, this focus moves them to take an avoidable risk that the fetus or newborn will expire. Although both parents may have the same hope for their offspring, they each have a different standpoint regarding the surgery. To ensure that Donna O'Donnell's request for the surgery is fully autonomous, consent should be obtained from her independently. Her standpoint is privileged vis-à-vis her husband's because she, not he, will undergo the pain and risks of the intervention.

If maternal-fetal surgery presented the only possible means by which the potential child's life could be saved, the case for surgical intervention prior to birth would be more compelling than it is for MMC. Even with regard to CCAM and CDH, however, affected infants occasionally survive considerably longer than anyone had anticipated. Just what span of life is necessary to warrant calling a condition from which one eventually dies "lethal" is unclear and subject to different interpretations by potential parents, investigators, and clinicians. As discussed in chapter 7, some think "lethal" means that death will occur within hours or days at most; others use the term for any condition for which those affected die within a year. "Life-threatening" may more accurately convey the notion that the condition does not always cause death within a very short time.

Case 4 illustrates the paternalistic tendency of many clinicians. Unless Janice is unable to understand that maternal-fetal surgery is an experimental treatment that is available elsewhere, the physician acts paternalistically in not disclosing this possibility to her. Although her standpoint, like everyone's standpoint, is limited, it is (or should be) privileged because she is in a nondominant position and more affected than her clinicians or her partner by the surgery. From that standpoint, she may be aware of resources for travel that the practitioners are not aware of. However, even if she is unable to travel to another medical center for the surgery, respect for her autonomy demands that she be told about the treatment.

This case also illustrates the need for justice in distribution of limited health care resources or options. From an egalitarian perspective, the opportunity to participate in experimental therapy for life-threatening conditions should be available to everyone. Admittedly, this is a moral ideal rather than a description of prevalent practice, but one whose pursuit is likely to extend the reach of justice in current practice.

Cloning and stem cell research

Cases

1. Hilary and Markus Kissinger would like to have children, but both are carriers of a life-threatening recessive gene. Rather than risk the 1 in 4 chance of having a child who will suffer a short and possibly painful existence, the couple considers the alternatives: to forgo parenthood, to adopt, to undergo prenatal diagnosis and abort an affected fetus; to use donor gametes free of the recessive trait, or to use the cells of one of them and attempt to clone a child. Although cloning to produce a child has never as yet proved successful, they opt to participate in a research protocol by which cloning may give them a genetically related child who is not at risk of the condition for which they are carriers. If development is triggered in tissue retrieved from one of them, they plan to have the embryo transferred to Hilary for gestation and birth.

2. The Langley family is in a terrible accident. Mark, the father, is killed, and his only child, Bernard, is dying. Dorothea Langley, a biologist, would like cells from her son to be used in an experimental program for somatic cell nuclear transfer to create another child who will be genetically identical to Bernard. This is the only way she can raise a child who is biologically related to her late husband.

3. The President's Council on Bioethics has been deputed to formulate guidelines for governmental regulation of stem cell research. Although all of the members support research with stem cells derived from nonembryonic sources, three different positions emerge during their deliberations about research with stem cells obtained from human embryos: (a) opposition to any research that involves destruction of the embryos; (b) permissibility only if the embryos were originally created for infertility treatment, are no longer desired by their progenitors, and would otherwise be discarded; and (c) support for the research regardless of how the embryos are derived. The last position includes support for research with embryos obtained through fertilization solely for research purposes, as well as those obtained through somatic cell nuclear transfer. The council chair is convinced that members will never agree on regulation of embryonic stem cell research and wonders, therefore, whether the council's deliberations should be limited to research on stem cells derived from other sources.

4. Umbilical cord blood from newborns is a potential source of stem cells that could provide effective treatment for conditions that develop later in their lives. ViaCord is a private blood banking company that potential parents can contact to arrange for retrieval and storage of the cord blood of their newborns. The company charges $1,800 for its processing service and $125 annually for storage of the cord blood.[13] The Rubins are an affluent couple who want to purchase ViaCord's services in order to maximize the health of their child throughout his or her lifetime. They wonder, however, whether their doing so is fair to those who cannot afford the service, especially those more likely than they to have children affected by diseases that can only be treated effectively through stem cells derived from their cord blood.

Empirical considerations

The desire to have children who are healthy and biologically related to both members of a couple is present in most adults and prevalently is fulfilled without requiring medical assistance. The desire is considered "natural" not only because it is common but also because it is usually triggered and sustained by biological (hormonal) factors in the partners. Obviously, satisfying this desire has very different consequences for men and women. The duration and risks associated with pregnancy, childbirth, and lactation explain why even the minimum parental investment of women in reproduction is considerably greater than that of men.[14] For men, on average, the drive to engage in sexual behavior is greater than the drive to parent.[15] For some women, however, the desire to be pregnant and give birth is even stronger than their desire to have a genetically related child.[16]

As discussed in the preceding section, the desire to have a healthy child leads some pregnant women to undergo risky and painful treatment that might otherwise have been avoided. If a couple are both carriers of a lethal recessive gene, as in case 1, reproductive cloning is a means by which they may avoid the high risk of having a child with this condition while also fulfilling their desire to have a child who is genetically related to one of them. By cloning the male partner, an embryo may be formed in vitro and transferred to the female partner for gestation and birth; the offspring is then biologically, but not genetically, related to both. If the female partner is cloned, the offspring can only be biologically related (genetically as well as gestationally) to one parent, the mother.

The process of cloning to produce another organism involves insertion of an adult cell into an ovum from which the nucleus has been removed. Development through cell division is then triggered by electrical or chemical stimulation, and the blastocyst that results may be transferred to a woman for gestation or used for derivation of stem cells. The latter use eliminates the possibility of further development. As yet, no transfer of a cloned human blastocyst has been reliably reported. Researchers who have derived stem cells from cloned human blastocysts have indicated their moral opposition to such transfer, and some have claimed that cloned embryos are unable to complete normal development if they are transferred for gestation.[17]

If and when human cloning leads to the birth of a child, the child will have the same genetic make-up (except for mitochondria) as the individual from which she is cloned.[18] However, since the phenotype (expression) of one's genetic make-up is determined not only by the genes themselves but by the interaction of multiple genes with environmental influences, the cloned individual would not express his or her genetic make-up in the same way as the individual from whom she is cloned. Characteristics, interests, and abilities of the clone would be different from those of the cloning source. If reproductive cloning were successfully employed in case 2, therefore, Dorothea could bear and give birth to a child who is genetically related to her deceased husband and genetically identical (except for mitochondria) to her previous child. The cloned child, however, would be different from his predecessor in ways that exceed the diversity present in identical twins born at the same time and raised together.

Stem cells are important to researchers because they are capable not only of perpetuating themselves but also of undergoing differentiation into one or more specialized cells. The ability to differentiate increases the likelihood that they may be used to successfully treat conditions for which effective treatment has previously been lacking, such as Alzheimer disease, Parkinson disease, and spinal cord injury. Although stem cells obtained from embryos hold promise of greater therapeutic effectiveness, those obtained from mature cells have already been used in successful treatment of some conditions.[19] Cloning embryos to produce stem cells affords the possibility of creating specialized tissue or organs that match the DNA of the recipient, greatly reducing the chance of rejection. However, unless and until researchers discover how to identify and remove or treat deleterious genes in the nuclear DNA of the donor, deleterious genes will also be transmitted through the organs or tissue developed from the stem cells.

Stem cells obtained from umbilical cord blood are less differentiated than those obtained from more mature sources. This factor alone makes them potentially more useful for treatment of certain disorders than stem cells obtained from more mature sources. Further, because umbilical cord blood matches the DNA of specific newborns, stem cells obtained from it are likely to provide a particularly effective source of treatment for those newborns if they acquire one of the treatable disorders during their life time. Not surprisingly, therefore, it has become a desirable option for some new parents who are affluent enough and knowledgeable enough to take advantage of this possibility. As with stem cells derived from cloned embryos, however, those obtained from cord blood not only match the DNA of the newborn but also carry the same deleterious genes with which the newborn came into the world.

Three options are available to potential parents regarding umbilical cord blood: the traditional route of disposal as medical waste, private family storage, and donor banking. As in case 4, the second option has been increasingly offered for a price by biotech companies. The third option is one whose therapeutic effectiveness has already been shown—for example, in cases of stem cell therapy for leukemia. Similar to traditional blood donor programs, it involves collection and analyses of cord blood from as many infants as possible, then making it available to those who are presently in need of stem cell therapy developed from the donated cord blood. This option avoids the risk that someone treated with stem cells from her own cord blood would face (transmission of the same deleterious genes) because the donor, while adequately matched for therapeutic effectiveness, is not genetically identical to the recipient.

Theoretical considerations

"Clones" are replications. In research, the term basically refers to a line of cells that is genetically identical to the originating cell.[20] Since the birth of the first mammal cloned from an adult member of the species was reported in 1997, "clone" has prevalently been used more restrictively for a newly developed organism formed from the nuclear DNA of a mature organism. The President's Council on Bioethics defines human cloning as "asexual production of a new human organism that is, at all stages of development, genetically virtually identical to a currently existing or previously existing human being."[21] Various ethicists and governmental commissions distinguish between "reproductive cloning" and "therapeutic cloning," using the former term for cloning intended to produce a child and the latter for cloning intended for therapeutic research. Because some people consider the production of embryos a reproductive function, and because research is not therapy, the President's Council on Bioethics prefers a distinction between cloning to produce children and cloning for biomedical research. Paul McHugh, a member of the council, has suggested that the organism formed through cloning be called a "clonote" or "nuclear transfer construct" instead of an embryo.[22]

Cases 1 and 2 illustrate why some have argued in favor of cloning to produce children: the main reasons are treatment for infertility or replacement of a child who has died.[23] Because these reasons reflect the standpoint and interests of potential parents, they are epistemologically and ethically relevant to decisions or policies about human cloning. From an egalitarian perspective, however, neither reason suffices to justify a practice with implications for others, including children born through cloning. Those whose starting point on the issue involves a minimal criterion for personhood oppose any method of reproduction that entails the destruction of embryos; for them, it would be better to transfer a cloned embryo to a woman for gestation than to use it for research that ends the possibility of further development.[24] Those who attribute no moral status or only partial moral status to in vitro embryos tend to support therapeutic cloning more strongly than reproductive cloning because the former carries greater promise of therapeutic effectiveness for those already born.

To avoid misunderstanding, practitioners who counsel the Kissingers in case 1 need to use language more explicit than "lethal" in informing them of a 1 in 4 chance of having a child affected by a deleterious gene. The couple should be told, for example, how soon the child is likely to die, with what degree of probability, and what treatment if any could possibly increase the child's chance of survival. They also should be informed about alternative means by which to become parents, both medical and social. Whether both Hilary and Markus provide ethically adequate consent to participate in cloning research depends, among other things, on their understanding that the potential child will be virtually genetically identical to one of them but not the other, the risks of participation to Hilary as well as the potential child, and the probability that participation will not lead to fulfillment of their goal: the birth of a healthy, genetically related offspring.

The rationale for human cloning in case 2 exaggerates the importance of the genetic link between a parent and offspring while neglecting the genetic newness that arises from having genetically unrelated parents. Advances in reproductive technology have been so extensive that it is difficult to believe that cloning will ever be the only means by which couples can have genetically related progeny. If and when this happens, however, cloning to produce one's "own" child shall reflect, even more than current reproductive technologies already reflect, a tendency to commodify children and underestimate their main need, which is to be nurtured as individuals. Arguably, adoptive parents are more likely than genetic parents to support the development of individuality in their children because their parenting is not influenced by expectations that their children will express their own genetic make-up.

Case 3 articulates the impasse that inevitably arises for policy makers who have different starting points about moral status when they address research on human cloning and embryonic stem cells. As the council chair probably recognizes, even if the council's recommendations were limited to research on non-embryonic stem cells, they might not be conscientiously supportable by those who believe the research should be completely unregulated because this would impede fulfillment of its therapeutic potential. To show respect for all of the different standpoints of members of the council, the only alternative is to acknowledge the impossibility of agreement on regulation and present as fully and clearly as possible the recommendations, if any, that arise from the different starting points of members. Morally justifiable consensus or unanimity cannot be achieved while respecting the legitimacy of these starting points. Nor should consultative bodies in a democratic society whose members have incompatible but defensible starting points be formed homogeneously to ensure consensus or unanimity.

Case 4 exemplifies the inequities of a health care system that provides opportunities to participate in the fruits of research for the "haves" but not for the "have nots." Paying subjects to participate in research that affluent individuals would not choose to participate in without substantially greater remuneration has long been a questionable mechanism for recruiting human subjects. In general, the poorer the potential subject or the more remunerative the participation relative to her financial status, the less likely she is to participate wholly autonomously. However, when the research is promising and carries little other-than-financial risk or inconvenience to potential subjects, affluent individuals such as the Rubins may seek the potential benefits of the research on their own behalf or on behalf of their children. Inequality thus occurs through overrepresentation as well us underrepresentation of nondominant groups in research. From an egalitarian perspective, the standpoint of parents whose children are more likely than others to be affected by diseases that are potentially treatable through research is privileged vis-à-vis the standpoint of parents for whom this is not the case. The standpoint of nondominant parents whose children are already affected by a condition that is effectively treatable through stem cells from cord blood banked by donor parents is even more compelling.

A rationale sometimes offered for limiting the availability of experimental or innovative treatment (e.g., reproductive technologies) to affluent individuals is that their support is necessary for further development of the therapy so that it will eventually be available to everyone as standard of care. In the context of a free enterprise system, this rationale justifies preservation of cord blood for an affluent couple such as the Rubins. An egalitarian ethic is nonetheless at odds with a system that facilitates the economic disparities that a free enterprise system perpetuates or exacerbates. According to that ethic, ViaCord should at least inform couples that banking their potential child's cord blood in no way ensures that their child will benefit from the banking and that other children can surely benefit from donating their child's cord blood.

Ethical concerns about research on human subjects have increasingly been addressed in laws and institutional policies throughout the world. As this chapter shows, however, research on women raises issues that are inapplicable to men, and women may still be unjustifiably excluded or included in research protocols. From an egalitarian perspective, the standard for inclusion or exclusion should be the same for both sexes, although different starting points regarding moral status may lead to different applications of this perspective to pregnant women. If potential children have the same moral status as those who are born, they must be treated as such, and women's decisions about the research may be overridden by concerns about them. If potential children lack moral status, women's decisions override these concerns. For all persons as such, the criteria for their participation in research should, in general, be more demanding than those applicable to treatment modalities that have already proved effective.

PART III

An Egalitarian Ideal

14

Virtue and Gender Justice in Health Care

In this chapter, I revisit the egalitarian perspective that threads through the preceding pages by explaining, albeit briefly, how this perspective is directed toward an ideal of justice. Since the book focuses on women's health care, this ideal is necessarily one of gender justice. Regardless of whether justice in general or gender justice in particular is considered, however, just what the ideal entails needs to be unpacked so that the perspective that aims toward it can be more fully understood.

Recapping the perspective

In chapter 1, I explain and defend standpoint theory as a means by which to remediate the inevitable nearsightedness of those who make decisions or formulate policies that affect others. While acknowledging that nondominant people are also nearsighted, I offer epistemological and ethical reasons for privileging their standpoints. The epistemological rationale involves recognition that the knowledge and experience of dominant policy and decision makers is limited, and this limitation can be reduced through the input of those whose standpoints are nondominant. The ethical rationale stems from the obligation to respect the autonomy of those who are nondominant, as well as the right of nondominant individuals to have their standpoints and interests included in decisions that affect them. The interests of individuals, as John Stuart Mill reminds us, can be best determined by the individuals themselves, from their own standpoints.[1] With regard to many issues in bioethics, these standpoints proceed from different starting points on moral status.

As mentioned at the outset, the starting point of an egalitarian perspective is the affirmation that every human person, while different in important ways from every other, has the same value as every other. Neither this starting point nor the perspective that proceeds from it settles the thorny question of whether some human beings, such as developing human fetuses and comatose or profoundly impaired adults, are persons. Even from different starting points, however, people can and do support the position that many human beings have the same value despite differences of class, gender, sexual orientation, race, age, talents, and abilities. This position is not only rationally defensible but relatively uncontroversial.

Another relatively uncontroversial position is that those who are capable of respecting the autonomy of others are morally obliged to do so. Because "respect" is not the same as compliance, this does not imply an obligation to agree with or implement the decisions that others make from different standpoints. But neither does it imply that it is impossible to resolve conflicts that occur when people operating from different standpoints arrive at incompatible positions on the same ethical question. By whatever conception of justice is invoked, the verity of justice serves a mediating role in these situations.

Justice is discussed in the preceding chapters as one of four basic principles applicable to bioethics. The others include beneficence and nonmaleficence, as well as respect for autonomy. Application of the principles, or verities, as I call them, in support or refutation of specific moral obligations is facilitated through maxims such as those listed in chapter 1. However, the egalitarian perspective I bring to issues and cases through consideration of verities, variables, and maxims may be criticized on grounds that it seldom leads to clear, definitive conclusions. My response to this anticipated criticism is that such conclusions can only rarely (possibly never) be drawn with certitude that they are morally right or good, as well as clear and definitive, because it is impossible to know all of the relevant variables and standpoints of those involved. There is no "recipe" that yields clear, definitive, and certainly right answers to all of the ethical quandaries faced in "real life" situations. Still, there are some routes that are more likely than others to lead to those answers.

Another response to the above criticism is that an egalitarian perspective is not only based on the principle or verity of justice but also on justice as a virtue or ideal. Considering justice in either or both of these ways sheds further light on how moral conflicts in women's health care may be resolved. The starting point of an egalitarian perspective does not determine its direction, however; indispensable to that determination is the end point—that is, the ideal toward which the perspective points.

The ideal of justice is a necessary supplement to an egalitarian ethic based on verities, with or without guidance through maxims. Pursuit of this ideal requires more than fulfillment of moral obligations; it calls for supererogatory or virtuous behavior. Moreover, just as justice is the verity by which priorities among other verities are determinable, justice is the virtue by which other virtues may be ordered.[2]

Obligations, virtues, and ideals

Most analyses of issues in bioethics distinguish between behavior that is obligatory and that which is not obligatory, with little or no consideration of virtuous or supererogatory behavior.[3] Beauchamp and Childress, for example, have long used their mantra of principles to examine a wide range of topics in support or refutation of specific moral obligations. In the earliest editions of their *Principles*, the four verities were presented and applied without addressing the relationship between virtue and moral decision-making. In the third and fourth editions, virtues and ideals were considered only in a final chapter, easily separable from the preceding, extensive, principle-based analyses. The fifth edition moves the discussion of virtue into the first part of the book but largely ignores this content in the chapters that follow.[4]

Analyses limited to determination of what is or isn't morally obligatory fail to take into account two important features of moral decision-making. One is that many (most, I think) moral agents are not concerned only about fulfillment of their moral duties or obligations; rather, they want to go beyond a minimal measure of morality by choosing alternatives that are morally more demanding—that is, supererogatory. To use an analogy with academic performance, they want to get better grades, not just passable ones. Or, like parents, they want to do more on behalf of their children than only what they are obliged to do. In the health care context, most practitioners want to provide even better care of their patients than they professionally, legally, or morally are obliged to provide.

The second feature of moral decision-making that obligation-based approaches tend to ignore involves the content of bioethical decisions. Often, several options available to the decision maker are morally justifiable; this is especially true in the context of health care. In tragic situations, for example, either allowing a patient to die or prolonging her life may be a morally justified decision. Recognizing this possibility allows parties to choose either alternative without judging those who choose the other as having failed to fulfill their moral obligations; it thus facilitates respect for the standpoints of others.

"Virtue" generally refers to a disposition or habit by which a person tends to perform moral actions or refrain from immoral actions.[5] While some habits are formed inadvertently, virtue can only be developed through persistent and deliberate repetition of moral behavior. The set of moral habits a person acquires constitutes her moral character. Because character affects all of a person's decisions, virtue is more comprehensive than obligation in its applicability to the moral dimensions of life. It focuses on the moral agent rather than on specific acts of the agent. Through this comprehensiveness and focus, virtue embraces the realm of supererogation. The end pursued through morally supererogatory behavior is a moral ideal. A virtuous person who seems to have reached this ideal is called a saint. As David Hilfiker observed, however, "not all of us are saints."[6] Even those who are virtuous do not always act virtuously.

As a virtue, justice entails the dispositional readiness to give everyone her due.[7] On a practical level, this definition raises the question of how to determine "what is due" for individuals who have different needs, desires, abilities, and talents. From an egalitarian perspective, an ideal of justice suggests an answer to this question because it identifies an end point that individuals with different starting points and standpoints, as well as capabilities, can simultaneously pursue without compromising their moral integrity. The ideal of justice allows each person to move toward this end point without impeding others' movement toward the same ideal. Affirming an ideal of justice is thus a means by which respect for people who make decisions from different standpoints may be maximized. To the extent that the same ideal is pursued, albeit from different standpoints, the pursuers tend to converge to form communities.[8] While their standpoints remain unique, the distances between them narrow as they approach the ideal.

This ideal of justice is at odds with the Rawlsian account of justice in health care developed by Norman Daniels.[9] Daniels maintains that health care resources should be distributed on the basis of whether they promote "normal species-typical function" (the set of functions that *most* people are able to perform) in those who would otherwise be unable to perform these functions. Specification of the normal functions is apparently determined by statistical averaging, but just what range counts as normal on either side of the precise average is disputable. Daniels's argument for the normal-function criterion relies on a conception of justice as a morally obligatory principle rather than virtue. From an egalitarian perspective, an obvious weakness of this criterion is that within any proposed range of normality there are inevitable disparities among individuals. Moreover, some people fall above rather than below the normal range. A Rawlsian strategy fails to address the possibility of tapping into this resource in order to promote a more equitable society for those below the normal range as well as in it.

Although this book stresses the verity or principle of justice, my discussion of issues and cases often points to an ideal of justice whose pursuit entails supererogatory or virtuous behavior. This ideal, supported in different ways by Amartya Sen, Martha Nussbaum, and Alasdair MacIntyre,[10] is one of human flourishing rather than functional normality. Justice as human flourishing is an ideal that can only be approximated by taking into account each one's different set of capabilities. These include not only abilities, disabilities, and preferences but also social variables (such as gender, race, and class) that may promote or hinder the expression of one's capabilities. To determine what constitutes flourishing for each person requires consideration of each as a unique individual rather than as belonging to a group on either side of what is "normal." By this standard, even those who cannot be brought into the range of normal species functionality are capable of flourishing to some degree. Someone whose mobility is impaired, for example, may develop outstanding academic skills, while someone who is cognitively impaired may develop outstanding physical skills. Because it is applicable to every person as such, the ideal of justice as human flourishing may require the flourishing of some to be reduced so that others may flourish. Human flourishing is thus maximized but not necessarily optimal for all individuals. Unlike the normative conception of justice endorsed by Rawls and Daniels, the ideal of justice applies to both those whose capabilities are already beyond the level of "normal functionality" and those who are below it.

An egalitarian perspective thus identifies the ideal of human flourishing as its end point, just as it identifies attribution of the same value to every person as its starting point. A normative principle of justice is thus a minimal requirement for morality, whereas the virtue of justice points to maximal expression as the ideal.

Individual decision-making and an egalitarian ideal

In chapter 2, I distinguish between guidelines and regulations and discuss the relationship between them and the verities. Guidelines are considered in the context of professional guidelines or policies that serve an advisory function; regulations are treated as laws or statutes that carry penalties if they are not observed. Professional guidelines, I suggest, tend to support maximization of the autonomy of practitioners so that they are free to deal with the nuances of cases as they see fit. This emphasis on autonomy relies on an idealistic conception of the practitioner as one who is steadfastly committed to the ideal of her profession, and who, in light of that ideal, wants to do more than what is obligatory for patients. Professional guidelines thus seem to assume that the professionals to whom they apply are virtuous practitioners.[11]

The emphasis on practitioner autonomy in professional guidelines should not be confused with an endorsement of a paternalistic model of the practitioner's role. Most guidelines acknowledge that a competent patient's autonomy with regard to refusal of treatment, even life-saving treatment, trumps the practitioner's obligations of beneficence and nonmaleficence toward the patient. This acknowledgment reflects the fact that governmental regulations require practitioners to comply with such refusals. The guidelines of professional organizations typically assume that the breadth of judgment they support for their members falls within the scope of what laws governing professional practice allow. Respect for autonomy, whether the patient's or the practitioner's, is nonetheless a paramount principle of health care guidelines, with beneficence and nonmaleficence toward the patient taking priority with regard to patients who are decisionally incompetent.

Although regulatory statutes or laws are intended to protect the autonomy of competent patients, they are also intended to promote the verity of justice by preventing undue risks or harms to patients and by mandating a basic level of health care for everyone. Because a basic level of health care is less than the level of care accessible by dominant members of society, it is more in accord with a Rawlsian conception of justice than an egalitarian ideal. Daniels, for example, supports this basic standard as one that should be ensured for everyone through governmental regulation. Ensuring it is thus obligatory rather than virtuous. A minimum of regulation serves to maximize individual autonomy while also reducing inequality in health care. However, this minimum permits inequality that, from an egalitarian perspective, is morally inadequate. A basic level of health care may suffice as a governmental or policy standard of justice, and maximization of practitioner autonomy may suffice as a criterion for professional guidelines, but neither of these mechanisms offers adequate moral guidance to practitioners or patients who are individually confronted with ethical quandaries about health care. For that, each one must look to her own moral starting point and end point, then attempt to make decisions consistent with the moral standpoint that stretches between the two.

The egalitarian perspective of this book is primarily applicable to individuals for whom guidelines and regulation are an inadequate moral guide. It is a more comprehensive guide than these because the range of decisions it encompasses is both quantitatively and qualitatively farther reaching. With questions that guidelines and legislation do not address, the verity of justice can determine where one's moral obligation lies; with regard to questions about the morally better course to follow, as opposed to the morally obligatory course, the ideal of justice is the relevant guide to virtuous behavior.

Virtue in women's health care

With regard to ethical questions in women's health care, gender justice is obligatory as a necessary subset of the verity or principle of justice, but gender justice may also be pursued as an ideal by practitioners and patients alike. Approximation to the ideal requires attention to the fact that women in general have a different set of capabilities than men in general. Paradoxically, some of the capabilities that women have and men lack impede rather than enhance women's ability to flourish. The obvious example of this is women's ability to gestate and nurse children. Men rarely if ever experience the lack of these abilities as an impediment to their flourishing. Another capability that most women have that most men lack is a lengthier life span. As discussed in chapter 12, however, a longer life span can impede rather than facilitate women's flourishing if the increased years entail an increased burden of care for themselves or others. If gender justice is a necessary subset of the ideal of justice, pursuit of the ideal requires efforts to reduce these impediments to women's flourishing.

In the health care setting, the verity of justice obliges practitioners to reduce the impediments to "normal" function caused by illness or impairment. The virtue of justice requires not only these efforts but also attention to factors that impede a patient's flourishing. To the extent that their own capabilities allow, practitioners who are virtuous foster whatever capacity for flourishing a patient has. Because women's health problems may be caused or exacerbated by social disparities, power differences, prejudices, and stereotypes, pursuit of the ideal of gender justice in health care requires attention to these factors also. With regard to eating disorders, for example, a virtuous clinician may exert efforts to change media images of women to healthy models of feminine beauty instead of models that can only be achieved through unhealthy, even life-threatening, behavior. With regard to health problems that arise because of domestic violence, a virtuous practitioner will not just treat the woman for the condition requiring immediate medical attention but try to help her avoid recurrence of the violence.

Although women as patients are nondominant, most women are moral agents who, as such, have moral obligations to others in the health care setting. Women as patients are obliged, for example, to respect the autonomy of clinicians who refuse to perform an elective procedure that they consider morally or medically inappropriate. Women in health care settings may also act virtuously—for example, by donating tissue or organs to others. When women act virtuously, however, they do so by choice rather than conformity to social expectations or pressures. No behavior is virtuous if it is coerced.

Women as patients also have different capabilities as individuals. In the language of standpoint theory, some who are dominant vis-à-vis other women already enjoy flourishing as individuals because their capabilities are relatively unimpeded, or much less impeded, in comparison with the capabilities of other women. Still, the ideal of justice pursued through the virtue of justice requires efforts on some women's part to reduce the impediments to flourishing of women whose capabilities are more impeded than their own. Those of us who stand on the fortuitous side of "normal species-typical functioning" are impelled by the virtue of justice to find ways by which to reduce the impediments to flourishing of others.

NOTES

CHAPTER 1

1. Cf. "Health-Related Quality of Life among Women," National Center for Chronic Disease Prevention and Health Promotion, *Chronic Disease Notes and Reports* (Winter 2003). Accessed 7/19/05 at http://www.cdc.gov/nccdphp/cdnr_winter0305.htm.

2. Van Rensselaer Potter, *Bioethics: Bridge to the Future* (Englewood Cliffs, N.J.: Prentice Hall, 1971), pp. vii–viii.

3. See M. B. Mahowald, "Biomedical Ethics: A Precocious Youth," in Joseph DeMarco and Richard Fox, eds., *New Directions in Ethics* (New York: Routledge and Kegan Paul, 1986), pp. 141–57.

4. William James described such decisions as "genuine options," which occur when the alternatives are living, forced, and momentous. James, "The Will to Believe," in *Essays on Faith and Morals* (Cleveland, Oh.: World, 1962), pp. 34–35.

5. Elements of my personal and professional background that contribute to my standpoint are ten years of elementary and junior high teaching, fifteen years as a philosophy professor, thirty-five years of mothering, and twenty-four years as a clinical ethicist at a major medical center (eight years in a department of pediatrics, sixteen years in a department of obstetrics and gynecology).

6. Cf. Albert R. Jonsen and Stephen Toulmin, *The Abuse of* Casuistry (Berkeley: University of California Press, 1989). The commission on which the authors served during the 1980s was a predecessor of more recent bioethics councils appointed by U.S. presidents. Its mandate was to address and make recommendations regarding access to health care, decisions to forego life-sustaining treatment, and the meaning and practice of informed consent. Highly informative reports on all of these issues were published by the U.S. Government Printing Office.

7. Because the terms "ethical" and "moral" are prevalently used interchangeably, I do likewise.

8. Drawing on Aristotle, Thomas Aquinas develops both natural law and virtue theory; Alasdair MacIntyre and Rosalind Hursthouse are contemporary proponents of virtue theory. Thomas Aquinas, *Summa Theologica* I–II, Questions LVI and XCIV, and Roger Crisp and Michael Slote, *Virtue Ethics* (New York: Oxford University Press, 2001). "Communitarianism," a recent coinage, describes diverse thinkers whose commonality is that they critique liberal individualism. This description generally applies to virtue theorists such as MacIntyre. Other prominent "communitarians" are Michael Sandel and Charles Taylor.

9. The most thorough and compelling work to date on "care ethics" is that of Virginia Held in *The Ethics of Care: Personal, Political, and Global* (New York: Oxford University Press, 2006). Held views this as a distinct moral approach that cannot simply be added to or included within other approaches.

10. Kathryn Montgomery Hunter, "Narrative," in Warren T. Reich, ed., *Encyclopedia of Bioethics* (New York: Simon and Schuster Macmillan, 1995), pp. 1789–94.

11. Beauchamp and Childress consider pragmatism an example of case-based reasoning without consideration of principles (p. 392), but I believe it combines theoretical and practical considerations. Tom Beauchamp and James Childress, *Principles of Biomedical Ethics*, 5th ed. (New York: Oxford University Press, 2001). As James would put it, truth (including moral truth) arises from the wedding between fact and theory, an "endlessly fertile" marriage. William James, *Pragmatism and Four Essays from the Meaning of Truth* (Cleveland, Oh.: World, 1965), p. 138. That Marx saw theory and practice as inseparable is evident from his critique of philosophers who "have only *interpreted* the world." "The point," he wrote, "is to change it." Lewis S. Feuer, ed., *Marx & Engels: Basic Writings on Politics & Philosophy* (Garden City, N.Y.: Doubleday Anchor, 1959), p. 245.

12. See Rosemarie Tong, *Feminine and Feminist Ethics* (Belmont, Calif.: Wadsworth, 1993), and Marilyn Friedman, "Care and Context in Moral Reasoning," in Eva Kittay and Diana Meyers, eds., *Women and Moral Theory* (Totowa, N.J.: Rowman and Littlefield, 1987), pp. 190–204.

13. Margaret Olivia Little, "Moral Generalities Revisited," in Brad Hooker and Margaret Little, eds., *Moral Particularism* (New York: Oxford University Press, 2000), p. 278.

14. See Catriona Mackenzie and Natalie Stoljar, eds., *Relational Autonomy: Feminist Perspectives on Autonomy, Agency, and the Social Self* (New York: Oxford University Press, 2000).

15. Carl E. Schneider, *The Practice of Autonomy* (New York: Oxford University Press, 1998).

16. Beauchamp and Childress, *Principles of Biomedical Ethics*, 5th ed., p. 63.

17. Ibid., pp. 114–15.

18. The term "topics" is based on Aristotle's use of the term to identify "bodies of experience that underlie the forms of argument that guide deliberation and discussion in the particular field." Jonsen and Toulmin, *Abuse of Casuistry*, p. 74, and Aristotle, *Topics*, Bk. III, chapters 1–6.

19. Albert R. Jonsen, Mark Siegler, and William J. Winslade, *Clinical Ethics*, 5th ed. (New York: McGraw-Hill, 2002), p. 147.

20. Who is to determine what counts as quality of life for another, and by what criteria, is obviously a controversial issue.

21. Beauchamp and Childress, *Principles of Biomedical Ethics*, 5th ed., p. 403.

22. Cf. Aristotle, *Posterior Analytics*, Bk. II, chapter 19.

23. Cf. John Rawls, "Justice as Fairness: Political Not Metaphysical," *Philosophy and Public Affairs* 14 (Summer 1985): 223–52.

24. Daniel Callahan apparently accords with my view in this regard: "I have yet to encounter a particularist who does not also have at least a few impassioned universalist commitments" and "I know of few universalists who will not admit some contextual or situational exceptions to their general principles." Callahan, "Universalism and Particularism," *Hastings Center Report* 30, no. 1 (2000): 41.

25. For example, the guidelines of different health care organizations or professional societies are not always in agreement with one another. The virtues that Beauchamp and Childress consider important for health professionals (e.g., trustworthiness, compassion, integrity) may also be considered "principles." The meanings of the virtues they name are variously interpretable and overlapping.

26. E.g., Beauchamp and Childress, *Principles of Biomedical Ethics*, 5th ed., pp. 15–19.

27. The "balancing" of justice, as I understand it, is comparable to John Rawls's account of "reflective equilibrium." See Rawls, *Theory of Justice* (Cambridge: Harvard University Press, 1971).

28. However, in the fifth edition of Jonsen, Siegler, and Winslade, *Clinical Ethics*, pp. 8–9, the authors, after contrasting their method with principle-based approaches, acknowledge that they refer to principles such as beneficence "as they become relevant to the discussion of the topics."

29. Cf. Jonsen and Toulmin, *Abuse of Casuistry*, pp. 253, 287.

30. In 1952, Case Western Reserve University Medical School launched a novel medical education program in which students were involved in the clinical setting from the first year on. Each was assigned a pregnant woman and expected to follow her through her pregnancy, delivery, and first year of her infant's life. Only recently have other medical schools in the United States imitated this method of training by introducing clinical experience into the first two years of medical school. Even in those schools, however, course work predominates before students start their clinical rotations in the third year.

31. Jonsen and Toulmin, *Abuse of Casuistry*, pp. 73–74.

32. "Rules" is often used as well to denote a lesser level of generality than principles. My argument that the "guidelines" of principlism are comparable to the maxims of casuistry could apply to "rules" also.

33. John Stuart Mill makes this argument in his essay *On Liberty* (Chicago: Henry Regnery, 1955), p. 111.

34. Admittedly, the distinction between failing to benefit another and harming her depends also on how the harm and benefit are valued by the individuals involved.

35. Jonsen, Siegler, and Winslade, *Clinical Ethics*, 5th ed., pp. 146–98.

36. See W. D. Ross's account of prima facie versus actual duties in *The Right and the Good* (Oxford: Oxford University Press, 1930), pp. 16–47.

37. For Plato, the just state is one in which the rulers (guardians) are rationally superior to those who are naturally more equipped to be warriors or craftsmen; correspondingly, the just individual is one whose reason rules her passion or ambition. See, e.g., *Republic*, Bk. V, 472–474, and Bk. IX, 580–582.

38. Beauchamp and Childress, *Principles of Biomedical Ethics*, 5th ed., p. 227. In Book V of the *Nichomachean Ethics*, Aristotle distinguishes between two senses of justice: universal justice, which involves virtue in its entirety, and particular justice, which may be distributive or retributive. Distributive justice necessarily involves equality and fairness; equity is a corrective to legal justice (chapters 2, 3, and 10).

39. In other words, health caregivers are mainly concerned with distributive rather than retributive or compensatory justice. Iris Marion Young critiques the tendency to consider justice too narrowly by focusing on the problem of distribution, ignoring questions of domination and oppression. As we shall see, however, the latter questions are related to the former problem when justice is defined as equal capability, as in Amartya Sen's account. See Young, *Justice and the Politics of Difference* (Princeton, N.J.: Princeton University Press, 1990), p. 9.

40. See John Rawls, *Political Liberalism* (New York: Columbia University Press, 1996). Rawls's theory of justice is also called contractarian because he supports it through the mechanism of a hypothetical social contract.

41. See Amartya Sen, *Inequality Reexamined* (Cambridge: Harvard University Press, 1992); Ronald Dworkin, "What Is Equality?" *Philosophy and Public Affairs* 10 (1981): 185–246, 283–345; Michael Walzer, *Spheres of Justice* (Oxford: Blackwell, 1983); Michael Sandel, *Liberalism and the Limits of Justice* (London: Cambridge University Press, 1982); Alasdair MacIntyre, *After Virtue* (London: Gerald Duckworth, 1985). Beauchamp and Childress distinguish between militant and moderate forms of communitarianism, imputing the moderate form to Walzer and the militant form to MacIntyre and Sandel. Beauchamp and Childress, *Principles of Biomedical Ethics*, 5th ed., p. 365.

42. Robert Nozick, *Anarchy, State and Utopia* (London: Blackwell, 1974).

43. Cf. Aristotle, *Posterior Analytics*, Bk. 1, chapters 1–3.

44. Sen has applied this model most famously to the issue of famine in India.

45. Simone de Beauvoir, *The Second Sex*, excerpted in Mary B. Mahowald, ed., *Philosophy of Woman* (Indianapolis: Hackett, 1994), p. 204.

46. H. Tristram Engelhardt, *Foundations of Bioethics* (New York: Oxford University Press, 1996), p. 381. However, the religious perspective that Engelhardt endorses leads to different positions than his libertarian account.

47. Decades ago, Diana Pearce coined the term "feminization of poverty" to highlight the economic discrepancy between men and women, citing the fact that a majority of the poor in the United States are women and their children. Pearce, "The Feminization of Poverty: Women, Work and Welfare," *Urban and Social Change Review* 11 (1978): 28–36. On the health risks of caregiving, see Mary B. Mahowald, Dana Levinson, Christine Cassel et al., "The New Genetics and Women," *Milbank Quarterly* 74, no. 2 (1996): 268–70.

48. Nozick, *Anarchy, State and Utopia*, p. 160.

49. Susan Okin, *Justice, Gender and Family* (New York: Basic Books, 1989).

50. Normal Daniels, *Just Health Care* (Cambridge: Cambridge University Press, 1985), p. 33.

51. Anita Silvers, "Formal Justice," in Anita Silvers, David Wasserman, and Mary B. Mahowald, *Disability, Difference, Discrimination* (Lanham, Md.: Rowman and Littlefield, 1998), p. 66.

52. Consider, for example, the difference between a woman of reproductive age who requires in vitro fertilization with her partner's sperm in order to conceive, and a healthy postmenopausal woman who already has children, who seeks egg donation, in vitro fertilization, and embryo transfer in order to bear another child.

53. Michael Sandel, *Liberalism and the Limits of Justice* (Cambridge: Cambridge University Press, 1982), p. 172.

54. Cf. Martin Buber, *I and Thou* (New York: Scribner's, 1958); Gabriel Marcel, *The Mystery of Being* (Chicago: Henry Regnery, 1960), and John McDermott, ed., *The Writings of William James* (New York: Random House, 1967), pp. 238, 216. Peirce develops his view on the reality and central importance of relationships in his triadic theory of signs and interpretation; see Justus Buchler, ed., *Philosophical Writings of Peirce* (New York: Dover, 1955), e.g., pp. 274–86.

55. In addition to Carol Gilligan and Nel Noddings, to be discussed next, these scholars include Joan Tronto, Marilyn Friedman, Sara Ruddick, Virginia Held, Annette Baier, and many others.

56. Nel Noddings, *Caring: A Feminine Approach to Ethics and Moral Education* (Berkeley: University of California Press, 1984).

57. Carol Gilligan, *In a Different Voice* (Cambridge: Harvard University Press, 1982).

58. Carol Gilligan, "Moral Orientation and Moral Development," in Eva F. Kittay and Diana T. Meyers, eds., *Women and Moral Theory* (Totowa, N.J.: Rowman and Littlefield, 1987), p. 31.

59. Virginia Held, *Justice and Care* (Boulder, Colo.: Westview, 1995).

60. With substantial revision, much of the material in this section is taken from Mary Briody Mahowald, *Genes, Women, Equality* (New York: Oxford University Press, 2000), pp. 14–23.

61. John Stuart Mill, *On Liberty* (Chicago: Henry Regnery, 1955), p. 111.

62. Thomas Nagel, *Equality and Partiality* (New York: Oxford University Press, 1991), pp. 10–20. In lectures published earlier, Nagel calls this "the view from nowhere." See Thomas Nagel, *The Tanner Lectures in Human Values* (Salt Lake City: University of Utah Press, 1980).

63. Charles Sanders Peirce, in Charles Hartshorne and Paul Weis, eds., *The Collected Papers of Charles Sanders Peirce* (Cambridge: Belknap Press of Harvard University, 1960), vol. 2, p. 654.

64. John Ladd, "The Ethics of Participation," in J. Roland Pennock and John W. Chapman, eds., *Participation in Politics* (New York: Lieber-Atherton, 1975), p. 101. Ladd imputes this view to Kurt Baier; see Baier's *The Moral Point of View* (New York: Random House, 1965), p. 107.

65. Ladd, "Ethics of Participation," p. 102.

66. Admittedly, utilitarian grounds for participation may also be invoked to curtail as well as demand participation by nondominant groups. Deontological arguments—for example, those based on the inalienable right of persons to participate in the development of social policies that affect them—also provide justification for a democratic form of participation.

67. Ladd, "Ethics of Participation," p. 103.

68. Ibid., p. 102.

69. Nancy C. M. Hartsock, *Money, Sex, and Power* (Boston: Northeastern University Press, 1985), and Hartsock, *The Feminist Standpoint Revisited* (Boulder, Colo.: Westview, 1998), pp. 105–32.

70. Charles Taylor, *The Ethics of Authenticity* (Cambridge: Harvard University Press, 1992).

71. Albert Camus, *The Rebel*, trans. Anthony Bower (New York: Knopf, 1956), p. 22.

72. Admittedly, the term "patient" also conveys nondominance, as passivity. But this term is even less likely to be changed to one that connotes greater autonomy, such as "client" or "consumer" (of health services).

73. See Mary B. Mahowald, "*Just* Caring: Power for Empowerment," in *Women and Children in Health Care: An Unequal Majority* (New York: Oxford University Press, 1993), pp. 255–69.

74. As a member of this panel for five years, I experienced first hand the benefits of inclusion of "consumers" in determination of research priorities. See Yvonne Andejeski, Erica Breslau, Elizabeth Hart et al., "Benefits and Drawbacks of Including Consumer Reviewers in the Scientific Merit Review of Breast Cancer Research," *Journal of Women's Health and Gender-Based Medicine* 11, no. 2 (2002): 119–36, and Yvonne Andejeski, Isabelle T Bisceglio, Kay Dickersin et al., "Quantitative Impact of Including Consumers in

the Scientific Review of Breast Cancer Research Proposals," *Journal of Women's Health and Gender-Based Medicine* 11, no. 4 (2002): 379–88.

75. Stephen H. Miles and Alison August, "Courts, Gender, and the 'Right to Die,' " *Law, Medicine, and Health Care* 18 (1990): 85–95.

76. Donna Haraway, "Situated Knowledges: The Science Question in Feminism and the Privilege of Partial Perspective," *Feminist Studies* 14 (1988): 584.

CHAPTER 2

1. Diana Pearce, "The Feminization of Poverty: Women, Work, and Welfare," *Urban and Social Change Review* 11 (Feb. 1978): 28–36. Poverty affects even more children than women because many poor women have children who are unsupported by their fathers.

2. Ruth Sidel, *Women and Children Last* (New York: Penguin, 1986), pp. 133–56.

3. For example, Ichiro Kawachi and Bruce Kennedy, "Socioeconomic Determinants of Health: Health and Social Cohesion—Why Care about Income Inequality?" *British Medical Journal* 314 (1997): 1037.

4. John M. Smith, *Women and Doctors* (New York: Atlantic Monthly Press, 1992).

5. ACOG Committee Opinion No. 289, American College of Obstetrics and Gynecologists, *Obstetetrics and Gynecology* 102 (2003): 2, citing Linda Emanuel and Ezekiel Emanuel, *Journal of the American Medical Association*, 1992.

6. Ibid., p. 3. Because this model suggests that the physician will simply do whatever the patient asks as long as she is fully informed, it is akin to what I have elsewhere called an instrumental model of the physician's role. M. B. Mahowald, *Women and Children in Health Care* (New York: Oxford University Press, 1993), p. 29.

7. For an excellent examination of how to respond ethically to situations in which autonomous patients are reluctant or opposed to making their own health care decisions, see Carl Schneider, *The Practice of Autonomy* (New York: Oxford University Press, 1998).

8. ACOG Committee Opinion No. 289, p. 3.

9. Ibid.

10. Albert R. Jonsen, Mark Siegler, and William J. Winslade, *Clinical Ethics*, 5th ed. (New York: McGraw-Hill, 2002).

11. Frank A. Chervenak and Laurence B. McCullough, "Perinatal Ethics: A Practical Method of Analysis of Obligations to Mother and Fetus," *Obstetrics and Gynecology* 66 (1985): 443. The authors elaborate on the meaning of "interests" and on "beneficence-based obligations" in obstetrics in Chervenak and McCullough, *Ethics in Obstetrics and Gynecology* (New York: Oxford University Press, 1994), pp. 25–42, 113–22.

12. In *Ethics in Obstetrics and Gynecology* Chervenak and McCullough indicate that the "interests of the male gamete provider, spouse, or partner are variably at stake in the pregnant woman's decision about whether the previable fetus is a patient" while also claiming that decisions about her pregnancy are "hers and hers alone to make" (p. 122).

13. When the difference between "embryo" and "fetus" is not relevant to the discussion, the term "fetus" may be used for the developing organism from fertilization onward.

14. John A. Robertson, *Children of Choice: Freedom and the New Reproductive Technologies* (Princeton, N.J.: Princeton University Press, 1994), pp. 22–23.

15. Ibid., p. 223.

16. Ibid., p. 23.

17. Carson Strong, *Ethics in Reproductive and Perinatal Medicine* (New Haven, Conn.: Yale University Press, 1997), p. 75.

18. Ibid., p. 72.

19. Ibid., p. 53.
20. Ibid., p. 6.
21. Ibid., p. 61.
22. Ibid.; italics added.
23. Ibid., p. 79.
24. Ibid., pp. 80–81.
25. Perinatologists are particularly prone to consider fetuses as separate patients; for example, Mark Evans, "Coercion for Fetal Therapy?" in F. K. Beller and R. F. Weir, eds., *The Beginning of Human Life* (Dordrecht: Kluwer Academic, 1994), p. 319.
26. See, for example, D. W. Bianchi, T. M. Crombleholme, and M. E. D'Alton, *Fetology: Diagnosis and Management of the Fetal Patient* (New York: McGraw-Hill, 2000); M. Harrison, M. Golbus, and R. Filly, eds., *The Unborn Patient* (Philadelphia: W. B. Saunders, 1991).
27. Margaret Olivia Little, "Abortion, Intimacy, and the Duty to Gestate," *Ethical Theory and Moral Practice* 2 (1999): 196.
28. The rationale for considering fetuses patients is that they are treatable as such through the woman's body. They may not be considered persons because they are as yet incapable of functions commonly attributed to those who are unquestionably persons.
29. F. A. Chervenak, L. B. McCullough, and D. Skupski, "An Ethical Justification for Emergency, Coerced Cesarean Delivery," *Obstetrics and Gynecology* 82 (1993): 1029–35.
30. Chervenak and McCullough, *Ethics in Obstetrics and Gynecology*, p. 101: "We take no position on this matter (i.e., when the developing human organism becomes a person)."
31. Chervenak and McCullough support treatment of the fetus without the pregnant woman's consent in cases of complete, well-documented placenta previa and when the urgency of the situation makes it impossible to obtain a court order for the medically recommended treatment.
32. I owe the term "entwinement" to Margaret Olivia Little who, like Judith Jarvis Thomson, is one of the few philosophers to focus discussion of abortion on this essential relationship rather than on the fetus alone. See Little, "Abortion, Intimacy, and the Duty to Gestate," 295–312, and Thomson, "A Defense of Abortion," *Philosophy and Public Affairs* 1, no. 1 (1971): 47–66.
33. Chervenak and McCullough, *Ethics in Obstetrics and Gynecology*, p. 102.
34. Thomas H. Strong, *Expecting Trouble: The Myth of Prenatal Care in America* (New York: New York University Press, 2000).
35. Chervenak and McCullough, *Ethics in Obstetrics and Gynecology*, p. 104; my italics.
36. Free Webster's Dictionary. Accessed 4/5/06 at http://www.hyperdictionary.com/search.aspx?Dict=&define=individual&search.
37. Although "previable" fetuses may also be described as "nonviable," the authors probably prefer the former term because it conveys the expectation that such fetuses will become viable.
38. Chervenak and McCullough, *Ethics in Obstetrics and Gynecology*, p. 102.
39. Ibid., p. 106.
40. Chervenak, McCullough, and Skupski, "Ethical Justification for Emergency, Coerced Cesarean Delivery."
41. Moral status is thus different from a status that may be conferred by others, as, for example, immigration or criminal status.
42. J. N. Kirkpatrick and M. B. Mahowald, "Golden Rule Reasoning and Clinical Medicine," *Journal of Clinical Ethics* 15, no. 3 (2004): 1–11.

CHAPTER 3

1. Concepts may also be developed from other concepts, but ultimately, in an Aristotelian account, all generalizations are derived from experience.

2. John D. Biggers, "When Does Life Begin?" *Sciences* (1981): 10–14.

3. For an excellent account of different definitions of death and criteria for determining it, see Robert M. Veatch, *Death, Dying, and the Biological Revolution* (New Haven, Conn.: Yale University Press, 1976). In light of ongoing controversy about the meaning of "death," Veatch suggests that individuals might choose the definition by which they wish their own deaths to be determined (pp. 72–73).

4. Ibid., p. 31.

5. For example, Plato, *Laws* 896a, *Timaeus* 46d, *Phaedo* 85e–86, 94c–95. In *Republic*, Bk. 4, Plato describes the tripartite soul as consisting of reason, courage, and appetite.

6. Cf. Aristotle, *On the Soul*, Bk. II, chapters 1–3.

7. John Haldane and Patrick Lee, "Aquinas on Human Ensoulment, Abortion and the Value of Life," *Philosophy* 78 (2003): 255–78.

8. Judith Jarvis Thomson and Baruch Brody, for example, use these terms interchangeably. Michael Tooley criticizes their doing so in "Abortion and Infanticide," in Susan Dwyer and Joel Feinberg, eds., *The Problem of Abortion* (Belmont, Calif.: Wadsworth, 1997), p. 43.

9. If and when human cloning can be successfully performed through transfer of adult DNA from any part of the donor's body, any human cell may be considered a potential embryo if its nuclear DNA is extracted and transferred to a woman's enucleated egg, inducing dedifferentiation before triggering the onset of new development.

10. "Moral status" and "moral standing" may be used interchangeably, but L. S. Sumner distinguishes between them. Moral status, for him, implies a continuum from no moral status to full moral status, whereas moral standing refers to the point along the continuum at which a specific entity stands. See Sumner, *Abortion and Moral Theory* (Princeton, N.J.: Princeton University Press, 1981), p. 26.

11. Mary Anne Warren elaborates and defends multiple criteria for full moral status in *Moral Status: Obligations to Persons and Other Living Things* (Oxford: Oxford University Press, 2000), chapter 6.

12. For a well-developed account of the relationship between respect and autonomy in the context of health care, see R. S. Calman and K. C. Calman, *Healthy Respect*, 2nd ed. (Oxford: Oxford University Press, 1994), chapter 4.

13. The term "vegetative" is unfortunate because it seems to prejudge the moral status of the entity to which it applies as less than that of other human beings.

14. The capacity of frozen embryos to develop is thwarted but not necessarily ended.

15. Judith Jarvis Thomson, "A Defense of Abortion," in Susan Dwyer and Joel Feinberg, eds., *The Problem of Abortion* (Belmont, Calif.: Wadsworth, 1997), p. 76.

16. A more recent account of abortion based on the uniqueness of the gestational tie as well as the life-altering event of motherhood is that of Margaret Olivia Little, *The Morality of Abortion* (New York: Oxford University Press, forthcoming).

17. See Mary B. Mahowald, "Person," in Warren Reich, ed., *Encyclopedia of Bioethics* (New York: Macmillan, 1995), pp. 1934–40.

18. See ibid. for the English translation, but for the Latin (*Persona est naturae rationalis individua substantia*), see Arthur C. Danto, "Persons," in Paul Edwards, ed., *Encyclopedia of Philosophy*, 8 vols. (New York: Macmillan, 1972), vol. 6, p. 111.

19. Bonnie Steinbock, *Life before Birth* (New York: Oxford University Press, 1992), pp. 53–54; Warren, *Moral Status*, pp. 94–95.

20. Robert P. George and Alfonso Gomez-Lobo, "The Moral Status of the Human Embryo," *Perspectives in Biology and Medicine* 48 (2005): 201–10. The President's Council on Bioethics, on which George and Gomez-Lobo serve, uses the term "cloned embryos" for those obtained through somatic cell nuclear transfer and refers to those obtained through fertilization simply as "embryos."

21. Brian Johnstone, *The Moral Status of the Embryo*, in William Walters and Peter Singer, eds., *Test-Tube Babies* (Oxford: Oxford University Press, 1982), pp. 49–56.

22. Alfonso Gomez-Lobo, "Does Respect for Embryos Entail Respect for Gametes?" *Theoretical Medicine and Bioethics* 25 (2004): 199–208.

23. Cf. Mary B. Mahowald, "Respect for Embryos and the Potentiality Argument," *Theoretical Medicine and Bioethics* 25 (2004): 209–14.

24. R. M. Hare, "Abortion and the Golden Rule," *Philosophy and Public Affairs* 4, no. 3 (1975): 201–22.

25. Helge Kuhse and Peter Singer, "The Moral Status of the Embryo," in Walters and Singer, eds., *Test-Tube Babies*, pp. 57–63.

26. Ibid., p. 59.

27. Frank A. Chervenak and Laurence B. McCullough, *Ethics in Obstetrics and Gynecology* (New York: Oxford University Press, 1994), 100–108.

28. E.g., H. Tristram Engelhardt, *The Foundations of Bioethics*, 2nd ed. (New York: Oxford University Press, 1996), pp. 135–51. This is a philosophical argument based mainly on Kant's account of person. Engelhardt also develops a personal view that differs from the philosophical position.

29. John T. Noonan, Jr., "An Almost Absolute Value in History," in John T. Noonan, Jr., ed., *The Morality of Abortion* (Cambridge: Harvard University Press, 1979), pp. 50–59. A more scientific definition of this process, called "syngamy," is provided by the President's Council on Bioethics: "the combining of paternally- and maternally-contributed haploid pro-nuclei to result in a unique diploid nucleus of a developing zygote." *Monitoring Stem Cell Research*, Report of the President's Council on Bioethics (Washington, D.C.: Jan. 2004), p. 76.

30. Congregation for the Doctrine of the Faith, Instruction on Respect for Human Life in Its Origin and on the Dignity of Procreation, *Donum vitae* (Feb. 22, 1987), I, No. 1:AAS 80 (1988), p. 79. Although the terms "conception" and "fertilization" refer to different points in development, they are often used synonymously, as is probable here. Technically, "conception" refers to the process by which pregnancy is established in vivo, whereas "fertilization" refers to the process by which sperm and ovum unite either in vivo or in vitro.

31. The primitive streak is the axis along which the spinal cord develops.

32. Norman Ford, *When Did I Begin?* (Cambridge: Cambridge University Press, 1988).

33. In a well-developed argument identifying brain function as determinative of a right to life, Baruch Brody allows that this may occur as early as the second week or as late as the twelfth week after conception. Brody, "Against an Absolute Right to Abortion," in Susan Dwyer and Joel Feinberg, eds., *The Problem of Abortion* (Belmont, Calif.: Wadsworth, 1997), p. 97.

34. A recent study claims that fetuses up to 29 weeks are probably unable to experience pain, but this study has been challenged as biased because the authors support late-term abortions without anesthesia on grounds of their claim. Denise Grady, "Study Finds Fetuses up to 29 Weeks Feel No Pain and Need No Anesthesia in Abortions," *New York Times*, Aug. 24, 2005, p. A8.

35. Hans-Martin Sass, "The Moral Significance of Brain-Life Criteria," in F. K. Beller and R. F. Weir, eds., *The Beginning of Human Life* (Dordrecht: Kluwer Academic, 1994), pp. 57–70.

36. Warren, *Moral Status*, pp. 215–16.

37. Ibid., pp. 19, 181.

38. Michael Tooley, "Abortion and Infanticide," in Susan Dwyer and Joel Feinberg, eds., *The Problem of Abortion* (Belmont, Calif.: Wadsworth, 1997), p. 57.

39. Peter Singer, *Practical Ethics*, 2nd ed. (Cambridge: Cambridge University Press, 1993), p. 97 (bracketed text added for clarity).

40. Norman C. Gillespie, "Abortion and Human Rights," *Ethics* 87 (1977): 238.

41. *Monitoring Stem Cell Research*, pp. 19–23.

42. A number of members of the President's Council on Bioethics support the view that the fetus occupies an "intermediate moral status." For a sampling of their diverse positions, see Mary B. Mahowald, "The President's Council on Bioethics, 2002–2004," *Perspectives in Biology and Medicine* 48 (2005): 159–171.

43. Steinbock, *Life before Birth*; Warren, *Moral Status*, p. 182.

44. John Robertson, *Children of Choice* (Princeton, N.J.: Princeton University Press, 1994), p. 55.

45. Ibid., p. 46.

46. Ibid., p. 53.

47. Carson Strong, *Ethics in Reproductive Medicine* (New Haven, Conn.: Yale University Press, 1997), p. 75.

48. Ibid., p. 53; see also Steinbock, *Life before Birth*, pp. 51–54.

49. Strong, *Ethics in Reproductive Medicine*, pp. 53–55.

50. Robertson, *Children of Choice*, p. 23.

51. Arguments against the postmodernist account have been well developed by others, and I will not repeat them here. But see, for example, David Detmer, *Challenging Postmodernism: Philosophy and the Politics of Truth* (Amherst, N.Y.: Humanity Books, 2003).

CHAPTER 4

1. Although I have fictionalized the identifiers, this case is one in which I was involved as an ethics consultant. For a more extended discussion, see Mary Briody Mahowald, *Genes, Women, Equality* (New York: Oxford University Press, 2000), pp. 23–27.

2. A "teratogenic" agent is one that causes malformation in the embryo or fetus; "microcephaly" means that the head is abnormally small and the brain is underdeveloped. E. Waisbren, B. D. Hamilton, P. J. St. James, S. Shiloh, and H. L. Levy, "Psychosocial Factors in Maternal Phenylketonuria: Women's Adherence to Medical Recommendations," *American Journal of Public Health* 85, no. 12 (1995): 1636.

3. Denise Grady, "Baby Spared Mother's Fate by Genetic Tests as Embryo," *New York Times*, Feb. 22, 2002, p. A16.

4. Cf. Sandra A. Carson and John E. Buster, "Biopsy of Gametes and Preimplantation Embryos in Genetic Diagnosis," *Seminars in Reproductive Endocrinology* 12, no. 3 (1994): 184–95.

5. An autosomal recessive disorder is transmitted through parents who are both nonsymptomatic carriers of the condition.

6. According to Glenn E. Smith, a neuropsychologist at the Mayo Clinic in Rochester, Minn., rare cases of Alzheimer's occur in patients between 30 and 40 years old. "Early-Onset Alzheimer's: An Interview with a Mayo Clinic Specialist." CNN.com Health Library (Feb. 28, 2005). Accessed 9/1/05 at http://www.cnn.com/HEALTH/library/AZ/00009.html.

7. "Disposition" of affected or extra embryos may not involve their destruction. They may be frozen, used in research, or donated to others. Moreover, they may be allowed to die

rather than directly terminated; these alternatives are analogous to the distinction between allowing born individuals to die versus killing them.

8. Glenn Schemmer and Anthony Johnson, "Genetic Amniocentesis and Chorionic Villus Sampling," *Obstetrics and Gynecology Clinics of North America* 20, no. 497 (1993): 515–16.

9. Rayna Rapp, *Testing Women, Testing the Fetus* (New York: Routledge, 1999), p. 223.

10. Cathleen M. Harris and Marion S. Verp, "Prenatal Testing and Interventions," in Mary B. Mahowald, Victor McKusick, Angela Scheuerle, and Timothy Aspinwall, eds., *Genetics in the Clinic: Clinical, Ethical, and Social Implications for Primary Care* (St. Louis, Mo.: Mosby, 2001), p. 62.

11. This figure may be higher if other risk factors are considered. Nancy Touchette, "Breast Cancer Susceptibility Genes: Overstating the Risk?" Genome News Network (Sept. 13, 2003). Accessed 9/2/05 at http://www.genomenewsnetwork.org/articles/09_02/cancer_breast.shtml.

12. Mahowald, *Genes, Women, Equality*, pp. 182–84.

13. Slightly modified versions of cases 1 and 2 and the data regarding them are taken from ibid., chapters 9 and 10.

14. Sally MacIntyre and Anne Sooman, "Non-paternity and Prenatal Screening," *Lancet* 338 (1991): 869; Marie-Gaelle Le Roux, O. Pascal, M. T. Andre, O. Herbert, A. David, and J. P. Maison, "Non-paternity and Genetic Counseling," *Lancet* 340 (1992): 607.

15. Mahowald, *Genes, Women, Equality*, p. 186.

16. American College of Obstetricians and Gynecologists and American College of Medical Genetics, *Preconception and Prenatal Carrier Screening for Cystic Fibrosis: Clinical and Laboratory Guidelines* (Washington, D.C.: ACOG, 2001).

17. Institute of Medicine, *Assessing Genetic Risks* (Washington, D.C.: National Academy Press, 1994), p. 6.

18. Benjamin E. Reubinoff and Joseph G. Schenker, "New Advances in Sex Preselection," *Fertility and Sterility* 66, no. 3 (1996): 343–48.

19. E.g., Bob Herbert, "China's Missing Girls," *New York Times*, Oct. 30, 1997, p. A23, and Sheryl WuDunn, "Korean Women Still Feel Demands to Bear a Son," *New York Times*, Jan. 14, 1997, p. A3.

20. Dorothy C. Wertz, "Society and the Not-So-New Genetics: What Are We Afraid Of? Some Future Predictions from a Social Scientist," *Journal of Contemporary Health Law and Policy* 13 (1999): 315.

21. Dorothy Wertz and John Fletcher, "Prenatal Diagnosis and Sex Selection in 19 Nations," *Social Science Medicine* 37, no. 11 (1993): 1362.

22. Herbert, "China's Missing Girls" and WuDunn, "Korean Women Still Feel Demands."

23. Herbert, "China's Missing Girls."

24. *American Heritage Dictionary of the English Language*, 4th ed., 2000. Accessed 4/27/06 at http://www.thefreedictionary.com/sexism.

25. Ethics Committee of the American Society for Reproductive Medicine, "Gender Selection for Nonmedical Reasons," *Fertility and Sterility* 75, no. 5 (2001): 861–64.

26. Christine Overall, *Ethics and Human Reproduction* (Boston: Allen and Unwin, 1987), p. 27.

CHAPTER 5

1. The incidence of infertility in couples of reproductive age is about 15 percent. Lisa A. Farah, "Infertility: Etiology and Evaluation," *Jacksonville Medicine* (May 2000). Accessed 4/17/06 at http://www.dcmsonline.org/jax-medicine/2000journals/may2000/infertility.htm.

2. "HIV-AIDS among Women." Centers for Disease Control (Dec. 2004). Accessed 4/17/06 at http://www.cdc.gov/hiv/pubs/facts/women/htm.

3. J. M. Karon, P. S. Rosenberg, G. McQuillan, M. Khare, M. Gwinn, and L. R. Petersen, "Prevalence of HIV Infection in the United States, 1984 to 1992," *Journal of the American Medical Association* 276 (1996): 126–31.

4. Julie Louise Gerberding, "Occupational Exposure to HIV in Health Care Settings," *New England Journal of Medicine* 348, no. 9 (2003): 827.

5. Annabel Kanabus, "HIV AIDS and Pregnancy." Avert.Org (Sept. 9, 2005). Accessed 4/5/06 at http://www.avert.org/pregnancy.htm.

6. Kristin Augustine, Carrie L. McMahon, and Eugene Pergament, "Organ Transplantation and Pregnancy," *Organ Transplantation and Pregnancy*, 9, no. 3 (Mar. 2002). Accessed 4/5/06 at http://www.fetal-exposure.org/?TRANSPLANT.htm.

7. Ibid.

8. Michael D. Lockshin, "Pregnancy and Lupus," Lupus Foundation of America (Feb. 3, 2005). Accessed 4/5/06 at http://www.lupus.org/education/brochures/pregnancy.html.

9. A. Sobczynska-Tomaszewska, "Genetically Determined Male Infertility Caused by the CFTR Gene Mutations" (in Polish), *Med Wieku Rozwoj* 6, no. 4 (2002): 335–47; accessed 12/2/2003 on PubMed.

10. Herbert J. Grossman, ed., *Classification in Mental Retardation* (Washington, D.C.: American Association on Mental Deficiency, 1983), p. 11.

11. The first reported instance of successful artificial insemination occurred in Britain in 1884. In this instance, not only was the donor anonymous but the procedure was performed without reporting the use of donor sperm to the infertile couple. Judith N. Lasker and Susan Borg, "Secrecy and the New Reproductive Technologies," in Linda M. Whiteford and Marilyn L. Poland, eds. (Boulder, Colo.: Westview, 1989), p. 134.

12. R. Klemetti, T. Sevon, M. Gissler, and E. Hemminki, "Complications of IVF and Ovulation Induction," *Human Reproduction* 20 (2005): 3293–300.

13. S. M. Plosker, "Refining Embryo Transfer," *Fertility and Sterility* 83 (2005): 710–14.

14. "Frequently Asked Questions about Infertility," American Society for Reproductive Medicine, (2006). Accessed 4/6/06 at http://www.asrm.org/Patients/faq.htm.

15. "Fee Schedule," Surrogate Alternatives, Inc. (2006). Accessed 4/6/06 at http://www.surrogatealternative.com/fees.htm.

16. "Frequently Asked Questions about Infertility," American Society for Reproductive Medicine.

17. I have put "compensation" and other terms in this section in quotation marks to suggest that their use in the context of assisted reproduction may be misleading. This problem is discussed briefly in what follows.

18. E.g., J. G. Thornton, H. M. McNamara, and I. A. Montague, "Would You Rather Be a 'Birth' or a 'Genetic' Mother? If So, How Much?" *Journal of Medical Ethics* 20 (1994): 87, and Amy J. Ravin, Mary B. Mahowald, and Carol B. Stocking, "Genes or Gestation? Attitudes of Women and Men about Biologic Ties to Children," *Journal of Women's Health* 6, no. 6 (1997): 1–9.

19. C. B. Coulam, S. C. Adamson, and F. J. F. Amyegers, "Incidence of Premature Ovarian Failure," *Obsetrics and Gynecology* 67, no. 4 (1986): 604–6.

20. A. L. Kalfoglou and J. Gittelsohn, "A Qualitative Follow-up Study of Women's Experiences with Oocyte Donation," *Human Reproduction* 15, no. 4 (2000): 800.

21. News Release, *Fertility and Sterility* (May 8, 2003). Accessed 9/22/05 at http://www.rand.org/hot/press.03/05.08.html.

22. Cf. "Disposition of Abandoned Embryos," statement of American Society for Reproductive Medicine Ethics Committee, accepted by Board of ASRM (July 20, 1996). Accessed 9/5/05 at http://www.asrm.org/Media/Ethics/abandon.html.

23. "Assisted Reproductive Technology (ART) Report," Centers for Disease Control and Prevention (2003). Accessed 4/6/06 at http://www.cdc.gov/ART/ART2003/section3.htm.

24. Definition of "disposal," Dictionary Information, Encyclopedia Index (2001). Accessed 4/6/06 at http://www.selfknowledge.com/27517.htm.

25. See, e.g., the meaning and synonyms of "destruction," *World Net Dictionary* (2005). Accessed 4/21/06 at http://www.hyperdictionary.com/dictionary/destruction. The synonyms provided in this entry are "death," "demolition," "devastation," and "end."

26. The contribution to research is less compelling than donation to an infertile couple if the research involves termination of the embryos, which is probable.

27. Cerclage is a surgical procedure intended to forestall premature labor.

28. This case is based on reports of the birth of the McCaughey septuplets and the Chukwu octuplets in the United States. Tribune News Services, "2 McCaughey Septuplets Being Monitored for Cerebral Palsy," *Chicago Tribune*, Apr. 26, 1999, sect. 1, p. 13, and Associated Press, "Work Just Begun for Octuplet Mom," *New York Times*, Dec. 31, 1998.

29. "Multiple Birth Rate for Older Women Is Sky-Rocketing," National Center for Health Statistics (Sept. 16, 1999). Accessed 09/6/05 at http://www.sciencedaily.com/releases/1999/09/990916074135.htm.

30. See K. R. Hammon, "Multifetal Pregnancy Reduction, *Journal of Obstetric, Gynecologic and Neonatal Nursing* 27 (1998): p. 338–39.

31. M. I. Evans, L. Littman, R. Richer et al., "Selective Reduction for Multifetal Pregnancy: Early Opinions Revisited," *Journal of Reproductive Medicine* 42 (1997): 772.

32. Cf. Richard L. Berkowitz, Lauren Lynch, JoAmye Stone, and Manuel Alvarez, "The Current Status of Multifetal Pregnancy Reduction," *American Journal of Obstetrics and Gynecology* 174, no. 4 (Apr. 1996): 1265–26.

33. At 6 weeks, which is earlier than the procedure is ordinarily performed, the developing organism is technically an embryo rather than a fetus.

34. Jodi Halpern develops this point, arguing that empathy with patients is therapeutically advantageous, in Halpern, *From Detached Concern to Empathy* (New York: Oxford University Press, 2001).

CHAPTER 6

1. D. K. Stevenson, L. L. Wright, J. A. Lemons et al., "Very Low Birth Weight Outcomes of the National Institute of Child Health and Human Development Neonatal Research Network, January 1993 through December 1994," *American Journal of Obstetrics and Gynecology* 179 (1998): 1632–39.

2. M. S. Bailey and A. B. Curtis, "The Effects of Hormones on Arrythmias in Women," *Currents in Women's Health Reports* 2, no. 2 (2002): 83–88.

3. *National Diabetes Fact Sheet, US* (2005). Accessed 4/17/06 at http://www.cdd.gov/diabetes/pubs/pdf/ndfs_2005.pdf.

4. Ketoacidosis is a metabolic disorder induced by insulin deficiency that involves an excess of ketone bodies in the bloodstream.

5. "Polyhydramnios" are excess amounts of amniotic fluid in the uterus.

6. "Diabetes Facts," U.S. Food and Drug Administration (Apr. 11, 2002). Accessed 9/23/05 at http://www.fda.gov/womens/taketimetocare/diabetes/fswomen.html.

7. *Diagnostic and Statistical Manual*, 4th ed. (Washington, D.C.: American Psychiatric Association, 1994).

8. Veronika Kolder, Janet Gallagher, and Michael T. Parsons, "Court Ordered Obstetrical Interventions," *New England Journal of Medicine* 316, no. 19 (1987): 1193.

9. Frank Chervenak and Laurence McCullough, "Justified Limits on Refusing Intervention," *Hastings Center Report* 21, no. 2 (1991): 12–17.

10. Charles Taylor, *The Ethics of Authenticity* (Cambridge: Harvard University Press, 1992).

11. Committee on Ethics, "Patient Choice in the Maternal-Fetal Relationship," *Committee Opinion* no. 214 (Washington, D.C.: American College of Obstetricians and Gynecologists, 2004), p. 36.

12. Moreover, recent data suggest benefits from maintaining it throughout the affected person's lifetime. R. Koch, H. Levy, W. Hanley et al., "Outcome Implications of the International Maternal Phenylketonuria Collaborative Study," *European Journal of Pediatrics* 155, Suppl. 1 (1996): S 162–64.

13. "Gestational Diabetes," *Medline Plus* (updated Apr. 13, 2006). Accessed 4/21/06 at http://www.nlm.nih.gov/medlineplus/ency/article/000896.htm.

14. "Diabetes Facts," U.S. Food and Drug Administration.

15. D. Kamalakannan, V. Baskar, D. M. Barton et al., "Diabetic Ketoacidosis in Pregnancy," *Postgraduate Medical Journal* 79 (2003): 454–57.

16. Liz Townsend, "Twins Born Healthy after Mother Wakes from 'Irreversible' Coma," National Right to Life (1999). Accessed 4/21/06 at http://www.nrlc.org/news/1999/NRL899/twins.html; Art Campos, "An Amazing Coma-Pregnancy," Scripps Howard News Service (1999). Accessed 4/21/06 at http://www.simplyfamily.com/display.cfm?articleID=000421_coma_pregnancy.cfm.

17. George Annas, "She's Going to Die: The Case of Angela C., *Hastings Center Report* 18, no. 1 (1988): 23–25.

18. M. B. Mahowald, *Women and Children in Health Care* (New York: Oxford University Press, 1993), pp. 131–32.

19. George Annas, "Forced Cesareans: The Most Unkindest Cut," *Hastings Center Report* 18, no. 1 (1988): 16.

20. Ibid.

21. "Cesarean Fact Sheet," Childbirth.org (1998). Accessed 4/21/06 at http://www.childbirth.org/section/CSFact.html.

22. Kolder, Gallagher, and Parsons, "Court Ordered Obstetrical Interventions."

23. Mahowald, *Women and Children in Health Care*, p. 132.

24. Cf. Richard T. Garner and Bernard Rosen, *Moral Philosophy* (New York: Macmillan, 1967), pp. 56–66.

25. Cf. Richard B. Brandt, "Some Merits of One Form of Rule-Utilitarianism," in Samuel Gorowitz, ed., *John Stuart Mill: Utilitarianism and Critical Essays*, University of Colorado Studies (Indianapolis: Bobbs-Merrill, 1971), pp. 324–44, and W. D. Ross, *The Right and the Good* (Oxford: Clarendon, 1930).

26. That what is prevalently described as "maternal-fetal conflict" is usually a conflict between physician and pregnant woman was well supported in a study by Ellen J. Stein. See Stein, "Maternal-Fetal Conflict: Reformulating the Equation," in Andrew Grubb, ed., *Challenges in Medical Care* (Chichester, UK: Wiley, 1992), 91–92.

CHAPTER 7

1. I first discussed both of the preceding cases in Mary Briody Mahowald, *Women and Children in Health Care: An Unequal Majority* (New York: Oxford University Press, 1993), pp. 125–28.

2. R. M. Pitkins, J. K. Perloff, B. J. Koos, and M. H. Beall, "Pregnancy and Congenital Heart Disease," *Annals of Internal Medicine* 112 (1990): 445–54.

3. N. Gleicher, J. Midwall, D. Hockberger et al., "Eisenmenger's Syndrome in Pregnancy," *Obstetrics and Gynecology Survey* 3 (1979): 721.

4. *Roe v. Wade*, 410 U.S. 113 (1973).

5. See Carol Gilligan's study of women's altruistic reasons for abortion. These are reported and analyzed in Gilligan, *In a Different Voice* (Cambridge: Harvard University Press, 1982), pp. 70–127.

6. The perineum in women is the region between the vulva and the anus.

7. An Apgar score is an assessment of the general physical condition of a newborn infant based on a rating of 0, 1, or 2 for each of five criteria: heart rate, respiration, muscle tone, skin color, and response to stimuli. A perfect score is 10.

8. The medically preferable type of C-section involves a low transverse incision that allows for vaginal deliveries in subsequent pregnancies. Classical cesarean section, which involves a vertical incision, is seldom performed but is necessary in some cases.

9. J. R. Scott, "Putting Elective Cesarean into Perspective," *Obstetrics and Gynecology* 99, no. 6 (2002): 967–68; W. B. Harer, "Patient Choice Cesarean," *ACOG Clinical Review* 5, no. 2 (2000): 1; S. Bewley and J. Cockburn, "The Unethics of 'Request' Caesarean Section," *British Journal of Obstetrics and Gynaecology* 109 (2002): 593–96.

10. Cf. H. P. Dietz and L. Schierlitz, "Pelvic Floor Trauma in Childbirth," *Australian and New Zealand Journal of Obstetrics and Gynaecology* 45 (2005): 3–11.

11. G. C. Smith, J. P. Pell, A. D. Cameron, and R. Dobbie, "Risk of Perinatal Death Associated with Labor after Previous Cesarean Delivery in Uncomplicated Term Pregnancies," *Journal of the American Medical Association* (2002): 2684–90.

12. "Multiparous" means that the woman has already given birth more than once. "Nulliparous" means that the woman has never given birth.

13. See K. Hofberg and I. Brockington, "Tokophobia: An Unreasoning Dread of Childbirth," *British Journal of Psychology* 176 (2000): 83–85.

14. This case occurred in 1982, was reported widely in the press, and gave rise to federal legislation regarding treatment of newborns with disabilities. See, e.g., U.S. Department of Health and Human Services, "Interim Final Rule 45 CFR Part 84, Nondiscrimination on the Basis of a Handicap," *Federal Register* 48 (Mar. 7, 1983): 9630–32, and "Child Abuse and Neglect Prevention and Treatment Program. Final Rule," *Federal Register* 50 (Jan. 11, 1985): 1487–92. See also Barbara J. Culliton, "Baby Doe Regs Thrown out by Court," *Science* 220 (Apr. 29, 1983): 479–80, and Mary B. Mahowald and Jerome Paulson, "The Baby Does: Two Different Situations," *Cleveland Plain Dealer* (Dec. 31, 1983), p. 9A.

15. Gestational age is measured in weeks from the first day of the woman's last menstrual cycle to the current date. A pregnancy of normal gestation is approximately 40 weeks, with a normal range of 38 to 42 weeks. Infants born before 37 weeks are considered premature. Infants born after 42 weeks are considered postmature.

16. This means that the fetus is smaller than 90 percent of all other babies of the same gestational age, a size that carries increased risks to its welfare.

17. Tertiary care centers are medical centers whose personnel are specially trained and equipped to care for critical conditions that do not routinely occur.

18. John Carey, "Trisomy 13 Facts," Support Organization for Trisomy 18, 13 and Related Disorders. Accessed 4/7/06 at http://www.trisomy.org/html/trisomy_13_facts.htm.

19. Robert G. Best and James Stallworth, "Patau Syndrome, *eMedicine* (2006). Accessed 4/7/06 at http://www.emedicine.com/ped/topic1745.htm.

20. About half of the children born with trisomy 21 live longer than fifty years. Congenital heart disease is the most common cause of death for them. See Harold Chen,

"Down Syndrome," *eMedicine* (2006). Accessed 4/7/06 at http://www.emedicine.com/ped/topic615.htm.

21. Cf. Mahowald, *Women and Children in Health Care*, pp. 65–66.

22. William Meadow, neonatologist and Professor of Pediatrics at the University of Chicago, in personal communication, September 14, 2005.

23. Intracranial hemorrhage (bleeding in the brain) is predictive of neurological impairment. The intestinal damage (necrotizing enterocolits) involves sloughing off of dead bowel tissue, requiring surgical removal.

24. R. A. Collacott, S. A. Cooper, D. Branford, and C. McGrother, "Behaviour Phenotype for Down's Syndrome," *British Journal of Psychiatry* 172 (1998): 85–89; Richard J. Robison, "Learning about Happiness from Persons with Down Syndrome: Feeling the Sense of Joy and Contentment," *American Journal on Mental Retardation* 105 (2000): 372–76; George Will, "Jon Will's Aptitudes," *Newsweek* (Mar. 3, 1993). Accessed 4/8/06 at http://www.epm.org/articles/willdown.html.

25. Cited in Mahowald, *Women and Children in Health Care*, p. 171, from *Federal Register* 50 (Jan. 11, 1985).

26. "Birth Defects—Ambiguous Genitalia," Murdock Children's Research Institute (Feb. 2002). Accessed 4/8/06 at http://www.disability.vic.gov.au/dsonline/dsarticles.nsf/(Pages)/Birth_defects_ambiguous_genitalia?OpenDocument. According to the Intersex Society of North America, however, the number is about 1 in 1500 to 1 in 2,000 births. See Intersex Society of North America, "How Common Is Intersex?" (2005). Accessed 4/8/06 at http://www.isna.org/faq/frequency.

27. V. Sobel, Y. S. Zhu, and J. Imperato-McGinley, "Fetal Hormones and Sexual Differentiation," *Obstetric and Gynecologic Clinics of North America* 31 (2004): 837–56.

28. "Phenotypic features" are the ways in which one's genetic make-up (genotype) are expressed.

29. Milton Diamond, "Sex Reassignment at Birth: A Long Term Review and Clinical Implications," *Archives of Pediatric and Adolescent Medicine* 151 (Mar. 1997): 298–304.

30. Diana W. Bianchi, Timothy M. Crombleholme, and Mary E. D'Alton, *Fetology: Diagnosis and Management of the Fetal Patient* (New York: McGraw-Hill, 2000), p. 570.

31. Ibid.

32. This is the same rationale that supports respect for parental decision-making in cases such as those addressed in the preceding section.

CHAPTER 8

1. I have discussed the requirements for moral decision-making in children in M. B. Mahowald, *Women and Children in Health Care: An Unequal Majority* (New York: Oxford University Press, 1993), chapter 11.

2. Cf. Ann Maradiegue, "Minor's Rights versus Parental Rights: Review of Legal Issues in Adolescent Health Care," *Journal of Midwifery and Women's Health* 48, no. 3 (2003): 170–77.

3. "U.S. Teenage Pregnancy Statistics with Comparative Statistics for Women Aged 20–24," Alan Guttmacher Institute (2004). Accessed 4/8/06 at http://www.guttmacher.org/pubs/teen_stats.html.

4. "Teenage Pregnancy," March of Dimes (2004). Accessed 4/8/06 at http://www.marchofdimes.com/msmres.asp?query=teenage+pregnancy+x=Hy=7.

5. Laurie Zabin, Marilyn B. Hirsh, and Mark R. Emerson, "When Urban Adolescents Choose Abortion: Effects on Education, Psychologial Status and Subsequent Pregnancy," *Family Planning Perspectives* 21, no. 6 (1989): 248–55.

6. "Teenage Pregnancy," March of Dimes; "When Children Have Children," No. 31, American Academy of Child and Adolescent Psychiatry (July, 2005). Accessed 4/8/06 at http://www.aacap.org/publications/factsfam/pregnant.htm.

7. "Trisomy 18 Facts," Support Organization for Trisomy 18, 13, and Related Disorders." Accessed 4/8/06 at http://www.trisomy.org/html/trisomy_18_facts.htm.

8. Susan Root and John C. Carey, "Survival in Trisomy 18," *American Journal of Medical Genetics* 49, no. 2 (1994): 170–74.

9. Patricia A. Baird and Barbara McGillivray, "Children of Incest," *Journal of Pediatrics* 104, no. 5 (1982): 854–57.

10. "Chlamydia," Fact Sheet approved by National Institute of Allergy and Infections Diseases, National Institutes of Health (Oct. 2002). Accessed 9/15/05 at http://www.hoptechno.com/bookchlam.htm.

11. "Suicide Facts and Statistics," National Institute of Mental Health (2004). Accessed 6/19/06 at http://nimh.nih.gov/suicideprevention/suifact.cfm.

12. Richard O'Connor, "Teen Suicide," Focus Adolescent Services (2000). Accessed 4/8/06 at http://www.focusas.com/Suicide.html.

13. Bruce E. Wilson, "Fact Sheet: Understanding Androgen Insensitivity Syndrome," eMedicine (July 11, 2003). Accessed 4/21/06 at http://www.emedicine.com/ped/topic2222.htm.

14. David S. Reitman and Wanda Gonzalez, "Sexuality: Sexual Orientation," eMedicine (2005). Accessed 9/15/05 at http://www.emedicine.com/ped/topic2773.htm.

15. American Academy of Pediatrics, "Confidentiality in Adolescent Health Care" (RE9151), *AAP News*, April 1989.

16. E.g., Immanuel Kant is often cited in support of an absolute moral prohibition against lying, while W. D. Ross argues instead that the prohibition against lying may be a prima facie obligation—one that may at times be overridden by other prima facie duties.

17. Scott Allen Miller, "U.S. Also Practices Genital Mutilation," *Collegian Archives* (May 3, 1996). Accessed 4/8/06 at http://www.kstatecollegian.com/issues/v100/sp/n145/opncircumcision-samiller.html.

18. This case and the next are adapted from Carol R. Horowitz and J. Carey Jackson, "Female 'Circumcision': African Women Confront American Medicine," *Journal of General Internal Medicine* 12 (1997): 491–99.

19. Ibid.

20. Carmen Retlaff, "Female Genital Mutilation: Not Just 'Over There,'" *Journal of International Association of Physicians in AIDS Care* 5 (1999): 28–37.

21. Regarding its illegality in the United States, see Federal Prohibition of Female Genital Mutilation Act of 1995, HR 941, 104th Congress, 1st session, Feb. 14, 1995.

22. Comfort Momoh, "Female Genital Mutilation: The Struggle Continues," *Practice Nursing* 10, no. 2 (1999). Accessed 4/8/06 at www.iamapeacekeeper.com/advocacy/2.8fgm.html.

23. Rebecca J. Frey, "Anorexia Nervosa," *Gate Encyclopedia of Medicine* (Dec. 2002). Accessed 4/8/06 at http://www.healthatoz.com/healthatoz/Atoz/ency/anorexia_nervosa.jsp.

24. P. F. Sullivan, "Mortality in Anorexia Nervosa," *American Journal of Psychiatry* 152, no. 7 (1995): 1073.

25. "Mental Health: A Report of the Surgeon General," Office of the Surgeon General, Washington, D.C. Accessed 4/8/06 at http://www.surgeongeneral.gov/library/mentalhealth/chapter3/sec6.html.

26. Mary Briody Mahowald, *Genes, Women, Equality* (New York: Oxford University Press, 2000), p. 164.

27. Cf. Krisha McKay, "Nurses of Hospice Patients Who Refuse Food and Fluids Report Peaceful Deaths," Swedish Medical Center, (July 2003). Accessed 4/8/06 at http://www.swedish.org/17601.cfm.

28. Tom Beauchamp and James Childress, *Principles of Biomedical Ethics*, 5th ed. (New York: Oxford University Press, 2001), pp. 81–82.

29. For example, a study of mass media magazines discovered that women's magazines had 10.5 times more advertisements and articles promoting weight loss than men's magazines did. "The Media, Body Image, and Eating Disorders," National Eating Disorders Association, (2002). Accessed 4/8/06 at http://www.nationaleatingdisorders.org/nedaDir/files/documents/handouts/MdiaBIED.pdf.

30. I first proposed this model in 1993 in Mahowald, *Women and Children in Health Care*, especially pp. 32–37.

CHAPTER 9

1. Jonathan Imber, *Abortion and the Private Practice of Medicine* (New Haven, Conn.: Yale University Press, 1986).

2. Moreover, the failure rate of male sterilization or vasectomy (1 in 700) is considerably lower than that of female sterilization (1 in 200).

3. The "morning after pill," also called "emergency contraception," is used much less often than other methods, mainly as a back-up to other methods. To some, this is an abortive agent rather than a contraceptive agent because it prevents implantation, not fertilization. Intrauterine devices have been called abortifacients for the same reason.

4. "Female Sterilization," Better Health Channel (Apr. 2001). Accessed 4/9/06 at www.betterhealth.vic.gov.au/bhcv2/bhcarticles.nsf/pages/Female_sterilisation?OpenDocument.

5. "Facts about Birth Control," Planned Parenthood Association of America (2004). Accessed 9/16/05 at http://www.plannedparenthood.org/pp2/portal/files/portal/medicalinfo/birthcontrol/pub-birth-control-06.xml.

6. "Cognitive impairment" has a broader meaning than "mental retardation" because it also includes memory loss, dementia, and other impediments to cognitive function. Mental retardation simply refers to the fact that the pace of learning in an individual is slower than that of those who are not similarly impaired. Because the term "retard" is sometimes used pejoratively, however, I prefer to use "cognitive impairment" instead.

7. As used here, "disability" is intended to convey recognition that the factors that tend to disable some members of society are constructed by members of society who do not have the specific impairments that other members have. "Impairment" refers to the condition of a person; "disability" to social impediments. All of us are impaired to the extent that our knowledge is inevitably limited.

8. The cases and discussion in this section are based on Mary Briody Mahowald, *Women and Children in Health Care: An Unequal Majority* (New York: Oxford University Press, 1993) pp. 60–61, 65–72.

9. P. G. Stubblefield, S. Carr-Ellis, and L. Borgatta, "Methods for Induced Abortion," *Obstetrics and Gynecology* 104, no. 1 (July 2004): 1174–85. In the United States, nine out of ten abortions occur during the first 12 weeks of gestation. For women's views on methods of early abortions, see K. Holmgren, "Women's Evaluation of Three Early Abortion Methods," *Acta Obstetricia et Gynecologica Scandinavica* 71, no. 8 (1992): 616–23.

10. Methods that ensure fetal demise include injection of potassium chloride into the fetal heart and dilatation and evacuation of a fetus after suction curettage; the latter method usually requires dismemberment of the fetus.

11. W. Cates Jr., K. F. Schulz, D. A. Grimes et al., "Dilatation and Evacuation Procedures and Second-Trimester Abortions," *Journal of the American Medical Association* 248, no. 5 (1982): 559–63.

12. I was involved as an ethics consultant in two cases involving survival of abortion performed through instillation during my years at Case Western University, from 1982 through 1990. After considerable time in the intensive care nursery, both infants went home with their parents.

13. U.S. Department of Health and Human Services, "Child Abuse and Neglect Prevention and Treatment Program; Final Rule," *Federal Register* 50, Jan. 11, 1985, pp. 1487–92.

14. J. Epner, H. S. Jonas, and D. L. Seckinger, "Late-term Abortion," *Journal of the American Medical Association* 280, no. 8 (1998): 124–29.

15. J. Preston, "Appeals Court Voids Ban on 'Partial Birth' Abortions," *New York Times* July 9, 2005, p. A11.

16. Robert Blum, "Contemporary Threats to Adolescent Health in the United States," *Journal of the American Medical Association* 257, no. 24 (1987): 3392.

17. F. C. Fraser and C. J. Biddle, "Estimating the Risks for Offspring of First-Cousin Mating," *American Journal of Human Genetics* 5 (1976): 522–26.

18. H. Fu, J. E. Darroch, T. Haas, and N. Ranjit, "Contraceptive Failure Rates: New Estimates from the 1995 National Survey of Family Growth," *Family Planning Perspectives* 31, no. 2 (1999): 56–63.

19. Some methods prevent pregnancy by preventing implantation in the uterus; this is not equivalent to prevention of fertilization, which can occur in vitro or in vivo. To be absolutely preventive of sexually transmitted diseases, there must be abstinence not only from sexual intercourse but also from any type of intimate contact between the sexes.

20. See, for example, *Williams' Obstetrics*, 20th ed., in which abortion is defined as "termination of pregnancy by any means before the fetus is sufficiently developed to survive" (Stamford, Conn.: Appleton and Lange, 1997), p. 582; *Stedman's Medical Dictionary*, 26th ed., which defines it as "giving birth to an embryo or fetus prior to the stage of viability" (Baltimore: Williams and Wilkins, 1995), p. 4; and *Dorland's Illustrated Medical Dictionary*, 28th ed., which defines it as "premature expulsion from the uterus of the products of conception" (Philadelphia: W. B. Saunders, 1994), p. 4.

21. Cf. Tom Beauchamp and James Childress, *Principles of Biomedical Ethics*, 5th ed. (New York: Oxford University Press, 2001), pp. 128–32.

22. Cf. Rayna Rapp, *Testing Women, Testing the Fetus* (New York: Routledge, 2000).

23. For a case illustrating this, see Mary B. Mahowald, "When a Mentally Ill Woman Refuses Abortion," *Hastings Center Report* 15 (1985): 22–23.

24. Although RU-486 is a drug that may be taken by women to terminate their pregnancies, its safe and effective use requires medical involvement.

CHAPTER 10

1. H. L. MacMillan and C. N. Wathen, "Violence against Women: Integrating the Evidence into Clinical Practice," *Canadian Medical Association Journal* 169, no. 6 (2003): 570–71.

2. Susan Moller Okin, *Justice, Gender and the Family* (New York: Basic Books, 1989), pp. 127–33; Iris Marion Young, *Justice and the Politics of Difference* (Princeton, N.J.: Princeton University Press, 1990), pp. 97, 120.

3. "What Is Child Abuse and Neglect?" National Clearinghouse on Child Abuse and Neglect Information, U.S. Department of Health and Human Services (updated June 3, 2005). Accessed 7/15/05 at http://www.nccanch.acf.hhs.gov/pubs/factsheets/whatiscan.pdf.

4. Ibid.

5. "Risk and Protective Factors for Child Abuse and Neglect," National Clearinghouse on Child Abuse and Neglect Information, U.S. Department of Health and Human Services (Jan. 2006). Accessed 4/9/06 at http://www.nccanch.acf.hhs.gov/topics/prevention/emerging/riskprotectivefactors.cfm.

6. "Child Abuse and Neglect Fatalities," National Clearinghouse on Child Abuse and Neglect Information, U.S. Department of Health and Human Services, (2004). Accessed 4/9/06 at http://www.nccanch.acf.hhs.gov/pubs/factsheets/fatality.cfm.

7. "What Is Child Abuse and Neglect?" National Clearinghouse on Child Abuse and Neglect Information.

8. Ibid.

9. "Elder Abuse and Neglect: In Search of Solutions," APA Online (2006). Accessed 4/9/06 at http://www.apa.org/pi/aging/eldabuse.html.

10. Ibid.

11. "Elder Abuse," eMedicine (updated June 5, 2001). Accessed 7/15/05 at http://www.emedicine.com/emerg/topic160.htm.

12. For an overview of the psychological and economic costs of informal caregiving by women, see Mary B. Mahowald, Dana Levinson, Christine Cassel et al., "The New Genetics and Women," *Milbank Quarterly* 74, no. 2 (1996): 268–70.

13. Stephen G. Post, "Women and Elderly Parents: Moral Controversy in an Aging Society," *Hypatia* 5, no. 1(1990): 83–85.

14. When a patient is cognitively able but unable to speak or write coherently, practitioners are obliged to facilitate communication in other ways, if possible, including the use of signs such as blinking or nodding in response to questions.

15. Admittedly, this rationale has the liability of preempting the possibility that the patient may have changed her mind.

16. "Intimate Partner Violence Fact Sheet," National Center for Injury Prevention and Control (Mar. 2006). Accessed 4/9/06 at http://www.cdc.gov/ncipc/factsheets/ipvfacts.htm.

17. "Domestic Violence during Pregnancy," Fact Sheet of the Program on Women, Health and Development (Nov. 2003). Accessed 4/9/06 at http://www.planetwire.org/files.fcgi/2368_violencepregnancy.pdf.

18. Carol Brady and Donna Buchanan, "Domestic Violence during Pregnancy," Jacksonville Medicine (May 2002. Accessed 4/9/06 at http://www.dcmsonline.org/jaxmedicine/2002journals/may2002/pregnancy.htm.

19. Melissa Farley, "Prostitution: Factsheet on Human Rights Violations," Prostitution Research and Education (Apr. 2000). Accessed 6/21/04 at http://www.prostitutionresearch.com/factsheet.html.

20. Ibid.

21. The exam generally includes swabbing of the genital area, combing and removal of pubic hair, examination of cuts and bruises in the vaginal area, and taking blood, urine, and fingernail samples. Cf. Diane K. Beebe, "Emergency Management of the Adult Female Rape Victim," American Academy of Experts in Traumatic Stress (June 1991). Accessed 4/9/06 at http://www.aaets.org/article130.htm. Regarding the backlog of unanalyzed rape evidence,

see "Backlog of DNA Evidence," President's DNA Initiative. Accessed 4/9/06 at http://www.dna.gov/basics/backlog.

22. It is also possible in case 1, but improbable in light of the patient's age.

23. Susan Brownmiller, *Against Our Will* (New York: Simon and Schuster, 1975), and Andrea Dworkin and Catharine MacKinnon, *Pornography and Civil Rights* (Minneapolis: Organizing against Pornography, 1988).

24. Nancy Wyatt, "Background on Sexual Harassment," *Information on Sexual Harassment*, Penn State University (Aug. 2000). Accessed 4/21/06 at http://www.de.psu.edu/harassment/generalinfo/background.html.

25. Ibid.

26. M. Komaromy, A. B. Bindman, R. Haber, and M. A. Sande, "Sexual Harassment in Medical Training," *New England Journal of Medicine* 328, no. 5 (1993): 322–26.

27. S. P. Phillips and M. S. Schneider, "Sexual Harassment of Female Doctors by Patients," *New England Journal of Medicine* 330 (1994): 1388–89.

28. Wyatt, "Legal Definition of Sexual Harassment," *Information on Sexual Harassment.*

29. This rationale is supported by W. D. Ross's account of prima facie versus actual duties in *The Right and the Good* (Oxford: Clarendon, 1930), pp. 16–47.

CHAPTER 11

1. "Uniting the World against AIDS," Joint United Nations Programme, May 2004. Accessed 4/10/06 at http://www.unaids/org.en.

2. "HIV Infection in Women," National Institute of Allergy and Infectious Disease, U.S. Department of Health and Human Services (May 2004). Accessed 4/10/06 at http://www.niad.nih.gov/factsheets/womenhiv.htm.

3. Ibid.

4. Julie L. Gerberding, "Transmission of HIV to Health Care Workers," U.S. Center for Disease Control and Prevention (Feb. 1998). Accessed 4/10/06 at http://hivinsite.ucsf.edu/InSite?page=kb-07&doc=kb-07-02-08-01.

5. Debra Baker, "Positively Truthful," *ABA Journal* 84 (1998): 38.

6. "Statement on the Surgeon and HIV Infection," American College of Surgeons (May 2004). Accessed 9/17/05 at http://www.facs.org/fellows_info/statements/st-13.html.

7. Professional organizations of surgeons have argued that the same confidentiality protections afforded patients should be applied to practitioners who are HIV positive, but this position is not endorsed by the American Medical Association or the Centers for Disease Control and Prevention. A. Halevy, "AIDS, Surgery, and the Americans with Disabilities Act, *Archives of Surgery* 135, no. 1 (2000): 51–54.

8. "Cancer Now Top Killer of Younger Americans," Associated Press (Feb. 11, 2005). Accessed 9/17/05 at http://www.msnbc.msn.com/id/6844751/. The data are from the American Cancer Society's annual statistical report for 2002.

9. "Cancer Facts & Figures 2006," America Cancer Society (2006). Accessed 4/28/06 at http://www.cancer.org/downloads/STT?CAFF2006PWSecured.pdf.

10. Ibid.; "Ovarian Cancer Control Initiative," National Center for Chronic Disease Prevention and Health Promotion (last reviewed Apr. 11, 2006). Accessed 4/28/06 at http://www.cdc.gov/cancer/ovarian/idex.htm.

11. "Screening Detects Breast, Ovarian Cancer in Women at Genetic Risk," American Cancer Society, Inc. (Feb. 4, 2004). Accessed 4/28/06 at http://www.cancer.org/docroot/NWS/content/NWS_1_1x_Screening_Detects_Breast_Ovarian_Cancer_in_Women_at_Genetic_Risk.asp.

12. "Cancer Facts & Figures 2006," American Cancer Society.

13. Ibid.

14. J. L. Kramer, I. A. Velazquez, B. E. Chen et al., "Prophylactic Oophorectomy Reduces Breast Cancer Penetrance during Prospective, Long-term Follow-up of BRCA1 Mutation Carriers," *Journal of Clinical Oncology* 23, no. 34 (2005): 8629–35.

15. Carol K. Sigelman and Elizabeth A. Rider, *Life-Span Human Development* (Toronto, Calif.: Wadsworth, 2006), p. 138. Accessed 9/17/05 at http://www.howtohavegoodsex.com/do_women_lose_their_sexuality_af.htm.

16. Cf. Patrice M. Buzzanell, Helen Stert, and Lynn H. Turner, *Gender in Applied Communications Context* (Thousand Oaks, Calif.: Sage, 2003).

17. V. M. Barnabei, D. Grady, C. W. Stovall et al., "Menopausal Symptoms in Older Women and the Effects of Treatment with Hormone Therapy," *Obstetrics and Gynecology* 101, no. 3 (2003): 619.

CHAPTER 12

1. *The American Heritage Dictionary of the English Language*, 4th ed. (2004). Accessed 5/10/05 at http://www.ansom/geriatrics&r=67. "Old" may be the bluntest designation among these, often connoting age-related weakness; "elderly" is more neutral and respectful, although it often suggests frailty also; "senior" is widely used as a euphemism to avoid less-positive connotations of "old" and "elderly."

2. "Health Care Professionals," American Association for Geriatric Psychiatry (2004). Accessed 4/10/06 at http://www.aagponline.org/prof/facts_mh.asp.

3. Daniel Brauner, M.D., a geriatrician at the University of Chicago, has reviewed the content of this chapter and made many helpful suggestions, for which I am thankful.

4. "Dealing with Older, Impaired Drivers," *ACP-ASIM Observer* (Apr. 2000). Accessed 4/19/05 at http://www.acponline.org/journals/news/apr00/dealing.htm.

5. Laura B. Brown, Brian Ott, George Papandonatos et al, "Predictors of On-Road Driving Performance in Patients with Early Alzheimer's Disease," *Journal of the American Geriatrics Society* 53 (2005): 94–98.

6. Ibid.

7. "Depression in Older Adults and the Elderly: Signs, Symptoms, Causes and Treatment," Helpguide (Feb. 2005). Accessed 4/10/06 at http://www.helpguide.org/mental/depression_elderly.htm.

8. *The American Heritage Stedman's Medical Dictionary*, Houghton Mifflin, (2002). Accessed 4/22/05 at http://www.answers.com/senile+dementia&r=67.

9. D. L. Bachman, P. A. Wolf, R. Linn et al. "Prevalence of Dementia and Probable Senile Dementia of the Alzheimer Type in the Framingham Study," *Neurology* 42 (1992): 115.

10. Charles Taylor, *The Ethics of Authenticity* (Cambridge: Harvard University Press, 1992).

11. Janet A. Clark and Katherine A. Weber, "Challenges and Choices: Elderly Caregiving," University of Missouri at Columbia (July 1997). Accessed 4/10/06 at http://www.muextension.missouri.edu/xplor/hesguide/humanrel/gh6657.htm.

12. Clark and Weber, "Challenges and Choices: Elderly Caregiving."

13. Cf. S. G. Parks and M. Pilisuk, "Caregiver Burden: Gender and the Psychological Costs of Caregiving," *American Journal of Orthopsychiatry* 61 (1991): 501–9.

14. Steven Gregory and Sheel Pandya, "Women and Long-Term Care," AARP Public Policy Institute (July 2002). Accessed 4/10/06 at http://www.aarp.org/research/reference/minorities/aresearch-import-679-FS77R.html.

15. Gregory and Pandya, "Women and Long-Term Care."

16. "Myth No. 3: Men and Women Age the Same Way," World Health Day (Apr. 7, 1999). Accessed 4/10/06 at http://www.who.int/docstore/world-health-day/en/pages1999/whd99_4.html.

17. "Information and Online Pancreatic Resources," National Coalition for Cancer, Oncology Nursing Society. Accessed 4/10/06 at http://www.deckerfund.tripod .com/links .html.

18. "Women and Stroke," Brigham and Women's Hospital (Feb. 2006). Accessed 5/3/05 at http://www.brighamandwomens.org/patient/womenandstroke.asp.

19. M. Astrom, R. Adolfsson, and K. Asplund, "Major Depression in Stroke Patients: A Three-Year Longitudinal Study," *Stroke* 24 (1993): 976–82.

20. John Jiang, David Matchar, and Gregory Samsa, "Stroke Burden—Especially in Elderly—Much Higher than Previously Estimated," American Heart Association (Dec. 1999). Accessed 4/10/06 at http://medicalreporter.health.org/tmr1299/stroke_burden.html.

21. "Cancer Fear?" CTRN, Inc. Accessed 4/10/06 at http://www.changethatsright now.com/problem_detail.asp?SDID=3980:1432.

22. "Chronic Obstructive Pulmonary Disease (COPD) Fact Sheet," *American Lung Association* (July 2005). Accessed 4/10/06 at http://www.lungusa.org/site/pp.asps?c=dvLUK 900E+b=35020.

23. Regarding substitute judgment, see Tom Beauchamp and James Childress, *Principles of Biomedical Ethics*, 5th ed. (New York: Oxford University Press, 2001), pp. 99–100.

24. Cf. Amy Sullivan, Katrina Hedberg, and David Fleming, "Legalized Physician-Assisted Suicide in Oregon: The Second Year," *New England Journal of Medicine* 342, no. 8 (2000): 598–604.

25. Although these are English expressions, I assume other languages have terminology that poses similar problems.

26. The Karen Ann Quinlan case is a well-known example of this: *In re Quinlan*, 70 N.J. 10; 355 A.2d 647; 1976 N.J. LEXIS 181; 79 A.L.R.3d 205.

27. The SUPPORT Principal Investigators, "A Controlled Trial to Improve Care for Seriously Ill Hospitalized Patients: The Study to Understand Outcomes and Risks of Treatments (SUPPORT)." *Journal of the American Medical Association* 274 (1995): 1591–98. Compare "Dying Well in the Hospital: The Lessons of SUPPORT," *Hastings Center Report* 25, no. 6 Suppl. (1995): S1–S36.

28. Cf. Willard Gaylin, Leon Kass, Edmund Pellegrino, and Mark Siegler, "Doctors Must Not Kill," *Journal of the American Medical Association* 259 (1988): 2139–40.

29. Cf. Mary B. Mahowald, "On Helping People to Die: A Pragmatist's Account," *Cambridge Quarterly of Healthcare Ethics* 9, no. 4 (2000): 532–41.

CHAPTER 13

1. This case is based on my experience with the Institutional Review Board at the University of Chicago in 1994. See Mary Briody Mahowald, *Genes, Women, Equality* (New York: Oxford University Press, 2000), p. 40.

2. "Research on the Fetus," National Commission for the Protection of Human Subjects of Biomedical and Behavioral Research (1975). Accessed 4/10/06 at http://bioethics .gov/reports/past_commissions/index.html.

3. Benjamin Freedman, "Equipoise and the Ethics of Clinical Research," *New England Journal of Medicine* 317 (1987): 141–45; Anne Drapkin Lyerly and Mary B. Mahowald, "Maternal-Fetal Surgery for Treatment of Myelomeningocele," *Clinics in Perinatology* 30 (2003): 155–65; and N. Johnson, R. J. Lilford, and W. Brazier, "At What Level of Collective

Equipoise Does a Clinical Trial Become Ethical?" *Journal of Medical Ethics* 17 (1991): 30–34.

4. A randomized clinical trial is a study in which the subjects are assigned by chance to separate groups that compare different types of treatment, placebo, or nontreatment to be compared for their effectiveness.

5. Hindbrain herniation refers to protrusion of the cerebellum into the base of the skull and neck; shunting refers to drainage and diversion of spinal fluid into the bloodstream.

6. A sacrococcygeal teratoma is a tumor originating in the development of the tailbone; congenital cystic adenomatoid malformation of the lung and congenital diaphragmatic hernia are described subsequently.

7. As used here, "nonlethal" means that the condition is not life threatening. However, anomalies associated with myelomeningocele may be life threatening in utero, as well as after birth.

8. N. S. Adzick, M. R. Harrison, A. W. Flake et al., "Fetal Surgery for Cystic Adenomatoid Malformation of the Lung," *Journal of Pediatric Surgery* 28, no. 6 (1993): 806–12.

9. M. Davenport, S. A. Warne, S. Cacciaguerra et al., "Current Outcome of Antenatally Diagnosed Cystic Lung Disease," *Journal of Pediatric Surgery* 39, no. 4 (2004): 549–56.

10. Gerben Stege, Alan Fenton, and Bruce Jaffray, "Nihilism in the 1990s: The True Mortality of Congenital Diaphragmatic Hernia," *Pediatrics* 112, no. 3 (2003): 532–35.

11. For newborns, extracorporeal membrane oxygenation (ECMO) is comparable to a heart-lung machine for adults.

12. E. Danzer, R. M. Sydorak, M. R. Harrison et al., "Minimal Access Fetal Surgery," *European Journal of Obstetrics and Gynecology and Reproductive Biology* 108, no. 1 (2003): 3–11.

13. Ad for ViaCord (2006). Accessed 4/18/06 at http://www.viacord.com/faq_viacord.htm#q7.

14. D. M. Buss, "Psychological Sex Differences," *American Psychologist* 50 (1995): 164–68.

15. Paul Okami and Todd Shackelford, "Human Sex Differences in Sexual Psychology and Behavior," *Annual Review of Sex Research* 12 (2001): 186–241.

16. Amy Ravin, Mary B. Mahowald, and Carol Stocking, "Genes or Gestation? Attitudes of Women and Men about Biological Ties to Children," *Journal of Women's Health* 6 (1997): 639–47.

17. Rudolf Jaenisch and A. Bird, "Epigenetic Regulation of Gene Expression," *Nature Genetics* 33 Suppl. (2003): 245–54.

18. The mitochondrial DNA, however, would come from the enucleated egg to which the nuclear DNA is transferred.

19. For example, childhood leukemia. See Janet McConnaughey, "Treating Leukemia with Stem Cells," CBS News (Nov. 2004). Accessed 4/30/06 at http://www.cbsnews.com/stories/2004/11/24/health/main657740.shtml.

20. President's Council on Bioethics, *Monitoring Stem Cell Research* (Washington, D.C., 2004), p. 146. Accessible at http://www.bioethics.gov.

21. President's Council on Bioethics, *Human Cloning and Human Dignity* (Washington, D.C., 2002), p. 54. Accessible at http://www.bioethics.gov.

22. Paul R. McHugh, "Zygote and 'Clonote': The Ethical Use of Embryonic Stem Cells," *New England Journal of Medicine* 351, no. 3 (2004): 209–10.

23. These arguments were presented by Dan Brock for President William Clinton's bioethics advisory panel, *Cloning Human Beings: Report and Recommendations of the*

National Bioethics Advisory Commission (Rockville, Md.: National Bioethics Advisory Commission, 1997), p. 79.

24. Robert P. George and Alfonso Gomez-Lobo, "The Moral Status of the Human Embryo," *Perspectives in Biology and Medicine* 48, no. 2 (2005): 201–10.

CHAPTER 14

1. John Stuart Mill, *On Liberty* (Chicago: Henry Regnery, 1955) p. 111.
2. Plato, *Republic*, Bk. IV.
3. Neither do these analyses distinguish between behaviors that are either more or less vicious than others.
4. Tom Beauchamp and James Childress, *Principles of Biomedical Ethics*, 1st through 5th eds. (New York: Oxford University Press, 1979, 1983, 1989, 1994, 2001).
5. The definition of virtue as a moral habit is found in Aristotle (*Nichomachean Ethics*) and in Thomas Aquinas (*Summa Theologica*, "Treatise on the Virtues"). Vice is then defined as an immoral habit. Beauchamp and Childress define virtue more broadly, as encompassing not only moral habits but also social and natural traits (5th ed., chapter 2).
6. David Hilfiker, *Not All of Us Are Saints* (New York: Ballantine Books, 1996).
7. Cf. Plato, *Republic*, Bk. I.
8. Cf. M. B. Mahowald, "Communities in Pursuit of Community," in Jason Bell, ed., *The Relevance of Royce* (New York: Fordham University Press, forthcoming).
9. See Chapter 1 in this volume and Norman Daniels, *Just Health Care* (Cambridge: Cambridge University Press, 1985).
10. Amartya Sen, *Inequality Reexamined* (Cambridge: Harvard University Press, 1992); Martha Nussbaum, *Women and Human Development* (Cambridge: Cambridge University Press, 2000), pp. 4–14 and 78–80; Alasdair MacIntyre, *After Virtue: A Study in Moral Theory* (Cambridge: Cambridge University Press, 1981), chapter 16.
11. See Edmund D. Pellegrino and David C. Thomasma, *The Virtues in Medical Practice* (New York: Oxford University Press, 1993).

INDEX

abortion
  definitions of, 56–7, 60, 166–7, 258 n.3, 259 nn.10–1
  and disabilities, 73, 78–84
  and previability, 45–6
  procedures, 164–5, 258 n.9, 259 n.10, 259 n.24
  women's reasons for, 163–70, 255 n.5
adolescents. *See* minors
adoption, 93, 101, 104, 142–5, 167
advance directives, 207–13
ageism, 201
Alzheimer disease. *See also* senile dementia
  and caregiving, 176–8
  meaning and incidence of, 201–2, 250 n.6
  and physician-assisted suicide, 208–9, 211–2
  and stem cell research, 225
  susceptibility testing for, 78– 81, 208–9, 250 n.6.
amniocentesis, 81–3
androgen insensitivity syndrome, 135, 147–8
Annas, George, 118
anorexia nervosa. *See* eating disorders
Aristotle. *See also* natural law
  on body/soul relation, 52–3, 64
  on knowledge, 14, 20, 248 n.1
  and maxims and topics, 16, 242 n.18
  on justice, equality, and virtue, 19–20, 243 n.38
  on potency, 60
artificial insemination, 74–7, 97–101, 182–4, 252 n.11
atrial fibrillation, 110–1
authenticity, 26, 113, 202–3
autoimmune deficiency syndrome, 74–8, 93–6, 187–90
autonomy
  and cultural differences, 151–3
  meanings of, 11–8, 202
  and physician/patient relationship, 35–6
  principle of respect for, 12–30

Beauchamp, Tom
  and pragmatism, 242 n.11
  and principles of biomedical ethics, 10–8, 37–9, 48, 235, 243 n. 27
  on virtue, 235, 243 n.25
beneficence, meaning and principle of, 12–8

bioethics, 3, 10–5
birth
  as beginning of life, 50–1, 59–60
  decisions at premature, 130–4
  mode of delivery at, 123–6
  moral significance of, 62, 64–6
  prevention of 123, 163–71. *See also* abortion
  sex assignment at, 123, 134–8
Boethius, 59
brain function, as criterion for personhood, 62–4
breast cancer
  incidence and treatment of, 186, 190–3
  susceptibility testing for, 81–5, 251 n.11
  research on, 27–8, 245 n.74
Brody, Baruch, 248 n.8, 249 n.33
Buber, Martin, 22
bulimia. *See* eating disorders

Callahan, Daniel, 243 n.24
Camus, Albert, 26
Case Western Reserve University, 243 n.30, 259 n.1
cancer. *See also* breast cancer
  cervical, 191–3
  meaning of, 208
  ovarian, 190–3
  pancreatic, 207–8
capabilities theory, 20–1, 236–9
care
  of the elderly, 198–203, 212
  ethic of, 11, 22–3
  of the dying, 121–2, 207–12
  and justice, 23–8
caregivers, 9, 23, 198, 203–7, 211
casuistry
  origin and meaning of, 10, 12–6
  maxims of, 16, 243 n.32
  modifications of, 37–40
  paradigms in, 16
  topics in, 13–4
cesarean section
  after maternal-fetal surgery, 221
  for nonmedical reasons, 126–30
  refusal of, 117–22
  types of, 255 n.8
  vaginal delivery after, 119, 128
Chervenak, Frank
  and coercive treatment of pregnant women, 112–3, 247 n.31
  and dependent moral status, 61–9
  on fetus as patient, 40–6, 246 n. 12, 247 n.30
  and principles of biomedical ethics, 37–46, 246 n.11
Childress, James. *See* Beauchamp, Tom
chorionic villus sampling, 82–3
chronic obstructive pulmonary disease, 207, 209, 211
cloning, 59, 223–7, 248 n.9
common morality, definition of, 14
communitarian theories, 19, 22, 242 n.8, 244 n.41
complicity, 138, 168, 184–5
conception, 166–7, 182, 249 n.30. *See also* fertilization
confidentiality
  and adolescents, 145–9, 168, 175
  and HIV testing, 187, 189–90, 261 n.7
  and misattributed paternity, 74, 85–8
  and sexual history-taking, 34, 168
congenital adrenal hyperplasia, 135
congenital cystic adematoid malformation of the lung, 221–3
congenital diaphragmatic hernia, 221–3
contraception
  methods of, 158–63, 166, 181–2, 258 n.3, 259 n.19
  failure of, 164, 166
cosmetic surgery, availability of, 32
cystic fibrosis, 74–7, 85–8, 95, 153–5

Daniels, Norman, 21–2, 236–7
death
  definitions of, 52–3, 66
  and embryos, 102–3, 107
  and aging, 208, 210
deBeauvoir, Simone, 20
decisional capacity, requirements for 140–1, 164–8. *See also* moral agency
depression
  in adolescents, 147, 154
  in caregivers, 178
  in the elderly, 208–10
  in conjunction with stroke, 208
deontology, 11, 121, 245 n.66
diabetes, 110–1, 114–7

disability
meaning of, 258 n.6, 258 n.7
cognitive, 28–9, 36, 161, 258 n.6. *See also* Down syndrome; senile dementia
and preconception decisions, 73–81
and pregnancy, 81–4, 94–7, 159–63
discrimination
meaning of, 183–4
and sexual harassment, 182–5
and sexual orientation, 146–7
dominance and nondominance, 20, 24–9
Down syndrome
and neonatal decisions, 130–4
prenatal testing for, 81–4, 164, 169
and life span, 255 n.20
double effect, principle of, 167
driving competence, 199–202
durable power of attorney for health care, 209, 211
Dworkin, Ronald, 19

eating disorders, 153–6
egalitarian perspective, explanation of, 17–24, 30–7, 234
egg "donation," 93, 97–101
Eisenmenger syndrome, 124–6
emancipated minor, 144
embryos
disposition of, 73, 96, 101–4, 250 n.7
and potential for personhood, 60–1
as separable from women, 38
Engelhardt, H. Tristram, 21, 61, 244 n.46, 249 n.28
Emmanuel, Linda, 35
Emmanuel, Ezekiel, 35
equality, meanings of, 17–23, 29–30
equipoise, 217, 219, 222
euthanasia, 169, 209
exencephaly, 124–6

fallacy of abstraction, 35, 38
female genital surgery, 149–53
feminism, 9, 11, 22–3. *See also* gender justice; standpoint theory
fertilization, 60–2, 181–2, 249 n.30
fetus. *See also* pregnancy
as inseparable from woman, 53
as living, 53
moral status of, 40–7, 55–7, 60–5
and pain, 249 n.34
and patienthood, 40–7, 247 n.28
and surgery on pregnant woman, 220–3
termination of. *See* abortion
thresholds of development in, 62–6
Ford, Norman, 63
futility, meaning of, 132–3

gender differences in health care, 9, 31–7
gender stereotypes, 32, 186, 258 n.29
gender justice
as feminist and egalitarian, 9, 19
and gender discrimination, 182–5
as ideal, 233, 238–9
meaning of, 3, 9–10, 20–1
gene therapy, 73
genetic testing
preimplantation, 73, 78–81
prenatal, 81–91
for late onset disorders, 190–3
for carrier status, 85–7
geriatrics, 198
gestation. *See* pregnancy
Georgetown mantra, 8, 37, 235. *See also* principles of biomedical ethics
Gillespie, Norman, 66
Gilligan, Carol, 22–3
golden rule, 47
Gomez-Lobo, Alfonso, 60
guardianship, 176–9, 199–203
guidelines
characteristics of professional, 47–8, 108, 243 n.25
as different from regulations, 31, 47–8
and maxims, 17, 243 n.32
as based on principles, 16–7, 238

Haraway, Donna, 28
Hare, R. M., 60–1
Hartsock, Nancy, 25–6
Held, Virginia, 242 n.9
Hilfiker, David, 235
Hellin's law, 105
herpes simplex virus, 127–9
human immunodeficency virus, 74–8, 93–6, 186–90, 261 n.7
Hippocratic dictum, 128. *See also* nonmaleficence
hormone replacement therapy, 194–7
human, meaning of, 53–4, 59

Huntington disease, 83
Hursthouse, Rosalind, 242 n.8

ideal
and virtue, 234–5
of justice, 5, 48, 233–9
of gender justice, 238
impartiality, 24
impairment. *See* disability
implantation, 63. *See also* conception
individual, definition of, 43
individuation, 63
infants, 53, 55, 64–5
premature, 123, 130–4
impaired, 123, 130–4
infertility, 92–6, 137, 251 n.1. *See also* reproductive technologies
informed consent. *See also* autonomy, principle of respect for
and patient choice, 15, 27, 35–6, 127
requirements for 11
interests, meaning of, 17
intracytoplasmic sperm injection, 93, 95
Institutional Review Board, 215–8, 220
intention, moral relevance of, 91–2, 167–9, 212
in vitro fertilization. *See* reproductive technologies

James, William, 22, 241 n.4, 242 n.11
John Paul II, 63
Johnstone, Brian, 60
Jonsen, Albert, 13–8, 39, 243 n.28. *See also* Toulmin, Stephen; casuistry
justice
in Beauchamp and Childress, 12
as blind, 24
in common parlance, 18
and equality, 18–9
as human flourishing, 5, 236–8
as normal species function, 21–2, 236, 238
mediating function of, 3, 15–8, 48, 212
in Plato and Aristotle, 19, 243 n.38
theories of, 18–23
as virtue or ideal, 5, 19, 48, 233–9
See also capabilities theory; Daniels, Norman

Kant, Immanuel
on lying, 257 n.16
on person, 55, 249 n.28
theory of, 11, 16, 121
ketoacidosis, 110–1, 253 n.4
Klinefelter syndrome, 19, 135–9
Kuhse, Helga, 61

Ladd, John, 24–6
lethal condition, 83, 130–2, 221–3, 264 n.7
liberalism, 19, 22
libertarianism, 19–22, 49
life, definitions of, 51–5, 212
Little, Margaret Olivia, 11, 40, 247 n.32, 248 n.16
living will, 209, 211
lupus, 93–6
lying, 148, 257 n.16

MacIntyre, Alasdair, 19, 236, 242 n. 8
Mahowald, Mary Briody, standpoint of, 241 n.5, 245 n.74
Marcel, Gabriel, 22
Marx, Karl, 11, 21, 242 n.11
"maternal-fetal conflict," 38, 254 n.26
maternal-fetal surgery, 41, 220–3
maxims
of casuistry, 16–7, 38
for prioritizing verities, 17–8, 40
as rules or guidelines, 16, 243 n.32
McCullough, Laurence. *See* Chervenak, Frank
medicalization, 32, 196
menopause
and hormone replacement therapy, 194–7
meaning and symptoms of, 194–5
as normal 32, 92, 186
and pregnancy, 92, 97–101, 196
menstruation, 194–5
Mill, John Stuart, 24, 233, 243 n.33
minors
definition of, 140
decisional capacity of, 140–1, 164–8
emancipated, 141
and confidentiality, 144–9
and mature minor status, 141
misattributed paternity, 74, 85–8
moral agency, 60–1, 65, 206, 235. *See also* personhood

moral status
and moral standing, 39, 248 n.10
meaning and significance of, 40, 46, 54–6
and personhood, 58–62
and thresholds of development, 55, 62–6
dependent and independent, 44–6, 61, 63, 68–9
and right to life, 50, 57
intermediate 46, 55–6, 63, 66–8, 250
and maximal or minimal criteria for, 120–1, 167–70
multiple gestation, 104–8
multiple sclerosis, 163, 166–70
myelomeningocele, 130, 220–3

Nagel, Thomas, 24, 245 n.62
narrative theory 11
natural law, 11, 242 n.8
Noddings, Nel, 22–3
nonmaleficence, principle of, 12–4, 17–8
Noonan, John, 62–3
normal species function, 21–2, 236, 238
Norplant, 160, 163
Nozick, Robert, 19–21
Nussbaum, Martha, 236

objectivism, criticisms of. *See* Ladd, John; standpoint theory; particularism
obligation, as less demanding than virtue, 5, 235–6
obstetrics and gynecology, 33–4, 40
Okin, Susan Moller, 21, 172

Pain, 14–5, 249 n. 34
paradigms in bioethics, 16–7, 39–40
parentalism, as antidote to paternalism, 156–7
Parkinson disease, 225
particularism, 11, 243 n.24
paternalism
as model for medical practice, 35–6
as unjustified, 156
voluntary, 12, 223
patient
meaning of, 33, 62, 41–7, 245 n.72, 247 n.28
couples as, 43–4
pregnant woman as, 41, 43. *See also* maternal-fetal surgery
Pearce, Diana, 32, 244 n.47
Peirce, Charles Sanders, 22–6, 244 n.54
pelvic inflammatory disease, 145
persistent vegetative state, 40, 55, 248 n.13
personhood. *See also* moral agency
definitions of, 53–9, 64–9
normative and descriptive, 39–40, 59, 67
maximalist and minimalist criteria for, 59, 62, 65
potential for, 40, 42–3, 58–62, 64
phenylketonuria, 74–8, 114–7
physician-assisted suicide, 209, 211–2
physician/patient relationship, models of, 12, 34–7, 48, 168, 246 n.6
Plato, 19, 52–3, 64, 243 n.16
postmodernism, 250 n.51, 250 n.69
Potter, Van Rensselaer, 10
poverty, feminization of, 32, 244 n.47
pragmatism, 11. *See also* James, William; Peirce, Charles Sanders
preembryo, 100
pregnancy
duration of, 255 n.15
as unique relationship, 31, 56–8, 247 n.32
in teenagers, 165–8
in menopause, 97–100
and patienthood, 41–6
noncompliance during, 109–22
preimplantaton genetic diagnosis, 78–81
premature ovarian failure, 97–101
President's Council on Bioethics, 41, 224–8, 249 n.20, 250 n.42
primitive streak, 63, 249 n.31
principles of biomedical ethics, 10–31, 243 n.28
principlism, meaning and modification of 10, 37–40
privacy, 34, 172
private/public distinction, 172, 185
procreative liberty, 39–40, 67, 162
profession, meaning of, 27
prostitution, 179–80

quality of life, 13, 14

rape kit exam, 179, 181, 260 n.21
randomized clinical trial, definition of, 264 n.4
Rawls, John, 19–28, 48, 236, 243 n.27, 244 n.40
relationships. *See also* pregnancy
and ethic of care, 11, 22–3

relationships (*continued*)
  and communitarianism, 22
  moral relevance of, 11–2, 61
  practitioner-patient, 12, 34–7
reproductive technologies, 32, 92–108, 215, 219–29
research, 214–29
  definition of, 217
  and women as subjects, 33, 215–23, 228–9
  on cloning and stem cells, 223–8
respect, concept of, 12, 55, 234
right
  definition of, 13
  to choose, 56, 68, 162, 170. *See also* autonomy
  to life, 50, 55–6, 68–9. *See also* life
  positive and negative, 13, 39, 55
Robertson, John, 38–9, 66–7
Ross, W. D., 243 n.36, 257 n.16
rules, as principles or maxims, 243 n.32

Sandel, Michael, 19, 22, 242 n. 8
Sass, Hans Martin, 64
Schneider, Carl, 12, 246 n.7
Sen, Amartya, 19–20
senile dementia, 199–201, 205, 208–9. *See also* Alzheimer disease
sentiency, 63–7
sexism, 20–1
sex selection, 74, 88–91
sexual harassment, 182–5
sexually transmitted disease, 141, 145–9
sexual orientation, 81, 146–7, 149, 182–5
sickle cell disease, 85–7
Siegler, Mark, 13–8, 38, 241 n.6, 243 n.28
Singer, Peter, 61, 65
somatic cell nuclear transfer, 59. *See also* cloning
soul, 52–3
spina bifida, 83, 130. *See also* myelomeningocele
spinal cord injury, 225
standard of care, 81, 214, 217, 221, 228
standpoint theory, 24–9
Steinbock, Bonnie, 59, 66–7
sterilization, 93–6, 158–63, 190–1
stroke, 207–8
Strong, Carson, 38–40, 67
suicide, 145–7, 202, 209, 211–2
Sumner, L. S., 248 n.10
supererogation. *See* virtue
surrogate decisions, 17, 178, 206, 211. *See also* advance directives
"surrogacy" in reproduction, 93, 97–101
syngamy, 249 n.29

Taylor, Charles, 26, 202, 242 n.8
Tay Sachs disease, 78–9
Thomas Aquinas, 53, 242 n.8. *See also* natural law
Thomson, Judith Jarvis, 57, 248 n. 8
tokophobia, 129
Tooley, Michael, 65
Toulmin, Stephen, 10, 16, 39, 241 n.6. *See also* casuistry
trisomy 13, 83,130–4, 143
trisomy 18, 83, 142–4
trisomy 21. *See* Down syndrome
truthtelling, 83, 136–7
Turner syndrome, 19, 135

umbilical cord blood, 224–8
universalizability, 121, 243 n.24
utilitarianism, 10–1, 25, 121, 245 n.66

variables, moral relevance of, 4,15–8, 29
Veatch, Robert M., 248 n.3
ventricular septal defect, 142–3
verities, as ethical principles, 15–8, 29
viability
  moral relevance of, 62, 64, 110, 112, 119
  as criterion for patienthood, 44–6, 64, 67
violence
  definition of, 172
  toward women, 172, 179–82
  toward children, 159–61, 164–9, 173–6
  toward elderly, 176–9
virtue
  meaning of, 235, 243 n. 25, 265 n.5
  and ideal of justice, 5, 48, 233–9
  and obligation, 234–7
  theory, 11
  in women's health care, 238–9

Walzer, Michael, 19
Warren, Mary Anne. 59, 64–6, 248 n.11
William syndrome, 159–63
Winslade, William. *See* Siegler, Mark

Young, Iris Marion, 172, 244 n.39